SPA MEDICINE

YOUR GATEWAY TO THE AGELESS ZONE

Graham Simpson, M.D.,
Stephen T. Sinatra, M.D., &
Jorge Suárez-Menéndez, M.D.

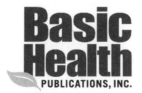

Basic
Health
PUBLICATIONS, INC.

The information contained in this book is based upon the research and personal and professional experiences of the authors. It is not intended as a substitute for consulting with your physician or other healthcare provider. Any attempt to diagnose and treat an illness should be done under the direction of a healthcare professional.

The publisher does not advocate the use of any particular healthcare protocol but believes the information in this book should be available to the public. The publisher and authors are not responsible for any adverse effects or consequences resulting from the use of the suggestions, preparations, or procedures discussed in this book. Should the reader have any questions concerning the appropriateness of any procedures or preparation mentioned, the authors and the publisher strongly suggest consulting a professional healthcare advisor.

Basic Health Publications, Inc.
8200 Boulevard East
North Bergen, NJ 07047
1-201-868-8336

The illustrations appearing on pages 10 and 11 are from *Wellness Workbook*, 3rd edition, John W. Travis, M.D., and Regina Sara Ryan, Celestial Arts, Berkeley, CA. © 1981, 1988, 2004 by John W. Travis. Reprinted with permission.

Library of Congress Cataloging-in-Publication Data

Simpson, Graham
    Spa medicine : your gateway to the ageless zone / Graham Simpson,
Stephen T. Sinatra, and Jorge Suárez-Menéndez.—1st ed.
        p. cm.
    Includes bibliographical references and index.
    ISBN 1-59120-128-4
    1. Middle-aged persons—Health and hygiene. 2. Older people—
Health and hygiene. 3. Self-care, Health. 4. Longevity. 5. Aging.
I. Sinatra, Stephen T. II. Suárez-Menéndez, Jorge III. Title.

    RA777.6.S584   2004
    613'.0434—dc22

                                        2004015606

Editor: Roberta W. Waddell
Typesetting/Book design: Gary A. Rosenberg
Cover design: Mike Stromberg

Printed in the United States of America

10   9   8   7   6   5   4   3   2

Contents

Appendices

Foreword

Cosmeceuticals

As a dermatologist, I know that, today, health and beauty go hand in hand; they are no longer separate entities, but are two sides of the same coin. To attain healthy, beautiful skin on the outside, we must first learn how to achieve health and balance on the inside, and these dual goals for both men and women can be accomplished in the very special medical-spa environment that has been created to help them.

The more we learn about our own bodies, the more we realize that the cell-to-cell communication system is vastly more complex than ever imagined. The skin is a unique organ derived from the same embryonic tissue as the brain, which gives both many similarities of structure and function. This means that what is therapeutic for the brain will also contribute to healthy and beautiful skin. And that is not all. The skin is not only our largest organ, but it also interacts with *all other* organ systems. The skin, however, is unique in that it is visible, and because of this very visibility, it can be used to assess health and disease throughout our bodies, as well as to indicate our age.

A key component of the medical-spa experience is to teach people how to implement strategies that can keep many of the signs of aging at bay. As readers of *The Perricone Prescription* and *The Wrinkle Cure* know, I have long held the theory that aging is a disease. And to successfully treat a disease we must begin by learning its etiology—its root cause.

However, with the disease of aging there is no one definitive cause, as for example, there is with a talc miner who might develop lung cancer after many years of breathing minute talc particles. The causes of aging, as outlined herein, are as diverse as they are fascinating, and they all work synergistically to break down our organ systems, ultimately resulting in death.

I believe that, regardless of the particular cause or causes, *inflammation on a cellular level* is at the very basis of aging. But there are many paths to inflammation and consequently, many methods at our disposal to stop it. Since we are responsible for creating much of the inflammation in our bodies by choosing the wrong diet and lifestyle, a few basic changes can greatly help us decrease the accelerated aging that inflammation can cause on our faces and bodies.

Armed with this knowledge, it becomes apparent that a total mind-body approach to health and well-being is mandatory, and nothing can be of more help to us in integrating this holistic approach than the introduction of spa medicine into our lives. With spa medicine we can learn how to safely detoxify our bodies and begin a targeted nutraceutical program proven to help delay the signs of aging and the mental and physical degeneration that too often accompanies it. With spa medicine, we can learn about the exciting world of cosmeceuticals—skin treatments containing highly active and efficacious ingredients that will help us delay, or avoid altogether, more invasive, potentially dangerous procedures.

Spa medicine can also make it possible to forever delete the word *diet* from our vocabulary and our daily life. Learning how to make the right food choices, while eliminating the bad food choices, will enable us to both look younger and live longer. In addition, the right foods—those with proven anti-inflammatory properties—will help feed the brain as well as the body, ensuring that our minds are sharp and clear, our memories are functioning at optimal levels, and our inner state is one of well-being, happiness, and serenity.

In introducing you to the basic tenets of spa medicine, we will make you aware of the latest mechanisms for slowing, preventing, and reversing the aging process. And with this new awareness, you will see that many of the conditions associated with aging are not inevitable, and you do not have to age at the same rate as your parents and grandparents did. Instead, we now have the means to remain healthy, independent individuals through the last few weeks, or last few hours, of our lives.

—Nicholas Perricone, M.D.
Author, *The Wrinkle Cure*

Foreword

Nutrition

I have a very simple definition of good medicine: it is any intervention that makes the patient feel better and can also be clinically verified. Although this is a much broader definition than most people are accustomed to, it also takes into consideration the true art of medicine. In the twentieth century, we associated medicine with drugs and surgery. Now, in the twenty-first century, we have to associate medicine with improved hormonal control. This is important since hormones can be more directly affected by diet and exercise than by drugs.

The reason hormonal control will have such a great effect on your future is that hormones control inflammation, which is not only the underlying cause of most chronic diseases but also the aging process itself. This is why this book is important. It ushers in a new era, showing how good medicine should be practiced. Current medical care is usually done in aseptic environments that are virtually guaranteed to increase stress because the tests will only (falsely) confirm how ill you really are. Spa medicine is the opposite. You find yourself in an extremely pleasant, nonstressful environment, taking tests that reflect your current state of wellness. And if they indicate that you are moving out of that zone of wellness, then your primary prescription will be one of diet and exercise to help those hormones drive you back toward wellness.

There are two distinct hormones that control your future: insulin and eicosanoids. Both are intimately connected with inflammation. Maintain these hormones in a therapeutic zone, and wellness is the result. Let them drift out of that therapeutic zone, and you have set the foundation for chronic disease. As you will learn in this book, insulin can best be controlled by diet and exercise, whereas eicosanoids can best be controlled by diet and nutritional supplements, especially purified fish oils.

The power of spa medicine is such that yo\
it. There are blood tests that measure these horm\
laserlike precision, your current state of wellnes\
not a philosophical feeling—it is a real physiolog

ing illness and inflammation under control. This is true for both the body and the outer skin. And here lies the evolution of spas. For years they have been considered a place where only the skin is pampered. Although that will still be true for spa medicine, skin wellness can now be maintained both topically and from within, at the same time that you are moving your body toward a clinically defined state of wellness.

If you are ready to experience a new type of medicine whose goal is achieving wellness, as opposed to treating symptoms, then spa medicine lies in your future. It is said that the average physician treats the symptoms of disease, whereas the superior physician maintains the wellness of the patient. In the future, you will be much more likely to find the superior physicians practicing spa medicine.

—Dr. Barry Sears
Author, *The Zone*

Preface

Researchers have long known that people in certain isolated villages around the world share an unusual feature. The Vilcabamba people of South America, the Hunzas of the Himalayas, the Okinawans of Japan, and the people living in the village of Orroli in Sardinia off the coast of Italy all boast an average life expectancy of a century, and their residents are astonishingly free of chronic age-related diseases. How do they do it? Research points to their unpolluted environments, stress-free lives, unprocessed whole-foods diets, and active lifestyles.

In our toxic, fast-food-driven, and stressful world, what can you do? Short of moving to a quaint village overseas and growing all of your own food, there is a solution. This book has been created to introduce you to an exciting new model of health—*spa medicine,* the future of wellness.

Spa medicine goes beyond pampering to a new way of life in which nutrition, exercise, nutraceuticals, and other healthy lifestyle practices can help you to not only survive but also thrive. This new body of medicine provides what our overburdened healthcare system cannot: healing and nurturing on all levels—nutritionally, physiologically, emotionally, and spiritually.

There are over 10,000 spas throughout the United States and Canada, and the number is growing every year. As microcosms of villages, these spas re-create stress-free, healthy lifestyles long known for well-being and longevity. The most forward-thinking spas now have physicians and other health professionals on staff to evaluate as well as educate their guests. In the future, many spas will be equipped with specialists in age-management, cardiology, dermatology, endocrinology, neurology, and plastic surgery. Eventually they will tackle hard-core medical issues like cancer and heart-disease prevention while providing creative ongoing care.

Spa Medicine was written to provide you with proven longevity strategies to counteract our stressful world on a daily basis and to give you a fresh perspective on how to restore balance in your life. In Part One, the four wellness pillars of detoxification, nutrition, exercise, and mind-body approaches will create the foundation to carry you through difficult times and brighten your future, and in Part Two, the four secrets of longevity will help you redesign your optimum self to feel and look your best. These chapters are followed by eight appendices with details of topics covered in the book, a glossary of the more technical terms, and finally, a listing of some of the better medi-spas.

You will benefit from the guidance of Doctors Graham Simpson, Stephen Sinatra, and Jorge Suárez-Menéndez, whose combined ninety years of medical and wellness knowledge take the principles of spa medicine into the twenty-first century and beyond. They will help you pinpoint the source of your stress, modify your diet, and support you in the most relaxed possible setting. Whether or not a spa visit is in your immediate future, this book will help you acquire the knowledge, resources, and inspiration to change, and will benefit you and your family for generations to come. Perhaps you, too, will write history when you reach the century mark.

Acknowledgments

I would like to thank a number of friends and colleagues who have helped make *Spa Medicine* possible, including Dr. Stephen Sinatra for his friendship and encouragement; Lee Rizzuto for his vision of CuisinArt Resort and Spa; Dr. Larry Dossey for his wisdom and inspiration; Dr. Barry Sears for his heartfelt commitment to improve the health of America; Bobby Waddell, our editor, Bobbie Lieberman, Marchann Sinatra, and Janice Lammers for their diligent work on the manuscript; Norman Goldfind, our publisher, a special thanks for recognizing the emerging field of spa medicine; Dion Friedland, a shining example of someone in the ageless zone; Phil Micans from International Anti-Aging Systems (IAS) for his contribution to the chapter on hormones; Dr. Howard Resh for his input on CuisinArt's hydroponic farm; Dr. Blake Tearnan for his useful comments on losing weight in the Zone; Francesca Bero, Ph.D., for her knowledge in cell therapy; Sim Van der Ryn, for introducing me to Jean Gebser; and the Zone Café team, especially George Jochum, Tom Morrell, Tony Kwok, Colin Smith, Justin Simpson, and Larry Henry.

Thanks also to my parents, Olive and Das, my three sons, Ryan, Justin, and Dylan; and lastly, my wife, Pam Simpson, for her keen insight and steadfast support over the years.

—Graham Simpson, M.D.

Spa Medicine has truly been a team effort, a work in progress for the last few years, ever since Dr. Graham Simpson and I held a wellness workshop at the CuisinArt Resort and Spa, Anguilla, British West Indies.

My sincere thanks to Dr. Mark Breiner, who helped us write the chapter on detoxification. One of Dr. Breiner's missions has been to increase public awareness of heavy metal toxicity, particularly mercury, and how it relates to illness. He is one of the world's leading biological dentists, and we appreciate the valuable information he has given us.

Thanks also to the following: Dr. Cass Terry for his insightful writings on growth hormone and testosterone. As a board-certified neurologist and former chairman for the neurology department at Marquette Medical School, Dr. Terry brings enormous credibility to the table; Graham and Pam Simpson for their endearing support and friendship; Bobby Waddell, our editor, who made our medical language much more manageable; Jo-Anne Piazza, President of Optimum Health International, for her invaluable assistance, and to all the employees at Zone Café and Zone Labs Inc., who have embarked on a mission to increase the awareness of an anti-inflammatory diet and targeted nutraceuticals as means for enhancing optimum health.

My heartfelt thanks go to my daughter, Marchann Kelly Sinatra, for her insightful comments, and meticulous editing and organizational skills. She was a great help to all of us.

Additional thanks go to Dr. Nicholas Perricone for contributing to the introductory comments and Dr. Barry Sears for reading the manuscript. Their pioneering work on inflammation continues to be a great contribution to medicine.

Lastly, I want to thank my wife, Jan Sinatra, R.N., M.S.N., A.P.R.N., for her continued support in fostering my passion for preventive and nutritional medicine.

—Stephen Sinatra, M.D.

Thanks to my parents who are the greatest—my father, Laurentino, and my mother, Aida, whom I was blessed to have during the good and bad times. They were always there for me, with unconditional love, support, understanding, and very wise answers, both in my growing years and now in my middle-age years. And I want to thank Suzanne, my beautiful and intelligent wife who has always been there for me with a smile and understanding. Also, I cannot forget my only brother, Tino, who has been a positive influence in my life.

There are three doctors, among many, whom I wish to thank, but in particular, my partner, Dr. Jacques Barth, who is the developer of the I.M.T. Heart Scan, and Dr. Dieter Kuster, who believed in me and encouraged me to write this book. Also, last but not least, Dr. Cass Terry, a renowned leader in the field of growth hormone therapies, and among the most brilliant scientific minds, who also influenced and encouraged me.

—Jorge Suárez-Menéndez, M.D.

Introduction

According to research on the subject, people are increasingly seeking out alternative practitioners. Who are these seekers? What is driving them, and why has there been so much distrust of practitioners of conventional medicine? What is motivating even conservative, doctor-knows-best types of people to seek out alternative forms of healing? Clearly, the medical consumer is searching for less invasive, more effective, and safer medical interventions.

Hungry for information, a significant percentage of our aging population is consulting alternative therapy practitioners, subscribing to health newsletters, visiting book and health food stores, and surfing the Web in record numbers. In the process, these people have created a whole new wellness industry outside the mainstream medical/pharmaceutical industry, which, in an attitude reminiscent of Nero fiddling while Rome burned, continues to promote drugs and surgery as *the cures* for soaring levels of chronic disease and premature aging.

I believe the medical profession must wake up, stop fiddling, and examine *all* options that have the potential to ease human suffering. And who is better qualified than the highly trained medical professional to assess the efficacy and safety of alternative/complementary therapies and protect the public from quackery and charlatanism? Who can best team up with individuals in their quest to take charge of their own health and well-being? Once empowered with the knowledge of a wide variety of healing methods, physicians and their patients can become true partners in healing with a common goal: to give and receive the best possible care.

These are the concerns of many forward-thinking physicians and health practitioners, and Graham Simpson, M.D., is a leader among them. He is a physician willing to embrace proven, complementary methods of nutritional, metabolic, and emotional medicine that will meet the needs of a new millennium. Using both the latest research and the wisdom of the ages, Simpson has tapped into a universal truth: optimal health involves much more than drugs or surgery, and true healing integrates the physical, mental, and spiritual aspects of human beings.

As a traditionally trained and grounded physician, Simpson has seen his share of disease, illness, pain, and trauma. He is highly credentialed, with board certifications in internal medicine and emergency room medicine. In these roles, Simpson has attended to thousands in internal medicine, and has worked tirelessly in emergency rooms.

But this unusual man's passion doesn't stop there. As a member of the new breed of *integrative* physicians, Simpson now blends the best of both conventional and alternative medicine. He is a founding member of the American Holistic Medical Association, is certified in acupuncture, holds a homeopathic license, and is the creator of The Wellness Game, a board game that allows people to learn more about wellness while having fun. Simpson's interest and expertise in executive medical programs, antiaging strategies, and whole-body health have placed him on the leading edge of the exciting new field of spa medicine.

Graham Simpson defines a compelling new wellness theory of *integral health,* which connects physical, mental, and spiritual energies. Striving to bring positive changes into people's lives, Simpson's goal is to transform the lives of the participants in his workshops where he offers an exciting model of preventive medicine and age management directed at reducing silent inflammation.

Over the next several years, I predict that what we are calling *medi-spas* are going to become the centers for health education, counseling, alternative methodologies, and other health strategies that are not available in most hospitals and HMOs today. Those healthcare organizations simply do not have the time, patience, or resources to offer all the integrative therapies that the now-aging baby-boomer generation is demanding. My first spa experience made me a believer in the importance of taking time out to nurture our bodies. In 1984, I lectured at Canyon Ranch in Tucson, Arizona, in a desert atmosphere where the flowering cacti and colorful rock formations encourage meditation and reflection, while the healthful surroundings ease allergies and other respiratory conditions. During this weeklong experience, I took extended bike rides, lost five pounds, participated in health-education seminars, and returned home with newfound alternative therapies to complement my traditional training as a cardiologist and psychotherapist.

In 1988, I discovered Gurney's Inn, a seaside resort in Montauk, Long Island, New York that features one of the world's purest saltwater pools, as well as an intensive program offering a dozen types of massage therapy. I wrote two of my books there, *Lose to Win* and *Optimum Health,* and developed a passion for fly-fishing.

Now I have discovered a third jewel in this triple crown of wellness: the CuisinArt Resort and Spa on the island of Anguilla in the Caribbean. CuisinArt offers a pristine oasis of wellness featuring exercise, massage, nutrition, yoga, and other body-oriented therapies. Guests enjoy a vast array of organic fruits and vegetables plucked daily from the spa's unique hydroponic farm (*see* Appendix D). They feast on fresh coldwater fish from the ocean, teeming with beneficial omega-3 fatty acids. The purity of the environment and the magnificent white beaches of Rendezvous Bay wash away stress and open up the body, mind, and spirit to a new way of living.

Guests at a typical medi-spa receive a comprehensive personal wellness profile from a wide variety of health professionals on the cutting edge of integrative medicine, and from world-class chefs, all teamed up to provide a blueprint for wellness like no other. They take home a priceless education on how they can help themselves survive, and thrive, on our planet today.

Engaging in the spa wellness experience nurtures the body in biochemical, emotional/spiritual, nutritional, and physiological dimensions. The key is to fully experience all the methods offered and then take the knowledge back home. For myself as a health practitioner, a hiatus at a health spa gives me a period of rest, renewal, and rejuvenation. For anyone, it can be the perfect jump-start in your search for an optimum health program tailored to your needs. Maybe you need to shed a few pounds, lower your blood pressure and/or cholesterol level, or nurture your emotional self. The wisdom gained from participating in such a total spa-medicine experience can significantly enrich your life—and your longevity.

Graham Simpson has added the spa experience to his considerable expertise in conventional and alternative medicine, catapulting him to heights beyond the normal health and wellness model, and making him a leader in this microcosm of health care. As a clinical and creative innovator in this emerging field, Simpson has listened carefully to the cries of the public, and, touched by the healing energies of the landscape of Anguilla, he envisioned the book you now hold in your hands as his way of answering their needs.

The creation of the spa MeSuá by Dr. Jorge Suárez-Menéndez offers a new, exciting model in preventive and antiaging medicine. Along with his team of health professionals, this highly talented plastic surgeon has used spa concepts of detoxification and rejuvenation to take the body, and especially the skin, to a new level of glowing radiance. Both Dr. Simpson and Dr. Suárez-Menéndez bring equal measures of caring and compassion into the healthcare picture.

. In Part One, you will find our blueprint for wellness. The key chapter here is detoxification (*see* Chapter 2). At the turn of the twentieth century, one out of thirty-three people developed cancer. Next year one out of three people will develop cancer, and it will soon surpass cardiovascular disease as the number-one cause of death in the United States. Medi-spas are ideally suited to lower the toxic load we are each exposed to and can thus help decrease the incidences of chronic disease and the number of cancer deaths.

Inflammation is the key chapter in Part Two, because it is emerging as the primary factor responsible for chronic diseases that are prevalent in aging, such as cancer and heart disease. You will soon see that stopping silent internal inflammation before it gets a foothold in the body is the key to healthy aging (*see* Chapter 7). Although many of you may not be able to avail yourselves of spa medicine in person, this book will provide you with all you need to practice the many spa concepts in your own home.

Antiaging medicine is not about achieving immortality or cheating death—promoting that would be pure snake oil, quackery, and charlatanism. There is not even any one successful formula for slowing down the ravages of aging, but there are some sound, scientifically strategic interventions that *can* slow down the inexorable decline that comes with the aging process. Our approach here combines ninety years of medical and wellness knowledge that carries the principles of age management into the twenty-first century and beyond.

—Stephen T. Sinatra, M.D., F.A.C.C.
Manchester, CT

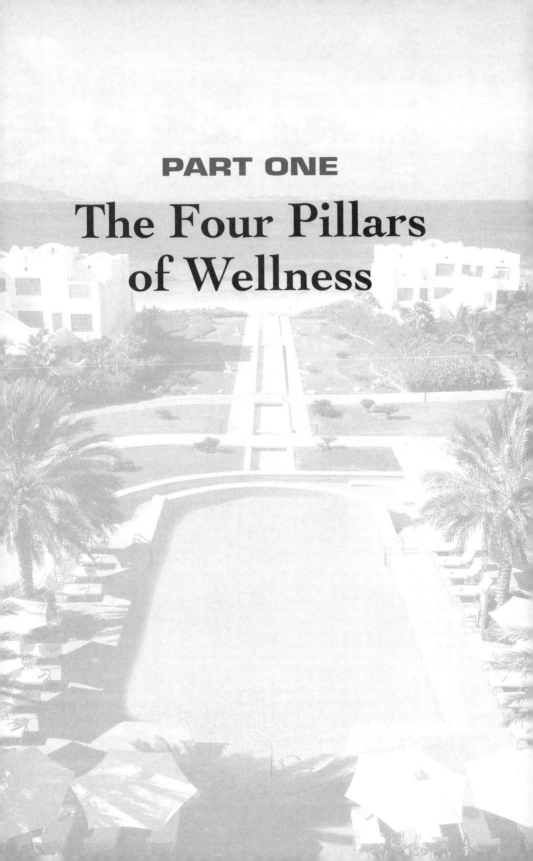

PART ONE

The Four Pillars of Wellness

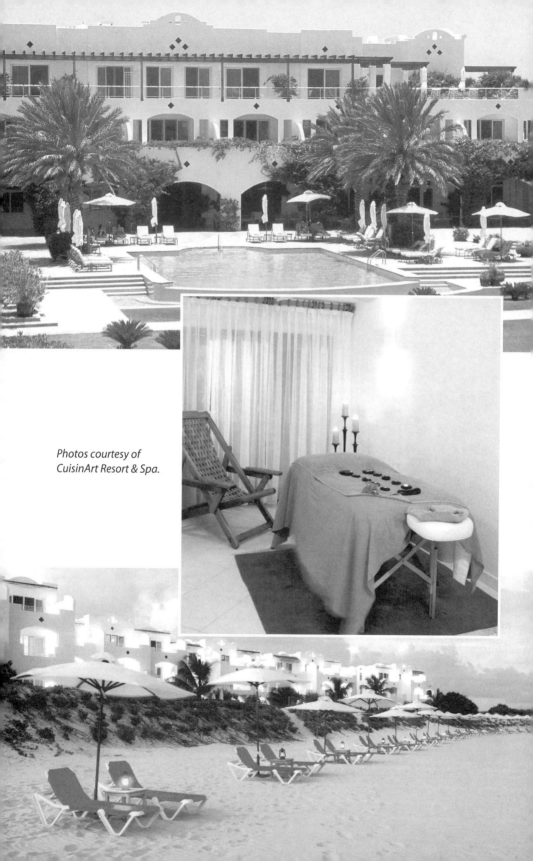

Photos courtesy of CuisinArt Resort & Spa.

Chapter 1

A Brief History of Wellness

Our state of health and happiness depends more upon our perception
of life events around us than on the events themselves.

—CHRISTIANE NORTHRUP, M.D., AUTHOR OF *WOMEN'S BODIES, WOMEN'S WISDOM*

I n the early 1900s, the germ theory—the notion that a single germ produced a certain disease and only a single drug would cure it—took hold of the American (and much of the developed world's) consciousness. As a result, pharmaceuticals became king with their promise of dramatic magic-bullet cures, and this resulted in huge economic incentives for the burgeoning pharmaceutical industry.

Conventional medicine is disease-oriented and diagnosis-driven. Establishment doctors are known to treat diseases, not people, using symptoms and medical tests to assess the problem and ascribe treatment, typically pharmaceutical drugs or surgery. More than forty years ago, faith in this conventional medicine began to erode. While it still has great value in treating trauma, and some value in treating acute infectious diseases, many of us began to observe its shortcomings when it came to cancer, heart disease, and other diseases of civilization. Furthermore, we started noticing the many harmful side effects of drug therapy. As Jay Cohen, M.D., pointed out in his book *Overdose,* over 300 Americans die *each day* from the side effects of *correctly prescribed* medications. And most people are unaware that, in this manner, physicians contribute to this fourth leading cause of death (after heart disease, cancer, and strokes) in the United States, an astonishing fact that was reported in the *Journal of the American Medical Association* in 1998 and again in 2003.

René Jules Dubos (1901–1982), microbiologist, experimental pathologist, and pioneering environmentalist, suggested in *Mirage of Health* that the advances made in the development of antibiotics and other medical technology had contributed far *less* to the improved health of the population of industrialized nations than had a variety of economic, social, behavioral, and lifestyle changes, such as improved sanitation, nutrition, and exercise.

Halbert Dunn, M.D., a Canadian psychiatrist, was the first to use the word *wellness* back in the 1950s. In his book, *High Level Wellness,* he tried to isolate those physical, emotional, psychological, and spiritual factors that he felt were essential to enjoying a high level of wellness.

Dunn's book influenced John Travis, M.D., to leave conventional medicine and open the first wellness center in Mill Valley, California, in 1975. Travis, a graduate of Tufts University School of Medicine, also completed a preventive medicine residency at Johns Hopkins University. It was there that he found Dunn's book and became one of the first to focus his professional career on the premise that health is more than the absence of disease, and that there are as many degrees of wellness as there are degrees of illness. Travis set about helping individuals grow into a higher state of wellness by caring for the body, using the mind creatively, channeling stress positively, expressing emotions instead of bottling them up, improving relationships, accepting responsibility, and getting in touch with the environment. Travis later published his findings in his *Wellness Workbook* (1981; updated in 1988 and 2004).

Dr. Simpson, who has known Dr. Travis for more than twenty years, says that many of the original concepts of wellness can be traced to this remarkable doctor's educational work. Dr. Simpson's own creation of the Wellness Game was a direct result of meeting Dr. Travis, who opened Dr. Simpson's eyes to many of the keys to optimum health. Wellness is a way of life, he learned, a lifestyle you can design in order to achieve your highest potential for well-being.

HOLISTIC HEALTH—PRELUDE TO ALTERNATIVE MEDICINE

In the late 1970s in California, another medical phenomenon—holistic health—was born. This antidote to conventional medicine focused on the whole person—body, mind, and spirit—and explored many alternative systems of healing. A core group of physicians interested in finding a better medical model founded the American Holistic Medical Association (AHMA) in Denver in 1978 to explore this new approach to healing and medicine. Although the holistic model was a much safer and more comprehensive approach, Travis felt that unlike wellness, which is about self-awareness, holistic health is about treatment or "fixing people."

The term holistic actually comes from Jan Smuts, a visionary South African statesman and philosopher who wrote *Holism and Evolution* in 1926. He believed that holism (from the Greek *holos,* or whole) formed the basis of evolution, which in turn was nothing more than the development of a progressive series of wholes, stretching from humble inorganic beginnings to the highest levels of spiritual creation. Smuts saw matter, life, and mind as parts of an active, creative process of the universe moving toward more and deeper wholeness. The concept of personality—considered the sum total of an individual's physical, mental, social, and emotional qualities—was put forth by Smuts as the latest, and supreme, whole that had arisen in the holistic series of evolution. He believed that humankind was evolving to a higher level and that the awakened human personality also reflected a whole that was greater than the sum of its parts.

The holistic health movement made an important contribution to the growing emphasis on wellness. In addition to highlighting the importance of looking at the whole person, it was the forerunner of alternative medicine, which has become an essential part of the medical landscape today.

ALTERNATIVE MEDICINE—A MAJOR SOCIAL FORCE EMERGES

In the 1990s, alternative medicine emerged as a major social force shaping medical care in the United States and abroad. Alternative medicine grants a major role to the mind and includes the spiritual dimension in health. In his article, "Why Patients Use Alternative Medicine," in the *Journal of the American Medical Association,* John A. Austin of the Stanford University School of Medicine says, "Users of alternative healthcare are more likely to report having had a transformational experience that changed the way they saw the world. They find in (alternative therapies) an acknowledgement of the importance of treating illness within a larger context of spirituality and life meaning . . . The use of alternative care is part of a broader value orientation and set of cultural beliefs, one that embraces a holistic, spiritual orientation to life."

As you may know, more people visit practitioners of alternative medicine today than visit conventional medical doctors. However, as with conventional medicine, one common pitfall with alternative therapies occurs when people focus on techniques—things that you do or have done to you—rather than on getting to know yourself and allowing the body's own healing mechanism to awaken. As a result, many of these techniques, such as acupuncture, biofeedback, and herbs, can become a hindrance when people ascribe so much power to the technique that they lose touch with their own innate healing ability.

We would like to introduce you to four key concepts of wellness (the first two by John Travis), which we believe to be the underpinning of health.

THE KEYS TO WELLNESS

Key Concept 1—The Illness/Wellness Continuum

As Dr. John Travis has stated, wellness is never a static state. No matter what your current state of health, you can begin to appreciate yourself as a growing, changing person, and allow yourself to move toward a more joyful and positive state of well-being.

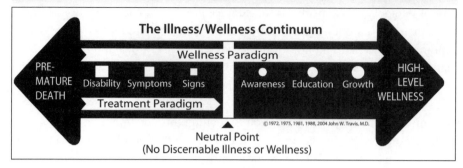

Figure 1.1. The Illness/Wellness Continuum

Illness is often the body-mind's attempt to get us to wake up and become more conscious of our unresolved issues in life. Wellness is an approach to health that encompasses a process of awareness, education, and growth. What matters most right now is the direction in which you are facing—is it toward high-level wellness, or toward premature death?

Moving from the center to the left of the continuum shows a progressively worsening state of health. Moving to the right of the center indicates progressively improving levels of health and well-being. The treatment paradigm can bring you to the neutral point where symptoms of disease have been alleviated. Moving toward wellness, however, which you can do at any point, takes you beyond the neutral point and encourages you to move as far to the right as possible. It is not meant to replace the treatment paradigm on the left side of the continuum, but to work in harmony with it.

One of the keys to wellness, as we show in Chapter 7, is the control of silent inflammation. The silent inflammation profile (SIP) is the first lab test that can monitor silent inflammation on a lifetime basis. At last, we have a *biomarker* (a predictive biological indicator and prognosticator of aging) that provides us with evidence-based wellness. The SIP allows us to see where we each fall on the illness/wellness continuum.

Key Concept 2—The Iceberg Model

Illness and health are only the tip of the iceberg. To understand their cause, as Dr. John Travis says, you must look below the surface.

Icebergs are interesting. They reveal only about one-tenth of their mass above the water. The remaining nine-tenths remain submerged, which is why they are such a nightmare to navigate around and why they are an apt metaphor when considering your state of wellness.

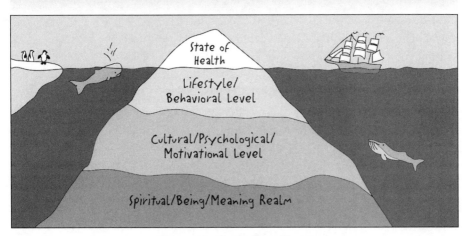

Figure 1.2. The Iceberg Model

Your current condition of health—be it one of disease or vitality—is like the tip of the iceberg. This is the apparent part—what shows. If you don't like your state of health, you can attempt to change it and chisel away at an unwanted malady. But, whenever you knock some of it off, more of the same comes up to take its place.

To understand what creates and supports your current state of health, you have to look underwater. As you can see in the iceberg above, the first level encountered below the waterline is the lifestyle/behavioral level—what you eat, how you use and exercise your body, how you relax and let go of stress, and how you safeguard yourself from the hazards around you.

Many people follow lifestyles that they know are destructive to their own well-being, to the people around them, and to the planet. Yet they may feel powerless to change the way they live. To understand why, it is necessary to look still deeper, to the next cultural/psychological/motivational level. Here we find what moves us to lead the lifestyle we've chosen. We learn how our cultural norms and our families influence us in subtle yet powerful ways from a very early age. Investigating this level, we also can become conscious of any ongoing psychological payoffs we have that are based on early life experiences and, ultimately, what their cost is to our physical and mental well-being.

Exploring down below the cultural/psychological/motivational level, there is the deepest spiritual/being/meaning level (a realm, actually, because it has no distinct boundaries). It includes the mystical, mysterious, metaphysical, and everything else in the subconscious mind, and concerns such issues as your reason for being, the meaning of your life, and your place in the universe. How you address these questions, and the answers you choose underlie and permeate all the layers above. This realm ultimately determines whether the tip of the iceberg, representing your state of health, will be one of disease or wellness.

Key Concept 3—Predictive Medicine

By comparing the ten leading causes of death in the United States in 1900 with those of today, we find that deaths in 1900 were mostly due to infectious disease, while most deaths today are attributable to lifestyle factors—diet, exercise, smoking, and so on. In fact, according to the U.S. Department of Health and Human Services, lifestyle is the main contributor to nineteen of the twenty-one major causes of illness and premature death today.

Even more important is that most diseases of civilization develop gradually (*see* Table 1.1 below), and that medical science has uncovered many of the key factors that contribute to particular diseases. Contrary to what the media proclaims, genetics (*nature*) accounts for less than 25 percent of modern illnesses—your environment and lifestyle (*nurture*) are much more important to your well-being. In most instances, genetic makeup is in the background as a tendency and is more likely to find expression when lifestyle factors (causing inflammation) give it the opportunity.

TABLE 1.1. The Increments of Chronic Disease

Age	Stage	Atherosclerosis	Cancer	Osteoarthritis	Diabetes	Emphysema	Cirrhosis
20	Start	Elevated cholesterol	Carcinogen exposure	Abnormal cartilage staining	Obesity	Smoker	Drinker
30	Discernible	Small plaques on arteriogram	Cellular metaplasia	Slight joint-space narrowing	Abnormal glucose tolerance	Mild airway obstruction	Fatty liver on biopsy
40	Subclinical	Larger plaques on arteriogram	Increasing metaplasia	Bone spurs	Elevated fasting-blood glucose	X-ray inflation	Enlarged liver
50	Threshold	Leg pain on exercise	Carcinoma in situ	Mild articular pain	Sugar in urine	Shortness of breath	Upper GI hemorrhage
60	Severe	Angina pectoris	Clinical cancer	Moderate articular pain	Hypoglycemic drug requirement	Recurrent hospitalization	Ascites (swelling in abdomen)
70	End	Stroke, heart attack	Metastatic cancer	Disabled	Blindness, neuropathy, nephropathy	Intractable oxygen debt	Jaundice, hepatic coma

With a comprehensive wellness assessment (also called a meta-analysis), physicians can often predict (using such biomarkers as the SIP) what types of problems are most likely to occur in an individual, and they can take appropriate action before clinical symptoms appear. Medi-spa programs offer this type of program. Participants can expand their health knowledge and their experiences and, in the process, get results that can identify, halt and, in many cases, actually reverse a number of chronic diseases.

Key Concept 4—Psychoneuroimmunology (PNI)

As recently as the 1980s, practitioners of conventional medicine still tended to treat the body and mind as separate entities. We now know that the mind and body are inextricably linked and that the health of one influences the other. The area of practice in which they converge is known as mind-body medicine.

Psychoneuroimmunology (PNI) is the study of the interrelation between the mind (psycho), the nervous and hormonal systems (neuroendocrine), and the immune system (immunology). Candace Pert, Ph.D., a pioneering researcher at Rutgers University, believes that as emotions fluctuate—from anger to pleasure, for example—neuropeptides (neurotransmitters) sweep through the body systems in response, causing such physical changes as a rise in blood pressure or a relaxation of the muscles.

Anxiety, depression, loneliness, and stress have all been shown to depress the immune system. On the other hand, writing in *Anatomy of an Illness,* Norman Cousins discussed how positive emotions, such as joy and laughter, can produce positive effects on the immune system, and how he believed these factors to be responsible for curing his own debilitating arthritis.

Relationships and social networks have also been shown to provide powerful protection against stress and disease. For example, a 1992 study of heart patients at Duke University showed that those without a spouse or confidante were three times as likely to die within five years of diagnosis as those who were married or had a close friend or animal companion.

Biofeedback is a practical way of showing how the mind mirrors and influences the body. As part of a medi-spa program, participants learn techniques to regulate physiological processes, such as heart rate, respiration, and brain-wave patterns.

In summary, every thought, mood, emotion, and feeling will cause a physiological reaction in the body that, in turn, has an impact, for better or worse, on your well-being. This realm is the more subjective and hidden part of the iceberg, but is, by far, the most important one for your health.

MEDI-SPAS—THE FUTURE OF WELLNESS

For the past decade or so, it has become obvious that a new approach to health care is needed. We no longer have to cling to the mechanistic, *fix-me* mentality traditionally advocated in health care. We now have the capacity to reverse the ever-increasing incidences of chronic disease, premature aging, and the shrinking quality of life by treating total individuals rather than treating only the diseases they evince.

We believe that our culture is ready for such a shift in perception. Humanity has evolved from simple consciousness to self-consciousness and is now poised for its next major transition, to what we call *integral consciousness*. As part of this new wellness-oriented spa medicine, the very nature of the interaction between physician and patient will change, with both working together as partners in healing.

The term *integral health* denotes:

- Integration of the body, emotions, mind, and spirit to enhance wellness and longevity;

- Integration of the best of conventional and alternative medicine;

- Expansion of consciousness (knowledge) and the intensification of consciousness (wisdom).

Such an approach deals with the person as a whole and views illness as a disruption of physical and mental well-being. As *clients* (in this new medicine, the word *client* replaces the less empowering *patient*) learn to adopt healthy lifestyle choices to stimulate the body's natural self-healing and self-regulating abilities; fewer drugs will need to be given and fewer surgeries scheduled. The present HMO-style practice offers little for either practitioner or patient beyond a drugstore. In most cases, drugs don't cure because they treat only symptoms; they don't get to the root cause, the bottom layer of the iceberg.

We feel strongly that medi-spas will become the natural delivery sites for this new wellness-oriented medicine. The spa of the future and the medical clinic of the future will be one and the same.

PIONEERS OF SPA MEDICINE

Dr. John Harvey Kellogg, the co-inventor of toasted flakes, was a pioneer in spa medicine in the 1920s and 1930s. At his sanitarium in Michigan, he advanced a revolutionary concept of health and fitness with his nutrition, exercise, fresh air, and different medical therapies of the day.

In 1940, Dr. Edmond Szekely and his wife opened Rancho La Puerta in Tecate, Mexico, adopting some of Kellogg's practices and adding many more innovative ideas of their own to enhance a person's well-being. Since then, the spa concept has greatly expanded, with more than 10,000 destinations and day spas spread across the United States, from the Caribbean to Hawaii. Most of these spas have focused primarily on pampering and beauty, providing massage, facials, body wraps, and some hydrotherapy.

Twenty Reasons for Spa Medicine

1. Marriage of beauty and health.
2. Increased interest in alternative medicine.
3. Recent science of antiaging medicine.
4. Aging boomer demographics.
5. Need for a new medical model.
6. Integration of body, mind, and spirit.
7. Self-care versus passive care.
8. More than 10,000 spas in the United States alone, and growing.
9. Power of the Internet and telemedicine.
10. Medi-spa provides a lifestyle coach for each client.
11. Central role of consciousness in the new medical model.
12. Multiple modalities available in a single location.
13. Desire of boomers to look good and feel good.
14. Medi-spas provide ideal healing environment.
15. Integral health model most inclusive one to date.
16. Spa medicine gives an individual the tools to take control of his or her health and well-being.
17. Spa medicine includes awareness of the infinite, indestructible, and immortal nature of our minds.
18. Spa medicine uses detoxification as a key factor in healing.
19. Boomers want convenience, service, excellence, and noninvasive health care.
20. Medi-spas help clients get in an ideal zone to control inflammation and extend longevity.

THE FUTURE OF SPA MEDICINE

Spas of the future will merge the best of the traditional spa therapies with the latest integrative medical practices. Spa medicine that is based on integral health (*see* Appendix A) has the potential to prevent most chronic disease and significantly improve not only the length of life, but more important, the quality of life.

Medicine as it is usually practiced today should be avoided whenever possible. We do not suggest abandoning Western medicine completely, but rather that you seek out spa medicine with its wellness and longevity focus, and use Western medicine only where it is at its best—in an acute crisis, such as an acute heart attack, a loss of consciousness, or a major trauma.

The nearby day medi-spa or the destination medi-spa each offer you the opportunity to reevaluate your health status and provide you with the information and tools to help jump-start your journey to longevity and well-being. The day medi-spa is ideal for providing ongoing wellness services and regular monitoring. For the more distant destinations, some clients use their annual vacation to go to a spa retreat where they can relax and renew their chosen wellness/anti-aging lifestyle.

Two-thirds of all the people age sixty-five and over who have ever lived on planet Earth are alive today, and it is no longer uncommon to have a family photo that includes six generations. Figure 1.3 below shows how dramatically the life span has increased in the last hundred years and what we can expect in the future.

Not so long ago, sixty-five was considered old. But now, many boomers consider eighty to be the start of old age, and this age wave is global. What then is

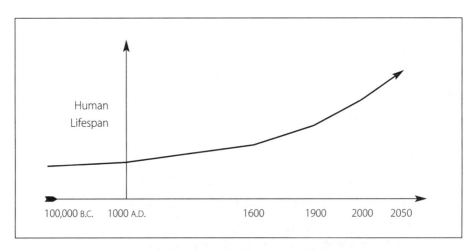

Figure 1.3. The Climbing Human Lifespan

the model for maturity? Unlike our parents, who went to school, then work, and finally retired (which means disappeared), the boomers of today choose to reinvent themselves at each stage. But, in order to move from their parents' linear lifestyles to the more circular lifestyles of today, they need to have health and vitality at the core of this new vision of maturity. Fortunately, we now have the key to preventing, and even reversing, many of the chronic degenerative diseases. This key is spa medicine based on integral health programs that can be found at select medi-spas throughout the world. Spa medicine is directed primarily toward detoxification and controlling silent inflammation that is at the center of aging and chronic disease; this is your gateway to the ageless zone. (*See Don't Retire, REWIRE!* by Jeri Sedlar and Rick Miners at www.dontretirerewire.com.)

SPA-MEDICINE PROGRAMS

Most spa-medicine programs include three distinct steps.

STEP ONE—Measuring

A four-part meta-analysis is completed on each person who is a client. A baseline set of biomarkers and laboratory tests provides objective markers to follow as the client becomes involved in the individually tailored program.

STEP TWO—Mentoring

A medi-spa coach assists the client with different wellness and longevity strategies and services. The client is provided with all the necessary tools and information to look and feel her or his best.

STEP THREE—Monitoring

Monitoring is important to document that the age-management strategies are working. Throughout the year, spa-medicine programs support and update clients via the Internet, sharing the latest medical breakthroughs, practical resources, and cutting-edge products. The medi-spa coach can respond to any questions and issues, and schedule necessary visits and services for the client.

Although every medi-spa is unique, all should provide a nurturing environment where each client is listened to and feels that all his or her health concerns (body-mind-spirit) have been addressed.

Sampling the wide variety of natural medi-spa services, medi-spa clients become active participants in their own health. Most of these services start clients out by helping them detox and control silent inflammation (*see* Table 1.2 on page 18).

Spa medicine is very different from the typical episodic, fragmented care that conventional medicine offers today. By giving a context in which to reframe health, medi-spas provide clients with important insights into the meaning of medicine and help them to learn how a supportive lifestyle and worldview can contribute to ultimate well-being.

TABLE 1.2. Sampling of Medi-Spa Services

Detoxifying	Nutrition	Exercise	Mind-Body	Beauty
Aquachi	Body analysis	Aerobics	Acupuncture	Botox
Aromatherapy	Cell therapy	Aquacise	Alexander	Color
Ayurvedic detox	Cooking	Basketball	Anthroposophy	Cosmeceuticals
Body wraps	Diet	Cycling	Art therapy	Cuts
Brushing	Eating out	Dancing	Autogenics	Dermabrasion
Candling	Fasting	Flexaball	Biofeedback	Electrical stimulation
Chelation	Food combining	Kickboxing	Breathing	Endermology
Colon therapy	Food composition 40/30/30	Personal training	Feldenkrais	Facials
Feng shui	Food preparation	Pilates	Heart-math	Hair removal
Holistic dentistry	Hormones	Qi gong	Hypnosis	Injections
Hydrotherapy	Hydroponics	Rowing	Imagery	Laser
Liver detox	Hyperbaric O2	Spinning	Lifelong learning	Makeup
Lymph drainage	Nutraceuticals	Stretching	Meditation	Manicures
Massage	Organic foods	Superslow Zone	Progressive relaxation	Mesotherapy
Nasal wash	RMR	Swimming	Psychoneuroimmunology	Pedicures
Reflexology	Serving size	Tai chi	Psychotherapy	Peels
Sauna (far infrared)	Shopping smart	Tai-bo	Relaxation response	Perms
Seaweed/mud	SIP	Walking	Rolfing	Skin analysis
Steam	Weight loss	Weight training	Universe story	Tanning
Stone therapy	Zone Rx	Yoga	Worldview well-being	Waxing

Chapter 2

Pillar One —
Detoxification

*The current level of chemicals in the food and water supply and indoor
and outdoor environment has lowered our threshold of resistance to
disease and has altered our body's metabolism, causing enzyme
dysfunction, nutritional deficiencies, and hormonal imbalances.*

—MARSHALL MANDELL, M.D.

Toxins are everywhere in our environment: carbon monoxide and other chemicals in our air, industrial chemicals in our water, mercury in our dental fillings, and pesticides in our food. Each year, we are exposed to literally thousands of toxic chemicals and pollutants that lace our air, food, soil, and water. As a result, we carry within us a veritable chemical cocktail of food additives, heavy metals, industrial wastes, pesticides, and pharmaceuticals. As Dr. Jay Cohen points out, more than half the drugs deemed safe by the FDA are subsequently found to have previously unrecognized, medically serious side effects, most of which are dose-related. This doesn't even count the residues from legal drugs, such as alcohol, caffeine, and tobacco; or illegal drugs, such as cocaine, heroin, and marijuana. The EPA conducted a National Human Adipose Tissue Survey (NHATS) in people across the entire country, and nearly every fat sample tested was loaded with multiple chemical toxins. We are all toxic and cannot escape the continual pollution that plagues the planet each and every day of our lives.

Over time, multiple factors and toxins strain a person's organs until there is eventually a total body overload (*see* Figure 2.1 on page 20). As mentioned earlier, it takes a long time for most diseases to develop; people don't suddenly get sick. In their book, *Vitality and Aging,* authors James Fries and Lawrence Crapo point out that people typically go through *increments* of disease, marked by progressively reduced function and increasing intensity of symptoms, which often go unrecognized until they develop into a diagnosed illness. A specialty known as *functional medicine* seeks to identify these increments in order to provide early

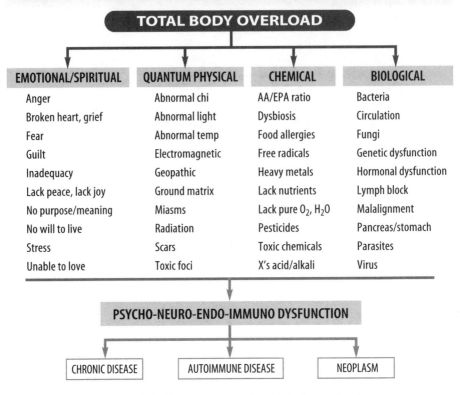

Figure 2.1. Consequences of Total Body Overload

intervention. As you'll see when answering the Ecology Screening Questionnaire on the following page, symptoms we often take for granted or just accept—a stuffy nose, itchy eyes, chronic coughing—may be harbingers of toxicity. One goal of spa medicine is to help you identify any abnormality at an early stage so the problem can be corrected before it leads to chronic disease.

To see if you might have any functional problems from toxic overload, take this simple test (*see* the Ecology Screening Questionnaire on page 21) from Jeffrey Bland, Ph.D., author of *The 20-Day Rejuvenation Diet Program*. If your points total less than 25, congratulations. Your toxic load is minimal. If your score is between 25 and 100, or you have a score of 10 or more in any single category, you have some degree of toxicity, but can expect your symptoms to improve by detoxifying your body with our advice in this chapter. A score over 100 indicates more serious symptoms, and you should make sure these symptoms are not associated with any medically definable disease. You may wish to copy this questionnaire for each family member and retake it every six months.

ECOLOGY SCREENING QUESTIONNAIRE

NAME _____ DATE _____ WEEK _____

Rate each of the following symptoms based upon your typical health profile. The initial test applies to instances of any of the following within the past seven days.

Point Scale: 0 = Never, or almost never, have the symptom
1 = Occasionally have it, effect is not severe
2 = Occasionally have it, effect is severe
3 = Frequently have it, effect is not severe
4 = Frequently have it, effect is severe

Head	_____ Headaches	
	_____ Faintness	
	_____ Dizziness	
	_____ Insomnia	**Subtotal** _____
Eyes	_____ Watery or itchy eyes	
	_____ Swollen, reddened, or sticky eyelids	
	_____ Bags or dark circles under eyes	
	_____ Blurred or tunnel vision (does not include near- or farsightedness)	**Subtotal** _____
Ears	_____ Itchy ears	
	_____ Earaches, ear infections	
	_____ Drainage from ear	
	_____ Ringing in ears, hearing loss	**Subtotal** _____
Nose	_____ Stuffy nose	
	_____ Sinus problems	
	_____ Hay fever	
	_____ Sneezing attacks	
	_____ Excessive mucus formation	**Subtotal** _____
Mouth/ throat	_____ Chronic coughing	
	_____ Gagging, frequent need to clear throat	
	_____ Sore throat, hoarseness, loss of voice	
	_____ Swollen or discolored tongue, gums, lips	
	_____ Canker sores	**Subtotal** _____

Skin	_____ Acne	
	_____ Hives, rashes, dry skin	
	_____ Hair loss	
	_____ Flushing, hot flashes	
	_____ Excessive sweating	**Subtotal** _____

Heart	_____ Irregular or skipped heartbeat	
	_____ Rapid or pounding heartbeat	
	_____ Chest pain	**Subtotal** _____

Lungs	_____ Chest congestion	
	_____ Asthma, bronchitis	
	_____ Shortness of breath	
	_____ Difficulty breathing	**Subtotal** _____

Digestive tract	_____ Nausea, vomiting	
	_____ Diarrhea	
	_____ Constipation	
	_____ Bloated feeling	
	_____ Belching, passing gas	
	_____ Heartburn	
	_____ Intestinal/stomach pain	**Subtotal** _____

Joints/ muscle	_____ Pain or aches in joints	
	_____ Arthritis	
	_____ Stiffness or limitation of movement	
	_____ Pain or aches in muscles	
	_____ Feeling of weakness or tiredness	**Subtotal** _____

Weight	_____ Binge eating/drinking	
	_____ Craving certain foods	
	_____ Excessive weight	
	_____ Compulsive eating	
	_____ Water retention	
	_____ Underweight	**Subtotal** _____

Energy/ activity	_____ Fatigue, sluggishness	
	_____ Apathy, lethargy	
	_____ Hyperactivity	
	_____ Restlessness	**Subtotal** _____

Mind	_____ Poor memory	
	_____ Confusion, poor comprehension	
	_____ Poor concentration	
	_____ Poor physical coordination	
	_____ Difficulty in making decisions	
	_____ Stuttering or stammering	
	_____ Slurred speech	
	_____ Learning disabilities	**Subtotal** _____
Emotions	_____ Mood swings	
	_____ Anxiety, fear, nervousness	
	_____ Anger, irritability, aggressiveness	
	_____ Depression	**Subtotal** _____
Other	_____ Frequent illness	
	_____ Frequent or urgent urination	
	_____ Genital itching or discharge	**Subtotal** _____
		Grand Total _____

In his book, Bland notes that problems with the digestive tract and liver (your major detoxifying organs) influence the hormonal, immune, and nervous systems, the primary control systems of overall health and balance. His approach to chronic toxicity is to:

- Identify and eliminate, or reduce, exposure to the exotoxins (from without) and endotoxins (from within) to which an individual may be sensitive (almost any substance produced outside our bodies is potentially an exotoxin, and substances produced inside our bodies, such as antibodies or hormones, are called endotoxins if they build up excessively);

- Improve the body's ability to detoxify and excrete those substances in nontoxic forms;

- Support the function of the individual's hormonal, immune, and nervous systems.

Since each person will respond differently to toxic exposures at different times, many physicians will not recognize chronic impairment until it becomes severe enough to produce a particular disease. For example, the usual American diet is notoriously high in fat and sugar (the average person consumes more than 150 pounds of sugar every year) and low in fiber. These factors can lead to a toxic bowel characterized by constipation and dysbiosis, which is an imbalance of intestinal flora that has been implicated in chronic fatigue, depression, digestive disorders, PMS, rheumatoid arthritis, yeast overgrowth, and even cancer.

Issues with dysbiosis and intestinal toxicity increase with age, as the mucous membrane lining that separates the intestine from the blood supply becomes even thinner. As Bland points out, a normal intestine is better able to absorb the good guys and get rid of the bad guys, but when the intestinal tract becomes overloaded with toxins (such as from refined sugar and flour, artificial food coloring, or chemical preservatives), its buffering ability—and its ability to discriminate friend from foe—diminishes, and a leaky gut results. Toxins then pass through the gut wall into the general circulation and begin to overload the liver, which contains important Kupffer cells, whose function it is to alert the rest of the body that exposure to toxins has occurred. This alert can cause the immune system to become overactive if too frequently repeated, which can, in turn, increase the risk of autoimmune diseases, such as arthritis. Table 2.1 below shows examples of common toxins that may adversely affect the body.

TABLE 2.1. Common Toxins	
Sources of Toxins	Harmful Examples/Results of Toxins
Food toxins	3,000 additives to foods and numerous pesticides, antibiotics, hormones
Water toxins	700 synthetic chemical compounds identified
Vehicle emissions	Carbon monoxide, benzene, sulphurs/increased chronic lung problems
Industrial waste	Oil refineries/harmful petrochemicals
Tobacco smoke	Dangers now accepted—secondhand smoke problems included
Drugs	Harmful side effects—legal or illegal drugs
Household appliances	Sick building syndrome
Household products	Cleaning agents and paints emit noxious gases
Personal care products	Mouthwashes, toothpaste, deodorants
Harmful metals	Cadmium, lead, aluminum cookware
Dental fillings	Mercury
Electromagnetic fields	Power lines, cellular phones
Radiation	X rays, radon

While your body is equipped to handle a certain level of toxins, a host of factors—polluted environment, poor diet, and stress, to name a few—can overtax the system. Once this occurs, toxins accumulate in the bloodstream and are then stored in the brain, fat, and other tissues. In the nervous system, toxins can cause brain fog and even seizures; toxins in muscle and cartilage can give rise to chronic fatigue and arthritis. Toxins can also disrupt hormonal activity or raise free-radical levels, increasing the risk of DNA mutations and cancer.

Whatever their target, the eventual result is ill health and accelerated aging. Over the past twenty-five years, a variety of terms have been used to describe individuals with these functional symptoms. Years ago, these walking wounded were described as having conditions ranging from distressed syndrome to hypoglycemia and adrenal exhaustion. Candidiasis, chronic fatigue, and food allergies are some other terms used to describe the results of toxic overload.

DETOXIFICATION PATHWAYS

In a healthy individual, the body's normal detoxification system is able to neutralize and eliminate toxins, minimizing tissue damage and preventing illness. When your body is unable to remove toxins, or is overwhelmed by their presence, you become more vulnerable to "silent inflammation" and chronic degenerative disease processes and accelerated aging.

The main components of the body's detoxification system include the:

- Gastrointestinal tract (small and large intestines);
- Liver;
- Lungs;
- Lymphatic system;
- Skin;
- Urinary system (kidney and bladder).

Your body's detoxification system relies upon two lines of defense. First, such organs as the skin and gastrointestinal tract prevent toxins from entering the body; then others, such as the kidney, the liver, and the lymphatic system, neutralize and excrete the toxins once they penetrate the initial line of defense. Obviously, it is always best to avoid toxins in the first place.

STEP I: REDUCE YOUR EXPOSURE TO TOXINS

Before getting started on a detoxification program, we suggest that you make an inventory of your habits and use the following recommendations, if necessary, to learn how you can prevent or minimize toxins in your environment and ensure that they will not be reintroduced into your body.

Eat a Healthy Diet

Start by selecting fresh foods that are organically raised or sourced; that is, free of antibiotics, artificial colorings and dyes, contaminants, herbicides, hormones, pesticides, and preservatives. Use a product derived from a natural source or use Clorox to wash the poisons off your nonorganic vegetables and fruits (*see* Appendix B).

Eat a diet high in antioxidant-rich phytonutrients (plant nutrients). This can be achieved by eating five to nine different kinds of fresh fruits and vegetables every day. These foods include citrus, cruciferous vegetables (broccoli, Brussels sprouts, cabbage, cauliflower), dark-green leafy vegetables, red-orange fruits and vegetables, garlic, and soy. This type of diet contains a broad and powerful array of what are known as *biological response modifiers,* food substances that change your body's ability to deal with toxins and other harmful substances.

Participants in spa wellness programs learn about these foods and the importance of a healthy, nontoxic diet, while world-class chefs at destination resorts, such as CuisinArt in Anguilla, give new meaning to gourmet dining. Additionally, our chapter on nutraceuticals will further discuss the exciting new science of antioxidants and supplements and their role in detoxification.

Avoid Xenoestrogens As Much As Possible

Xenoestrogens are biological compounds that mimic estrogens. They can stimulate estrogen receptors in the cells and trigger new genetic messages that cause abnormal growth of cells and tissues. There is mounting evidence that xenoestrogens set the stage for, and are playing a role in, the epidemic rise in breast, prostate, and other cancers. Be aware that these compounds are found high up on the food chain, in hormone-fed poultry, cattle, and cows. To avoid this potential problem, choose only organic dairy products and use only natural range-fed beef, bison, and poultry.

Beware of Xenobiotics

Xenobiotics are synthetic petrochemical-based compounds that are related to xenoestrogens. They can be found everywhere—in dry cleaning, gasoline vapors, hair spray, household cleaners, perfumes, plastic food containers, plastic wrap, soaps, and industrial toxins, such as DDT, and insecticides.

Xenobiotics also mimic estrogen and can be transported to the breast. Once there, they can lock on to receptor sites and cause abnormal cell division. While it's impossible to avoid all of these products, the more you become aware of their potential impact on your health, the more ways you can come up with to circumvent the problem. For example, try to buy as many foods as possible from small markets that use good old-fashioned butcher paper to wrap meats and seafoods. If that's not possible, remove the plastic wrap from your foods as soon as you get home. Don't use a microwave to heat any food wrapped in plastic because it magnifies the leaching of toxins from the plastic. You should also consume squalene, a substance in extra-virgin olive oil, rice bran oil, shark liver oil, and wheat germ oil. The squalene in these oils, available in health food stores, can neutralize many petrochemicals, and for that reason alone, *all women over forty should consider adding squalene to their diets.*

Olive oil is one of the safest and most beneficial oils you can consume. The research on its ability to counteract cancer and heart disease is overwhelming. In fact, one of the reasons that Mediterranean cultures have fewer incidences of cancer is because they regularly consume olive oil. Put one tablespoon a day on salads and vegetables.

Drink Pure Water

Drink at least six to eight glasses of pure, filtered water each day to help you hydrate and flush toxins out your body. You can use a home water filter or purchase water bottled in glass from a reliable source. Water bottled in plastic can leach out cadmium and phalates (plastic toxins). If you must use water bottled in plastic, use a filter or check the bottom of the bottle. If there is a #7 in a triangle, it's the best container. Lower numbers indicate potential toxicity, while a number above 4 is safe (most plastic bottles in stores are a #1). Up to 70 percent of toxins enter the body through the skin, which means that a filter for the bathtub or shower is as important as one for kitchen drinking water.

Use Natural Cleaning Products

Substitute natural cleaning products for toxic ones. In their place, use baking soda, Borax, castille soaps, citrus cleaners (nonpetrochemical), distilled white vinegar, lemon juice, and ecologically safe commercial products.

Breathe Clean Air

Since most people spend more time indoors than out, consider purchasing an air purification device for your home and/or office. Houseplants can also be used as filters to help remove indoor air pollution. Ferns, English ivy, philodendrons, and spider plants all make good natural purifiers.

Beware of formaldehyde fumes from carpeting, cabinetry, floor coverings, new furniture, and upholstery. Cysteine, MSM, taurine, thiamine, and vitamin B_6 can help detox formaldehyde.

Table 2.2 sets forth the pollutant standards index (PSI) developed by the U.S. Environmental Protection Agency (EPA) to measure pollution levels for major air pollutants. PSI figures are reported daily in metropolitan areas.

TABLE 2.2. Effects of Air Quality on Health

Pollutant Standards Index (PSI)	Degree of Effect	General Health Effects	Cautionary Statements
500 400 300	Hazardous	Premature death of ill and older people. Healthy people will experience adverse symptoms that affect their normal activity.	Everyone should remain indoors, keeping windows and doors closed. People should also minimize physical exertion and try to avoid sitting in traffic.
200	Very unhealthy	Premature onset of certain diseases in addition to significant aggravation of symptoms and decreased exercise tolerance in healthy persons.	Older people and those with existing diseases should stay indoors and avoid physical exertion. General population should avoid outdoor activity.
100	Unhealthy	Significant aggravation of symptoms and decreased exercise tolerance in anyone who has heart or lung disease, with widespread symptoms in the healthy population.	Older people and those with existing heart or lung diseases should stay indoors and reduce physical activity.
50	Moderate	Mild aggravation of symptoms in susceptible people, with irritation of symptoms in the healthy population.	People with existing heart or respiratory ailments should reduce physical exertion and outdoor activity.
0	Good	None	None

Source: U.S. Environmental Protection Agency, Washington D.C. 20460

Protect Your Hearing

Just as excessive sound levels can cause hearing-related damages (*see* Table 2.3 on page 29), they can also cause stress-related illnesses, such as hypertension. By contrast, gentle sounds can be one of the easiest ways to relax and prevent such stress-related illnesses as anxiety, headaches, and high blood pressure. Noise pollution can also result in cardiac arrhythmias caused by magnesium depletion. Healthy sounds range from peaceful music to gentle environmental sounds, types of sound often experienced at medi-spas.

Take in the Right Kind of Light

As light enters the eyes, it speeds along neurochemical pathways to the pineal and

TABLE 2.3. Sound Levels in Decibels and Human Response

This decibel (dB) table compares some common sounds and shows how they rank in their potential harm to hearing. Note that 90 dB is the point at which noise begins to harm hearing. To the ear, each 10 dB increase seems twice as loud.

Common Sounds	Noise Level (dB)	Effect
Carrier-deck jet operation Air raid siren	140	Painfully loud
Jet takeoff (200 feet)	120	Requires maximum vocal effort
Thunderclap Discotheque Auto horn (3 feet)	115	Very loud and uncomfortable
Pile drivers	110	Very uncomfortable
Garbage truck	100	Uncomfortable
Heavy truck (50 feet) City traffic	90	Very annoying Hearing damage (8 hours)
Alarm clock (2 feet) Hair dryer Noisy restaurant Freeway traffic	80	Annoying
Man's voice (3 feet)	70	Telephone use difficult
Air conditioning unit (20 feet)	60	Intrusive
Light auto traffic (100 feet)	50	Quiet
Living room Bedroom Quiet office	40	Quiet
Library Soft whisper	30	Quiet
Broadcasting studio	20 10 0	Quiet Just audible Hearing begins

Source: U.S. Environmental Protection Agency, Washington, D.C. 20460

pituitary glands, the master controllers of the endocrine (hormonal) system. The right amount of light and the right type (full-spectrum) is important for well-being. John Ott, a pioneer in photobiology, suggests you spend time outside every day and make use of natural light whenever possible. Full-spectrum lights, which simulate natural light, are available for use indoors and can be especially useful during the winter months.

Attend to Dental Care

You may not realize the enormous impact your dentist can have on your life. The more we research the subject, the more convinced we are that the mouth is a major indicator of overall health. If our eyes are the windows of the soul, then our teeth are the windows of the body, and especially the heart. There are many common dental problems that can have a negative impact on your health, and doctors are becoming increasingly aware of the mouth-body link. The most common problems include the following:

- Allergic reactions to dental materials;

- Cavitations: holes in the jawbone where teeth previously were;

- Electrical currents caused by dissimilar metals in the mouth;

- Focal points of infection in or under old root canals and sites of extraction;

- Mercury fillings;

- Periodontal disease, which weakens the immune system.

Amalgams, root canals, and cavitations can cause increased oxidative stress in the body. And half of all amalgam fillings are mercury, which is very toxic, especially to the brain (the amount of mercury in the brain directly relates to the number of fillings in your mouth), the heart, and the immune system. It leaks out of the fillings and goes to every tissue in the body. Many dentists believe that the mercury present in amalgam fillings can be a source of chronic toxicity that can push some people over the edge of good health and lead to chronic medical problems (it can take more than six months for the body to clear out the mercury after amalgam fillings have been removed).

Detecting heavy metals, including mercury, can be easily accomplished with a provocative urine test done by Doctors Data Lab. In this test, urine is collected for twenty-four hours after the client ingests DMSA (dimercaptosuccinic acid). DMSA pulls mercury out of body tissue and into the bloodstream, where it is then filtered through the kidneys, into the urine, and out of the body. Mark Breiner, D.D.S., offers important insights on this subject in his book, *Whole Body Dentistry.*

To see if you might be mercury toxic, fill out the Mercury Screening Questionnaire on page 31. You can also contact the International Academy of Oral Medicine and Toxicology (IAOMT) or the American Academy of Biological Dentistry to locate a holistic dentist.

An average 4-foot fluorescent bulb has 22 milligrams of mercury in it, and according to the EPA, it should be treated as toxic waste. An average molar amalgam has 1,000 milligrams of mercury in it. If you were to throw this into a five-acre lake, the EPA would declare the lake toxic and prevent your eating any fish from it. We have often seen dramatic improvement in certain chronically diseased patients when mercury is removed and, on this subject, we would again encourage you to read Dr. Mark Breiner's book.

MERCURY SCREENING QUESTIONNAIRE

NAME _____ DATE _____ WEEK _____

Rate each of the following symptoms based upon your typical health profile. The initial test applies to instances of any of the following within the past seven days.

Point Scale: 0 = Never   2 = Often
                    1 = Rarely   3 = Always

Head		
	_____ Headaches	
	_____ Migraine headaches	
	_____ Stuffy sinuses	
	_____ Vision problems	
	_____ Hearing difficulties	
	_____ Memory loss	
	_____ Lack of concentration	
	_____ Insomnia	**Subtotal** _____

Mouth/ throat		
	_____ Chronic hoarseness	
	_____ Sore throats	
	_____ Cold sores	
	_____ Bleeding gums	
	_____ Painful gums	
	_____ Swollen glands in throat	
	_____ Thyroid problems	**Subtotal** _____

Cardiopulmonary		
	_____ Asthma	
	_____ Bronchitis	
	_____ Chest pains	
	_____ Irregular heartbeat	
	_____ Tachycardia	
	_____ High blood pressure	**Subtotal** _____

GI tract	_____ Bloating	
	_____ Constipation	
	_____ Crohn's disease	
	_____ Diarrhea	
	_____ Gastrointestinal problems	
	_____ Irritable bowel syndrome	
	_____ Stomach ulcers	
	_____ (*Helicobacter pylori*)	**Subtotal** _____

| Kidneys/ | _____ Frequent urination | |
| bladder | _____ Bladder infection | **Subtotal** _____ |

| Neuromuscular | _____ Muscle tremor | |
| | _____ Numbness anywhere | **Subtotal** _____ |

Sensitivities	_____ Allergies	
	_____ Skin disorders	
	_____ Dry peeling skin at ends of fingers (acrodynia)	**Subtotal** _____

| Metabolism | _____ Lack of energy | **Subtotal** _____ |

Personality traits	_____ Anxiety	
	_____ Bad temper	
	_____ Depression	
	_____ Dizziness	**Subtotal** _____

Major signs	_____ Metallic taste in mouth	
	_____ Metallic smell from urine	
	_____ Metallic smell from feces	**Subtotal** _____

Have You Ever Had?	_____ Kidney disease	
	_____ Kidney failure	
	_____ Multiple sclerosis	
	_____ ALS (amyotrophic lateral sclerosis)	
	_____ SLE (systemic lupus erythematosus)	
	_____ FM (fibromyalgia)	
	_____ CFIDS (chronic fatigue syndrome)	**Subtotal** _____

NOTE: *Score 3 points for each condition you have currently or have had in the past.*

Grand Total _____

Score:

1–20   You may have some degree of toxicity, but it isn't enough for major concern.

21–40   You are somewhat toxic and should reduce your exposure to mercury and other heavy metals such as lead and cadmium.

40+   You are highly toxic. See a clinical ecologist, naturopath, or your regular doctor immediately.

Avoid Excess Radiation

Excessive radiation causes enormous premature aging to the body. People exposed to excessive radiation, such as radiologists, airline pilots, and flight attendants have been known to develop inflammatory situations that can result in more disease and cancer. Probably the most famous recent radiation accident occurred at Chernobyl in what was then the Soviet Union. Although many of the adults in Chernobyl developed various cancers, particularly thyroid cancer, the children of Chernobyl not only developed thyroid problems, but have also been left with extremely high oxidized cholesterol in their bodies. Since radiation is forever, it can continuously oxidize the LDL cholesterol, which is a problem because it can eventually lead to greater inflammation and result in heart attacks and strokes.

One of the most common forms of silent radiation in our homes is radon, an odorless radioactive substance coming from deep within the earth. If your home is built on large stores of radon, then its insidious radioactive gases can literally engender disease and even premature death. Dr. Sinatra had a tragic case in his cardiology practice when one of his patients contracted lung cancer even though he had never smoked. Turned out he was unknowingly living on a base of radon rock, and it had slowly poisoned him over time.

Radiation, whether from radon or other sources, is not to be taken lightly, and we need to be more aware of its highly toxic, invisible nature. We also need to beware our x-ray–happy medical society. Before you submit to another set of dental radiographs, a chest x-ray, or another type of radiograph, ask yourself and your doctor, "Is it really necessary?" Remember, even in small amounts, radiation is cumulative and remains in your tissues for life.

Remove Electromagnetic Fields (EMFs)

Even simple household appliances—bedside clocks, computers, heating blankets, TVs, and other products that have electromagnetic fields—can alter the function of cells, change biorhythms (including heart rate variability), decrease melatonin, and promote tumor growth.

One case study showed that the heart rhythm of a woman wearing a twenty-four-hour monitor to detect a second-to-second analysis of her heartbeat went suddenly out of rhythm after she was jolted awake by an alarm clock (noise pollution can also be potent). Unfortunately, she died, and the Holter monitor revealed that the cause was a sudden erratic heartbeat (ventricular fibrillation) at the time of her abrupt awakening. We know now that many of these situations of sudden death that occur during *startle reactions* are actually precipitated by a depletion of potassium and magnesium in the body. Magnesium and potassium are vital cardiac nutrients, and when depleted, as they were in this case, the heart is extremely vulnerable to arrhythmia.

As physicians, we constantly hear people tell us they can't sleep, and we know that one of the major factors in insomnia is the abundance of EMFs in bedrooms. If insomnia is a problem for you, it is absolutely essential that you remove all electronic equipment from your sleep area, and that includes bedside clocks, computers, electric blankets, stereos, and TVs.

Medical illnesses, such as chronic fatigue syndrome and fibromyalgia, as well as cancer, have been related to electromagnetic fields coming from outside, as well as inside, the home. Sometimes, for example, wiring next to a bedroom wall can contain an enormous amount of EMFs that can slowly poison the body.

The problem with EMFs is the same as for radiation—you cannot see or feel either. Many people now use small EMG detectors or Gaussmeters to check out the amount of EMFs in different areas of the home. Although you cannot escape all EMFs, your awareness of the need to keep the exposure minimal can only improve your quality of life and may well extend it as well.

Take in Positive Emotions

Negative emotions and stress can oxidize your blood fat (LDL) just as much as a poor diet or smoking can, which makes it vital that you develop ways to detox mentally as well as physically. Take the Emotional Longevity Screening Questionnaire in Chapter 5 to find out if you need to mentally detox.

STEP II: DETOX BY DESIGN

As you can see, it's an ocean of chemicals out there, and toxic substances are bombarding your body day after day. When you take steps to remove the toxins circulating in your bloodstream, clogging your important organs, and lodging in your soft tissues, you'll be on your way to reducing silent inflammation and recapturing your vitality and well-being. A detoxification program to accomplish this is an important facet of spa medicine. Here are some components of a typical, highly regarded spa program, which you can also do at home.

Body Therapies

Bathing

About one-third of the toxins can be eliminated through the skin by bathing or sweating during exercise. Soaking in Dead Sea salt, diluted hydrogen peroxide, or Epsom salts will help clear toxins more quickly than normal bathing (*see* Appendix B). Alternating water temperatures between cold and hot helps to activate the lymphatic system, which is designed to help the body carry and remove toxins (as is the bloodstream). Spas have a variety of healing water treatments that incorporate essential oils and botanicals, as well as seawater (thalasso) therapy principles to help increase excretion of toxins, and there are even water spas that specialize in hydrotherapy. For example, Cathy Rogers, N.D., the former dean of Bastyr University, is considered the queen of naturopathic hydrotherapy, and she owns the Chico Water Cure Spa in Bremerton, Washington.

Skin Brushing

Using a loofah sponge or soft brush made of vegetable fiber during your bath or shower, or doing ten minutes of dry-skin brushing before a shower or bath, at least twice a week, can be very effective for detoxification.

Bodywork

Massages and other types of bodywork assist lymph and blood flow. Activating these areas can also help relax the abdominal muscles and encourage normal peristalsis to prevent any buildup of fecal material. Bodywork acts to decrease leels of stress hormones, which can weaken your immune system, and spas offer a range of bodywork treatments, from relaxation to deep tissue therapy and aromatherapy.

Lymphatic Drainage and Massage

Cleansing the lymphatic system is a key step in reducing the total toxic load on the body. Exercise can increase lymphatic flow fourteen times over resting rates, and the higher the flow rate, the better it can detoxify. Bouncing on a trampoline (rebounder) is especially helpful, as are gentle aqua aerobics. In addition, light beam therapy, which uses light circular pumping and draining movements and a special blue light that stimulates the lymphatic channels, can help unclog the lymphatic system. Manual lymphatic drainage—gently stroking the right places with light pressure—also improves lymphatic flow. We recommend that you consult a qualified massage therapist who knows this technique and can teach it to you.

Body Wrapping

Body wraps are prepared by mixing the essential oil of selected herbs with a vegetable oil base, such as sunflower or almond oil (they can also be mixed with aloe or seaweed gels). A variety of body wraps, including eucalyptus, juniper, rosemary, and sage, can enhance detoxification by stimulating the circulatory and lymphatic system—stimulating the circulation helps to move stagnant lymph and, as an added bonus, improves the condition of the skin. Spa clients can choose treatments for exfoliation or for skin-enhancing with a nourishing seaweed body wrap.

Saunas and Steam Rooms

Heat forces toxic materials out of cells so they can be excreted through the sweat glands. Use heat therapies with caution, and consume plenty of fluids to keep your body well hydrated during the process.

Far-Infrared Sauna

Unlike current convection-heat saunas, which operate at temperatures well above 180°F, the far-infrared sauna provides a comfortable environment with temperatures as low as 110°F. As this gentle warmth penetrates all parts of the body, it:

1. Exercises the cardiovascular system;

2. Deep-cleanses the body of toxic wastes;

3. Relieves muscle aches and pains;

4. Reduces fatigue and tension;

5. Helps weight control by burning calories;

6. Helps inflammation and edema;

7. Helps hypertension and cardiomyopathies.

(In this, as in all saunas, it is important to periodically wipe the sweat and toxins off your body.)

By raising our body's temperature, the sauna is the perfect instrument for opening our sweat pores and allowing toxic metabolites to escape. When our temperature rises, the skin begins to expire, and the toxins, pesticides, and petrochemicals, stored for years in our subcutaneous fat, come to the surface and get excreted through our pores via the sweat. Saunas also promote microcirculation, which provides more oxygen to injured tissues, cartilage, joints, and musculoskeletal areas, and leads to a decrease of inflammation. When chronic inflammation recedes, not only do chronic degenerative diseases—cancer and heart disease, for example—decrease, but overall health, energy, and well-being improve. We've even had people with chronic insomnia show remarkable improvements with the use of a sauna.

A sauna will also help rid the body of a toxic metal overload. Toxic metals, including petrochemicals, can literally block the cells' ability to receive oxygen and vital nutrients. Toxins also limit the cells' energy, as well as hinder the elimination of toxic metabolic waste. As more and more toxins gradually build up, the toxic burden on your body overwhelms the immune system, causing chemical alterations that eventually result in disease. One of the best ways to rid your body of toxic metals, including mercury, is to use a sauna.

Sweating out mercury has a long history. For example, this technique was employed in Spain in the 1950s and 1960s; miners who showed mental confusion and tremors, both clinical signs of mercury toxicity, were placed in hot environments and forced to sweat to get rid of the mercury.

Many of our contemporary patients have sweated their way out of cancer and heart disease. In a Japanese study, sauna therapy has been reported to lower blood pressure. In fact, anyone who has an elevated score on intramedial thickness of the carotid arteries (IMT) could benefit from routinely using saunas to help reduce the chances of having a stroke. Some of our patients are convinced that their use of a sauna has been a vital factor in their battle against cancer. But you don't have to have cancer or heart disease to get the benefits of a sauna.

Free-radical stress is at an all-time high in our society, with more than 75,000 chemicals plaguing us on a daily basis. And now, with an average of more than 3,000 chemicals added to the daily food supply, it is nothing short of mandatory that you regularly detoxify if you wish to preserve your health and retard the aging process. Sauna therapy is available at spas, or you can even put a sauna in your basement or outside your home. We highly recommend the far-infrared sauna, in particular, because we feel it offers a multitude of medicinal benefits (*see* Resources and Medi-Spa Directory).

Hyperbaric Oxygen

Hyperbaric oxygen chambers are being increasingly used to help with detoxification and to help oxygenate tissues. In spas, a client is introduced into a sealed chamber where oxygen is delivered under pressure, usually for about an hour.

W have seen good results with certain chronic conditions, such as strokes, some chronic infections, chronic fatigue syndrome, and others. We generally recommend a series of ten or more treatments.

Gastrointestinal (GI) Therapies

Modified Fast or Meal Skip

Meals consisting solely of fruits, raw vegetables, nonprocessed juices, water, and organic yogurt can help eliminate toxins. You can replace your regular meals with these foods several times each month.

Small Bowel Therapy

Hydrochloric-acid production in the stomach decreases with age, resulting in reduced nutrient absorption, inefficient breakdown of proteins, decreased release of bile, and reduced levels of pancreatic enzymes. These deficiencies can eventually lead to microbial overgrowth and the flourishing of certain parasites in the small bowel. Eating plenty of raw vegetables takes much of the digestive burden off all of these organs. Taking digestive enzymes (including protease, amylase, and lipase) during each meal further aids digestion and also preserves vital organs.

Colon Cleansing

In addition to dietary changes, many programs recommend the periodic use of a cleansing supplement, typically one containing a combination of enzymes, herbs, nutrients, and toxin absorbers, which are designed to help remove the false mucous membrane that lines the GI tract and sequesters toxins. Many health practitioners use periodic enemas and colonic irrigations to augment colon cleansing. Soluble fiber, such as crushed flaxseed, pectin (found in apples), or psyllium, and stimulating botanicals, such as cascara, rhubarb, senna, or triphala, will usually help promote bowel health.

Liver Cleansing

The liver is the body's main organ of detoxification. You can overcome mild toxicity by improving your diet and avoiding alcohol, drugs, and saturated fats. A combination of unprocessed citrus juice, garlic, ginger, and olive oil—best taken in the morning—can periodically be used as a natural liver flush. There are numerous nutritional supplements that support healthy liver function, including alpha-lipoic acid, carnitine, chlorophyll, choline, dandelion root, globe artichoke, glutathione, hesperidin, inositol, milk thistle, Oregon grape root, psyllium, quercetin, and taurine.

Lymphatic Stimulation

The often-overlooked lymphatic system is the virtual superhighway of your immune system. About a dozen quarts of lymphatic fluid (twice the amount of blood) flows through your body, bathing every cell as it sifts out chemicals and waste products. The lymphatic fluid carries these toxins and metabolic byproducts back to your liver via a series of switching stations, known as lymph nodes, where impurities are filtered out, detoxified, disarmed, and excreted through the kidneys.

Gerald M. Lemole, a cardiovascular surgeon, researcher, and the author of *The Healing Diet,* has uncovered an intriguing link between the lymphatic system, the heart, breathing, and your emotions. In fact, his research has led him to believe that lymphatic detoxification is one of the most important ways to prevent cancer and heart disease.

This fits exactly with Dr. Sinatra's experience as a cardiologist. He has found that his patients with heart disease often don't breathe deeply. Breath work, to increase lymph flow in the chest, consists of deep breathing designed to open the chest and encourage emotional release.

According to Dr. Lemole, the more lymphatic flow there is coursing through your heart's surface arteries, the more any LDL (bad) cholesterol will be filtered out, thereby reducing the potential for coronary-artery damage. But, since the lymph system is largely passive, it takes an active approach to maximize the benefits of this key internal detox system. As it happens, those activities that promote deep breathing—exercise, yoga, and massage, for example—all significantly increase lymph flow, and for this reason alone we would encourage you to begin incorporating deep breathing, exercise, and all forms of massage into your spa-medicine program.

Special Detoxifying Conditions

Parasites

Internal parasites can make it harder for the liver, intestines, and kidneys to detoxify and eliminate waste products. If you have been diagnosed with parasites via a stool exam or a medical screening, you may need to:

- Cleanse the intestines, using natural substances like agar-agar, beet root, bentonite, clay, papaya, psyllium, and extra vitamin C;

- Do a colonic irrigation, using garlic juice and vinegar; this is best done under the care of a healthcare professional;

- Use antiparasitic herbs, such as aloe vera, artemisia, citrus seed extract, garlic, and goldenseal, again under the supervision of a healthcare provider.

Lyme Disease

Some researches believe that as many as 60 million people in the United States are infected with *Borrelia,* the spirochete responsible for Lyme disease. Ticks are not the only culprit for transmitting the disease—blood transfusions, fleas, mosquitoes, sexual intercourse, and unpasteurized milk have also been implicated. Lyme disease can masquerade as a multitude of diseases. As the toxic load on the body increases, the immune system breaks down, leading to many subtle expressions of Lyme disease. For this reason, it is important to find a physician knowledgeable in the disease, as it is often misdiagnosed and mistreated (over 50 percent of the people with Lyme disease have a negative blood test for it).

Lyme disease has been named the Great Imitator because its symptoms are so extensive and widespread that it's all too easily diagnosed as another medical problem. Lyme causes a cluster of physical signs similar to that of mercury intoxication for one, and its symptoms can include brain fog, confusion, constipation, decreased immune response, diarrhea, headaches, or joint pain. Investigators in one study found that, of thirty-one patients diagnosed with chronic fatigue syndrome, twenty actually had Lyme disease. The disease has been documented in cases of autism, and the *Borrelia* spirochete has been observed in the cerebrospinal fluid of people with both multiple sclerosis (MS) and amyotrophic lateral sclerosis (ALS). Lyme disease has additionally been diagnosed in those with Alzheimer's disease, attention deficit disorder, candidiasis, chronic fatigue syndrome, Crohn's disease, Parkinson's disease, and TMJ (temporomandibular joint) syndrome. The list goes on and on. In one medical conference we attended, a Dallas-based neurologist said he personally found that 90 percent of the unexplained headaches he observed were associated with a chronic Lyme infection.

One of the major problems with Lyme disease is that the *Borrelia* organism is almost impossible to kill. It is tenacious and digs deep into our muscles and mesenchyme (connective tissue) and invades our blood cells and tissues. Since many of the spirochetes lie outside the bloodstream and are found inside the cells, these organisms literally hide from the eyes of our immune systems.

Researchers feel this could be one of the great plagues of the twenty-first century. And the reasons are obvious. First, the illness can be spread by many hosts and, as stated, the diagnosis is difficult. The disease mimics many other illnesses and the treatment requires an integrative approach, including antibiotics, as well as cat's claw, diet therapy, enzymes, and even psychosocial and emotional support.

A recent study by Drs. William Cowden and Luis Romero using cat's claw for the treatment of Lyme disease has shown great promise, and one of the best physicians in the country for treating the disease is JoAnne Whitaker, M.D., in Palm Harbor, Florida, who uses all the above therapies. Furthermore, the Bowen technique, developed in the 1950s by Tom Bowen, an Australian therapist, helps people deal with the psychosocial and emotional stress, which often accompanies a chronic infection such as Lyme disease. For more information on the Bowen technique, please visit www.bowen.org.

Anyone who is looking to get her or his life back from Lyme disease needs to address four specific areas of concern. They are:

1. Detoxifying and cleansing the body;

2. Repairing the overstimulated immune system;

3. Healing the neurological damage;

4. Removing the emotional and spiritual drain that accompanies any chronic disease, such as cancer or Lyme disease.

You can complete the Lyme Disease Screening Questionnaire on page 42 to see if you are at risk.

Heavy Metals

Chelation therapy with EDTA (a weak synthetic amino acid that chelates lead and other heavy metals out of the body) is FDA-approved for the treatment of lead and heavy metal toxicity. Since the 1940s, several hundred thousand patients have safely (and successfully) taken this treatment. DMSA (oral) or DMPS (IV) are also effective chelating agents, which must be administered under the supervision of a healthcare practitioner. If you decide to undergo chelation therapy, prior to treatment, it is important to take a variety of the core vitamins and minerals, as described in Chapter 8.

Fungal Infections

Fungal infections are often the sign of a compromised immune system. Recovery from one of them, chronic candidiasis, can take several months. A sugar-free diet together with lactobacillus acidophilus will rebalance the system and help to halt fungal overgrowth. Sometimes an antifungal medication, such as Nystatin, may be required.

Viral Illness

Certain viruses, such as *Chlamydia*, cytomegalovirus, and herpes, have been implicated in many chronic diseases, from cancer to heart disease. In our experience, a person who has a high toxic burden is often immune suppressed and has indications of high levels of viruses. As part of our spa-medicine detox program, we will often attempt to neutralize this viral load with various treatments and select nutraceuticals that improve the immune system.

LYME DISEASE SCREENING QUESTIONNAIRE

	Yes	No
1. I have lived in the Northeastern United States.		
2. I have been bitten by, or exposed to, a tick.		
3. I have had a red rash.		
4. I have had joint pain or swelling.		
5. I often suffer from fatigue.		
6. I suffer from depression.		
7. I experience a stiff, aching neck.		
8. I experience tingling or numbness in my extremities.		
9. I have difficulty with my memory.		
10. I have noticed enlarged lymph nodes.		
11. I experience changes with my vision.		
12. I get confused or dizzy at times.		
13. I experience being in a mental fog.		
14. I experience frequent urination.		
15. I have difficulty concentrating.		
16. I have experienced episodes of fever.		
17. I suffer from fibromyalgia or chronic fatigue.		
18. I have had a facial nerve paralysis.		
19. I experience muscle twitches.		
20. I get heart palpitations.		
TOTAL OF "YES" RESPONSES:		

Score:

Add the number of YES answers for your total.

0–5	unlikely infection
5–15	possible infection
15–20	probable infection

Nutraceuticals

Our top twelve scientifically proven nutraceuticals for detoxification and immune support are:

1. Coenzyme Q_{10}

2. Omega-3 EFAs

3. L-carnitine

4. Alpha-lipoic acid

5. N-acetyl cysteine

6. Flavonoids

7. Garlic

8. Vitamins E and C

9. Carotenoids (lutein, lycopene)

10. Calcium, magnesium, and selenium

11. Vitamin A

12. B vitamins

Another important group of nutrients essential for detoxification are enzymes—the life energy of all organisms. In Part Two, we will cover their important role in inflammation and the immune system. Enzymes are catalysts—they make things work faster—and they can only be formed from organic living matter. To date, there are only about 3,500 known enzymes in the human body, but within a single cell there are roughly 100,000 genes, the majority of which code for enzymes, so that means there are probably thousands more still to be identified. Treatment with enzymes has increased the activity of macrophages (scavenger white blood cells of the immune system) by up to 700 percent, and that of natural killer (NK) cells (infection-fighting white blood cells) by 1,300 percent shortly after taking them. Such an increase in activity will often rocket the immune defenses of the person. Enzymes also assist in the detoxification process by helping break down the *protective* proteinlike coatings many microbes have around them.

Detoxification is a major step in achieving optimum health. Now that you are protecting yourself from toxins and beginning to eliminate them, you can move on to perhaps the most important pillar of wellness: Nutrition.

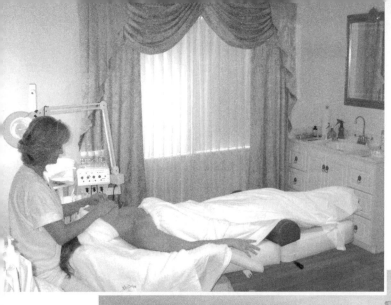

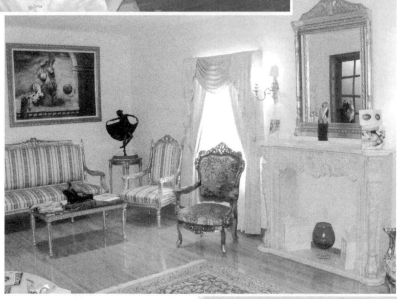

*Photos courtesy of MeSuá
Dermocosmetic Spa.*

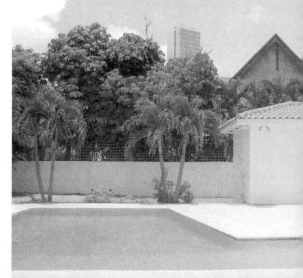

Chapter 3

Pillar Two —
Nutrition

*A healthy diet teamed up with regular exercise and no smoking can
eliminate 80 percent of heart disease and 70 percent of some cancers.*
—WALTER C. WILLETT, M.D.
CHAIRMAN, DEPT. OF NUTRITION, HARVARD SCHOOL OF PUBLIC HEALTH

THE ROLE OF NUTRITION IN WELLNESS

From detoxification we move forward into nutrition, the second of the four pillars of wellness. Exercise and mind-body health, which we'll discuss in the next
two chapters, are the other primary factors that can directly enhance your health
and longevity.

The quality and quantity of scientific information on diet and health has
grown enormously over the last two decades. Most doctors have had little or no
training in nutrition in medical school, and only recently have medical students
been exposed to evidence of the vital role that nutrition plays in our health. Other
than the oxygen you inhale, the only other source of healthy input for your body
comes from what you eat and drink.

When we talk about nutrition, we are including *macronutrients* (protein, carbohydrates, and fats) and *micronutrients* (vitamins and minerals). Both types of
nutrients—and water, of course—are essential for life and health. Let's begin by
taking a brief look at each of these elements of nutrition.

Macronutrients

Protein

The word protein comes from the Greek *proteios,* meaning primary. Our bodies
are composed chiefly of protein; specifically twenty-two amino acids that are
required to build all the proteins necessary for humans. Of these, fourteen can be
produced by the body (nonessential) while eight (essential) must be obtained
from food. A food source in which all eight essential amino acids are present is
called a complete protein and includes cheese, eggs, fish, meat, (organic) milk,

nuts, poultry, soybeans, and yogurt. In this chapter, you'll learn why protein is the most neglected nutrient and why it should compose up to 30 percent of the calories you ingest each day.

Carbohydrates

Carbohydrates are the most common source of energy in the diet. However, not all carbohydrates are created equally. There is a significant difference between *unrefined* (healthy) carbohydrates, such as fruits, vegetables, and whole grains, and *refined* (unhealthy) carbohydrates, such as bleached flour, white rice, and sugar. Refined carbohydrates generally rank on the high end of the glycemic index (*see* Appendix C), which signals rapid spikes in blood sugar and insulin levels, followed by an equally precipitous decline, and leading to rebound cravings for even more carbs.

A significant number of people have, or develop, an exaggerated insulin response to refined carbohydrates. Many researchers believe this vicious cycle is responsible for much of today's epidemic of obesity and cardiovascular disease in the United States. Whenever possible, select foods with a lower glycemic index to avert the refined carbohydrate trap and preserve the health of your insulin receptors. In this chapter, we'll show you how to team up healthy unrefined carbohydrates with fat and protein to blunt your appetite, manage your weight, and enhance health.

Fats

Fats contain twice the energy of proteins and carbohydrates per unit weight and are essential for proper nutrition. Fatty acids are the building blocks of fat and come in three types: saturated, monounsaturated, and polyunsaturated.

The problem with fat is not that we eat it at all, but that we eat too much of the wrong kind. Where we get into trouble with fats is through the process known as hydrogenation. Partially hydrogenated fats start life as polyunsaturated oils, which are then hardened into solid fats, such as margarine and shortening, when hydrogen is bubbled into them. The end result is stable fats with a long shelf life, which is why these are the fats you see on the labels of most packaged baked goods, cookies, crackers, french fries, frozen convenience foods, microwave popcorn, pancake mixes, salad dressings, and so on. In fact, these so-called killer fats are believed to be in 75 percent of all foods consumed by Americans today. Such fats, which create an unhealthy ratio between omega-6 and omega-3 fatty acids, the two main types of polyunsaturated fats, are now thought to trigger inflammatory processes and cause free-radical damage to cell membranes. Later in this chapter, we'll show you how to strive for a 2:1 to 4:1 ratio of omega-6 to omega-3 fats in your diet.

Your overall fat intake should not exceed approximately 30 percent of the total calories you ingest, and saturated fat should make up less than 10 percent of this total. To make this happen, it is important to increase your awareness of poly- and monounsaturated fats, which are found in avocados, flaxseed, nuts, olive oil, and salmon. Table 3.1 shows you which fats are considered healthy.

Largely due to the misguided belief of the past two decades that *all* fats are bad for us, most of our bodies are now starving for omega-3 fatty acids, a type of polyunsaturated fat that increases healthy cholesterol and decreases triglycerides. Americans consume only about 120 milligrams of omega-3 fats per day, in contrast to the average Japanese who consumes a whopping 600 milligrams daily, primarily from fish, tofu, and seaweed. It's no coincidence that the Japanese who follow a traditional Japanese diet have far lower rates of arthritis, cancer, and heart disease than we Americans do.

TABLE 3.1. Healthy Fats	
Monounsaturated	Polyunsaturated
Avocado oil	Black currant oil
Nut oils (almonds)	Borage oil
Olive oil	Flaxseed oil
	Pumpkin-seed oil
	Walnut oil

Healthy omega-3 fatty acids can be challenging to work into your diet because there are few natural sources. These include dark green leafy vegetables, flaxseed, hemp, tofu, and pumpkin-seed and walnut oils. Certain fish are also rich in omega-3 fatty acids, but the Cadillac of all omega-3 oils is found in coldwater fish, especially wild salmon. That's because these fish convert the main omega-3 building block, alpha-linolenic acid, into two highly beneficial end products for your health: eicosapentaenoic acid (EPA) and docosahexaenoic acid (DHA). Fish has all the protein of beef and less that half the fat (*see* Table 3.2 on page 48).

Remember to choose healthy fish and not unhealthy fish. What do we mean by this? Although heavy metal toxicity can come from dental mercury amalgams, as we discussed earlier, a greater source of mercury comes from the fish we eat. The chain of events works something like this. The burning of coal in the world creates an industrialized waste that ascends into the atmosphere. Mercury residues are formed there, and when it rains, the mercury falls back to the earth and into our streams, lakes, rivers, and oceans. Much of this organic mercury is then taken up by algae, which is, in turn, eaten by small fish. Bigger fish eat the small fish, with the result that the highest mercury concentrations are found in the largest fish, such as shark, swordfish, tilefish, and tuna, to mention a few. Even grouper and large Pacific halibut contain high levels of mercury, as do all freshwater fish, also a major problem.

So, not all fish are healthy. In a Finnish study, cardiologists showed that men

TABLE 3.2. Levels of Omega-3 Fatty Acids in Fish

Type of Fish	Omega-3 grams per 4-oz serving	Type of Fish	Omega-3 grams per 4-oz serving
Sardines	5.5	Pollack	0.6
Chinook (king) salmon	3.6	Crab	0.5
White (albacore) tuna	2.6	Ocean perch	0.5
Sockeye salmon	2.3	Shrimp	0.5
Mackerel	1.8–2.6	Halibut	0.4
Herring	1.2–2.7	Scallop	0.4
Rainbow trout	1.0	Cod	0.3
Squid	1.0	Flounder	0.3
Striped bass	0.9	Lobster	0.3
Whiting	0.9	Sole	0.3
Mussel	0.8	Clam	0.2
Channel catfish	0.7	Haddock	0.2
King crab	0.6	Northern pike	0.2

who ate freshwater fish had higher levels of toxic metals in their bodies than those who didn't, with subsequent higher coronary artery disease. The study also revealed that heavy-metal contamination was much worse in freshwater fish than in the saltwater varieties. The same is true in this country. Farmed freshwater fish not only contain higher quantities of heavy metal residues, such as mercury, but also contain insecticides and pesticides as well. We recommend using great caution when eating any farm-raised fish because it can also contain toxins from chemical residues, such as dioxin and petrochemicals.

Small migratory fish, such as Atlantic halibut, cod, and wild salmon from the Aleutian Islands in Alaska, are the healthiest fish around. For shellfish, the best choice is scallops. Remember, fish does contain healthy omega-3 essential fatty acids that will protect your body from oxidative stress (free radicals), but you must choose wisely.

Micronutrients

Vitamins

Vitamins are essential for the proper regulation of metabolism as they control the way in which ingested foods are assimilated and distributed throughout the body. Most vitamins must be obtained from the diet or from supplements. For example, while most animals make some of their own vitamin C, humans must get vitamin C from the diet, as we are unable to synthesize it. Eating a variety of raw fruits and vegetables is your best bet, since boiling vegetables destroys most vitamins and the rest of them are dissolved in the water, which is usually tossed away. The next best option is lightly steaming or low-fat stir-frying vegetables to preserve vitamin content. Table 3.3 below lists our recommended minimal daily doses for many of the essential vitamins and the foods in which they are found.

TABLE 3.3. Vitamins—Benefits, Sources, and Recommended Doses

Vitamins	Benefits	Sources	Recommended Daily Dose
Vitamin A and beta-carotene	Growth, especially skin, hair, nails, teeth; healthy condition of mucous linings and membranes; maintenance of glandular activity; resistance to infection	Carrots; fish-liver oils; liver; parsley, spinach, and other green vegetables; sweet potatoes	5,000 IU
Vitamin B_1 (thiamine)	Appetite; growth; digestion and assimilation; muscle tone; nervous system; normal red-blood count; protein, carbohydrate, and fat metabolism; vitality	Beans; brewer's yeast; grains; nuts; soybeans; wheat germ	1.5 mg
Vitamin B_2 (riboflavin)	Breakdown of fatty acids; cell respiration; control of infection; healthy eyes; nerve tissues	Beans; brewer's yeast; dried milk; fruits, grains; green vegetables; liver; wheat germ	2 mg
Vitamin B_6 (pyridoxine)	Enzyme and brain; enzyme system; nervous system and brain; protection from infection; protein and fat metabolism	Avocados; bananas; bran; Brewer's yeast; green leafy vegetables; pecans; wheat germ	2 mg
Vitamin B_{12} (cobalamin)	Enzymatic process; prevention of anemia; production and regeneration of blood cells	Brewer's yeast; dark green leafy vegetables; nuts	300 mcg
Vitamin C	Appetite; defense against bacterial toxins; glandular activity; growth, especially teeth; protection of vascular system; tissue respiration	Brussels sprouts; citrus fruits; green vegetables	200 mg
Vitamin D	Bones, teeth, tissue; regulation of blood calcium	Sunshine; butter and dairy products; egg yolk; salmon; tuna	800 IU
Vitamin E	Circulation; keeps red blood cells from being destroyed; sexual glands and reproductive skin	Eggs; milk; corn, peanut, sun-flower-seed oils; wheat-germ oils; green vegetables; wheat germ; whole grains	200 IU
Folic acid	Healing; prevention of infection; protein metabolism; red blood cells; RNA and DNA	Cheese; eggs; liver; orange juice; oysters; sunflower seeds	800 mcg

Reference: Zone Café

Minerals

Minerals such as sodium (table salt) and potassium are needed in relatively large amounts; others, like copper and chromium (trace minerals), are necessary in much smaller amounts (*see* Table 3.4 below).

Sodium is an important mineral found mainly in body fluids. One teaspoon of salt provides 2 grams of sodium. The average person consumes between 3 and 7 grams daily, mostly from salt already present in food. About 30 percent of those with high blood pressure are salt-sensitive and should eat a diet low in salt (less than 2.3 grams per day). It is important to read the labels and learn how much sodium, and what other ingredients, have been added to packaged foods.

TABLE 3.4. Sodium Content of Foods

Low-Sodium Foods	mg per 100 grams	Moderate-Sodium Foods	mg per 100 grams	High-Sodium Foods	mg per 100 grams
Apples	1	Milk	50	Salmon, canned	521
Asparagus	1	Light meat chicken	70	Graham crackers	686
Grapefruit	1	Dark meat chicken	90	Cornflakes	914
Pineapple	1	Eggs	118	Potato chips	1,000
Egg noodles	5	Celery	125	Cured ham	1,310
Shredded wheat	10	Tomato juice, canned	200	Processed cheese	1,450
Raisins	12	Cottage cheese	404	Sauerkraut	1,750
Sweet potato	16			Bacon	1,957
Broccoli	19			Olives, green	2,018

Commonly needed minerals are listed in Table 3.5 on page 51, with their benefits for the body, their dietary sources, and the recommended doses.

Water

The human body is close to 90 percent water, and its total body weight is 70 percent water. We rely on water for digestion, cooling, waste elimination, and to help circulate nutrients to every cell in the body. The exact amount of water required will depend on the type of food you eat, the air temperature, humidity, the amount of exercise you do, and your individual metabolic rate. We recommend a minimum of 6–8 glasses of water per day.

Fiber

Fruits, vegetables, and whole grains all contain abundant fiber, which helps

TABLE 3.5. Minerals—Benefits, Sources, and Recommended Doses

Minerals	Benefits	Sources	Recommended Daily Dose
Calcium	Acid/alkaline balance; bones and teeth; coagulation of blood; enzyme stimulation; heart and nerves; skin tone; vitamin metabolism	Cheese; green vegetables; milk products; oranges	1,500 mg for women; 500 mg for men
Chromium	Helps protein and fat metabolism; important for control of blood sugar	Meats; whole grains; wine and beer	120 mcg
Copper	Conversion of iron into hemoglobin; red blood cells	Broccoli; garlic; leeks; parsley; radishes	2.0 mg
Iodine	Circulation; oxidation of fats and proteins; prevention of goiter; size and activity of thyroid gland	All sea plants; iodized or sea salt; seafood; spinach	150 mcg
Iron	Blood cells; hemoglobin; liver; oxygen transmission; tissue respiration	Beans; blackstrap molasses; bran; dried apricots; eggs; grains; liver meats; nuts	18 mg (for children and premenopausal women)
Magnesium	Heart rhythm; lung tissues; nervous system; stimulation of enzymes; structure of bones; relaxation	Almonds; bran; cabbage; lettuce; spinach; tomato; wheat germ	400 mg
Manganese	Nervous system; red blood cells; tissue respiration	Vegetable foods which contain iron	1–2 mg
Potassium	Cell activity; counteracts constipation; elasticity of muscle tissues; purification of blood in kidneys	Cabbage; celery; kale, lettuce; tomatoes	1–2 g
Selenium	Antioxidant that decreases risk of free-radical damage to blood vessel walls	Tortilla chips; Brazil nuts; tuna	100 mcg
Zinc	Circulation; healing; normal growth; preventing high blood pressure; sexual development; tissue respiration	Brewer's yeast; eggs; liver; oatmeal, oysters; pumpkin and sunflower seeds; wheat germ	15 mg

Reference: Zone Café

regulate digestion and metabolism, and stabilizes blood sugar. High-fiber diets assist the digestive process, adding bulk to stools and helping the body rid itself of toxic waste more quickly. When Dr. Graham Simpson worked as an intern at Baragwanath Hospital in Johannesburg, South Africa, in the early 1970s, he saw very little diverticular disease, inflammatory bowel disease, gallbladder disease, appendicitis, hemorrhoids, or colon cancer. This, as we now know, is due to the South African penchant for eating a high-fiber diet, which normalizes pressure in the intestines and decreases the transit time of waste elimination. Dennis

Burkitt, M.D., a British researcher working in Africa, is credited with recognizing the important role of fiber in health. His 1974 paper, "Dietary Fiber and Disease," was published in the *Journal of the American Medical Society* and is considered a classic.

BESTSELLER DIETS—DO ANY OF THEM REALLY WORK?

We have all been exposed to the latest advances in nutrition, whether it was a new fad supplement or a vogue diet, and you've probably figured out by now that much of the media hype has heretofore been based on thin evidence. In the last decade, however, we have seen a convergence in thinking from the world's leading nutritional scientists, with additional information supplied by research from paleontologists and anthropologists, and some of the newer bestseller diets are now backed by their evidence-based research.

Back in 1992, the USDA Food Pyramid—advising us to eat two or more servings from each of four food groups: meat and fish, vegetables and fruits, milk and dairy products, and breads and cereals—was built on very shaky scientific research. We stand to learn much from our ancestors who lived before the development of agriculture and animal husbandry (over 10,000 years ago) and derived all their nutrients from just the first two food groups. They apparently consumed cereal grains rarely, if at all, had no dairy products, and obviously no refined, processed foods. Fortunately, since its inception, the Food Pyramid has undergone significant testing and revision by the Harvard School of Public Health (*American Journal of Clinical Nutrition,* December 2002) and is now similar to the OmegaRx Zone Food Pyramid, by Dr. Barry Sears.

The updated pyramid moves us a step closer to making the general public more aware of how a preventive diet can be effective against cancer, heart disease, and a range of other chronic diseases. (*See* Figure 3.1 on page 53.) We offer the following general guidelines for cultivating a healthy diet and lifestyle.

- Eat fewer bad fats and more good fats.
- Eat fewer refined-grain carbohydrates and more whole-grain, low-glycemic carbohydrates (avoid bread whenever possible).
- Choose healthier sources of protein (for example, sea salmon, free-range organic meat, or poultry).
- Eat plenty of organic vegetables and fruits.
- Drink plenty of pure, filtered water.
- Take nutraceuticals for insurance.
- Use alcohol in moderation.

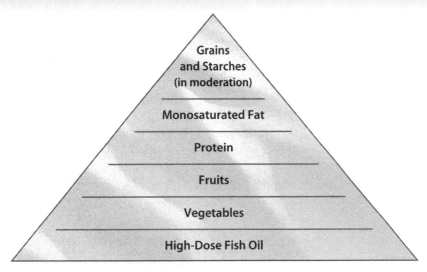

Figure 3.1. Food Pyramid

RETHINKING WHAT AND HOW WE EAT

For the past twenty years, the American people have been unwitting participants in a massive scientific experiment, the goal of which was the reduction of excess fat in the American diet. Largely due to the association between the high cholesterol found in saturated fats and an increased incidence of heart disease, all of us—health professionals, nutritionists, and the government—were guilty of encouraging people to eat more carbohydrates and less fat. The sad truth of our counsel is now apparent: Americans have gotten fatter—there has been a 32 percent weight increase in the past ten years, and nearly two-thirds of the American population is now considered overweight.

Let's examine a few of the diets that we believe have significant merit.

The Paleolithic Diet—Culinary Lessons from Our Ancestors

We recognize most diseases today as the so-called diseases of civilization. Although our Paleolithic ancestors had many health problems, they were not plagued by our modern maladies. Interestingly, since 99 percent of our genetic heritage dates to well before our ancestors became human, most of our genes are ancient, attuned to living conditions that existed more than 100,000 years ago, long before human beings became farmers. When we deviate from what we have genetically adapted to over millions of years, the result is biological maladjustment and discord. We can utilize the wisdom of our Paleolithic ancestors, not by imitating them, but by using several key elements of their diet uncovered by modern science.

In his book *The Paleolithic Prescription,* anthropologist Boyd Eaton, M.D., explains further: "With genetic makeups essentially out of synch with our lifestyles, an inevitable discordance exists between the world we live in today and the world our genes 'think' we live in still. This mismatch—referred to as the 'discordance hypothesis'—can account for many of our ills, especially the chronic 'diseases of civilization' that cause 75 percent of the deaths in industrial societies."

Currently, atherosclerosis is by far the most deadly disease in the United States, yet cardiologist Paul Dudley White, M.D., found it was virtually nonexistent before 1920. Studies of men in their twenties killed in World War II, Korea, and Vietnam show that the layering of atherosclerotic plaques had already begun. Autopsies of men in pre-industrial societies fail to show similar results. The absence of atherosclerosis in these studies, Eaton observes, corresponds to the absence of any signs of it in groups presently living a Paleolithic lifestyle, such as the Arctic Eskimos, Australian Aborigines, Kalahari San (Bushmen), Kenyan Kikuyu and Masai, Navajo Indians, New Guinea Highlanders, Solomon Islanders, and Zairian Pygmies, which would indicate that, by re-creating a modified Paleolithic-style diet free of processed, refined foods, we could expect to reverse or prevent atherosclerosis in our lives. Under this hypothesis, any other diseases of civilization, including chronic obstructive lung disease, diabetes, diverticular disease, hypertension, and obesity, can also be healed or prevented by altering our diet and lifestyle.

Eaton summarizes and compares the prehistoric diet of our ancestors with the decades-old diet of today's Americans.

- They ate only half the fat, but significantly more protein than we do. Although their cholesterol intake equaled or exceeded our intake, the fat they ate was more polyunsaturated than saturated, the reverse of our proportions.

- They ate very few refined carbohydrates and far less sugar than we do.

- Their sodium intake averaged only a quarter of ours, and they consumed more potassium than sodium.

- Their diet provided an abundance of essential micronutrients, particularly ascorbic acid, essential fatty acids, folate, iron, and vitamin B_{12}.

- They ate five to ten times our levels of fiber, mostly from fruits and vegetables rather than from grains.

- Their foods were bulky and filling, while ours are calorie-dense, due to higher levels of fat, refined carbohydrates, and lower levels of fiber.

- They probably had little or no alcohol and, in any case, could never have consistently obtained 7 to 10 percent of their calories in this form, as average adult Americans now do.

History can provide us with insight for creating a better future. Those of you who are interested in eating more like the ancient hunter-gatherers can visit the Internet to download hundreds of bean-free, dairy-free, grain-free, potato-free, and sugar-free recipes from www.paleofood.com or www.thepaleodiet.com.

The Zone Diet

Barry Sears, Ph.D., creator of the popular Zone diet, agrees with the Paleolithic prescription. In fact, a 1985 *New England Journal of Medicine* article shows that the neo-Paleolithic diets have the same protein-to-carbohydrate ratio as his Zone diet. Sears points out that eicosanoids, glucagon, and insulin are the key hormones affected by our metabolic response to food.

Eicosanoids evolved as one of the first hormonal-control systems to enable living organisms to interact with their environment. They are powerful biological agents that include leukotrienes, lipoxins, prostaglandins, and thromboxanes, all of which act on inflammation and blood flow. Sears believes, and we agree, that eicosanoids provide a universal link to virtually every major disease—including arthritis, cancer, and heart disease. Since dietary fat is the only source of essential fatty acids to form the building blocks for all eicosanoids, it becomes clear that some fats are indeed essential in the daily diet.

Ultimately, at the molecular level, disease can be viewed as the body simply making more bad eicosanoids and fewer good ones. Sears's definition of wellness is the body making more good, and fewer bad, eicosanoids. (*See* Table 3.6 below.)

TABLE 3.6. Good and Bad Eicosanoids	
Good Eicosanoids	**Bad Eicosanoids**
Act as anti-inflammatories	Act as proinflammatories
Decrease pain transmission	Increase pain transmission
Inhibit cellular proliferation	Promote cellular proliferation
Inhibit platelet aggregation	Promote platelet aggregation
Promote vasodilation	Promote vasoconstriction
Stimulate immune response	Depress immune response

Lean meats, nuts, and vegetables are part of a menu that's in harmony with our genetic makeup, which has not changed substantially for the past 1 million years.

It is interesting to note that O was the predominant blood group at this time. Peter D'Adamo, M.D., suggests that people with blood group O—the oldest known blood type—feel best when they eat diets comprised mainly of meat and fish.

Transformation of this dietary and genetic harmony began about 10,000 years ago with the agricultural revolution and the development of farming. Agriculture introduced two entirely new food categories, grains and dairy products, to the human diet, and by and large, humankind has not been genetically able to cope well with these foods.

Note: This change from a hunter-gatherer to a more domesticated agrarian lifestyle also brought a new blood type—A. Blood type B also developed about the same time in the areas of the Himalayan highlands that are now part of Pakistan and India. The newest of the blood types, AB, is rare (less than 5 percent)—the result of type A Caucasians intermingling with type B Mongolians—and is rarely found in European graves prior to A.D. 900. Dr. D'Adamo believes that these newer blood types evolved due to certain stressors, including food availability; he also believes that the different blood types do better on different dietary regimes. The science supporting this theory remains uncorroborated, but it is, nevertheless, an interesting observation.

Sears believes that, by using food like a drug, you can manipulate the hormones of the body to achieve a state of optimal health, physical performance, and mental alertness. He postulates that, if you change *what* you eat at each meal, you can be far less concerned about *how much* you eat. In other words, weight loss has more to do with balancing your protein, carbohydrates, and fats in the proper ratios than with your willpower. (*See* Figure 3.2 below.) Please recognize that this is not a diet prescribed to you by a doctor or a government agency, but rather one derived from 2 million years of evolutionary wisdom. In the absence of this wisdom, we may find the source of our dietary woes to be all the alcohol, dairy products, fatty meats, killer trans fats, processed foods, refined carbohydrates, salts, soft drinks, and sugars that simply did not exist in Paleolithic times.

As in athletics, there is an optimum state (the Zone) that can be achieved when the correct proportions of macronutrients are ingested. Dr. Sears believes

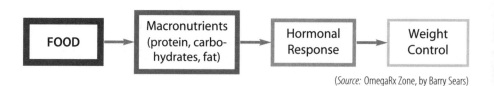

(*Source:* OmegaRx Zone, by Barry Sears)

Figure 3.2. Food as a Drug

that protein is the most neglected nutrient and should make up approximately 30 percent of the calories we ingest each day. He states that the ideal meal should contain:

- Carbohydrates: 40 percent
- Fats: 30 percent
- Proteins: 30 percent

Sears asserts that most diet advice has been wrong because most experts do not understand how body fat is influenced by the macronutrient content of the food we eat. For example, a high-carbohydrate intake will increase your insulin levels (too much insulin is believed to be primarily responsible for inflammation, the underlying cause of most chronic diseases and aging). High insulin levels also increase the levels of stored fat. We now know that the conventional wisdom of the past twenty years—including the USDA's original, now-defunct, food pyramid—has been misguided.

One of the best indications that you are making too much insulin is if you are overweight and shaped like an apple. Recent research indicates that waist size may be a quick, simple, and effective predictor of heart-disease risk because it measures intra-abdominal fat, the most dangerous kind of body fat. For men, waists over forty inches indicate increased risk; for women, it's thirty-five inches. This abdominal fat acts like an endocrine gland, with its fat cells releasing a host of proinflammatory molecules.

Dr. Sears's OmegaZone Dietary Program is the first anti-inflammatory nutritional program designed to reduce body weight, slow aging, and reverse chronic disease. Meals based on this anti-inflammatory diet are served at Zone Cafés and Zone Expresses, a chain of healthy fast-food restaurants based on Dr. Sears's Zone Diet, being developed throughout the United States.

The Carbohydrate-Addict's Diet

Drs. Rachael and Richard Heller, authors of *The Carbohydrates Addict's Diet,* believe that most (90 percent) of obesity today is due to what they term *carbohydrate addiction*. The Hellers define carbohydrate addiction as "compelling hunger, craving or desire for carbohydrate-rich foods; an escalating or recurring need or drive for starches, snack foods, or sweets."

We now know that frequent and excessive intake of refined carbohydrates is the primary reason people are overweight. The carbohydrate load leads to insulin resistance in these individuals, resulting in excessive amounts of insulin circulating in the blood. This biochemical imbalance sets off a vicious cycle that leads to obesity. Insulin is known as the hunger hormone because it stimulates people to eat. The mechanism is shown in Figures 3.3 and 3.4 on page 59.

High levels of insulin are correlated with a decrease in the number and sensitivity of insulin receptors in muscle and fat cells. When there is too much insulin in the blood, the cells paradoxically let less blood sugar into the tissues. The liver converts the extra glucose left in the blood to glycogen and triglycerides. A continued sense of hunger is maintained, so greater and more frequent quantities of carbohydrates must be consumed, which results in weight gain without any feeling of gratification.

This insulin resistance is what characterizes most adult-onset diabetes. Interestingly, recent work by Edward Lichten, M.D., one of the top fifty doctors listed in the *Sinatra Health Report,* has shown that testosterone will help to reverse adult-onset diabetes, especially in men. Most people with adult-onset diabetes have normal or elevated levels of insulin. Testosterone increases the use of glucose in the muscles and, used with caution, can provide a solution to reversing diabetes for many such men.

In addition to diabetes, extra insulin tends to increase adrenaline levels, promote atherosclerotic plaques, increase blood clotting, and constrict blood vessels. Perhaps most important, all of this increases blood pressure, and the resulting hypertension (high blood pressure) is a direct result of this underlying insulin dysfunction. This is the central theme in Dr. Sinatra's book *Lower Your Blood Pressure in Eight Weeks,* which says there is no doubt that the higher your blood sugar, the higher your blood pressure, the faster you age.

In her book *Going Against the Grain,* author Melissa Diane Smith writes that essentially all the grain-based foods we eat (breads of all types, pasta, rice, etc.) are the true culprits in obesity and heart disease. As she points out, 99 percent of all carbohydrates are grain, and our culture is overwhelmingly grain based. Cereal grains, she says, also contain opioid substances that are addictive and allergenic for up to 60 percent of people.

In addition, gluten-containing grains, such as wheat, can cause delayed food allergies, bloating, and other GI ailments, excess mucus production, fatigue, headaches, hyperactivity, mood swings, unexplained irritability, and weight gain, to name a few. If any of these symptoms sound familiar, you might consider cutting way back on *all* grain-based products (even unrefined, healthy ones), limiting your intake to once or twice a week, and see if it makes a difference.

The Mediterranean Diet

How do we know that people in a particular area of the world have a healthier diet than a typical Western diet? Epidemiology, the study of disease patterns, can

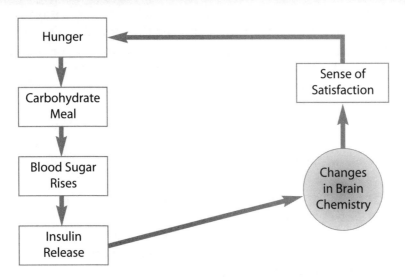

Figure 3.3. Normal Metabolism

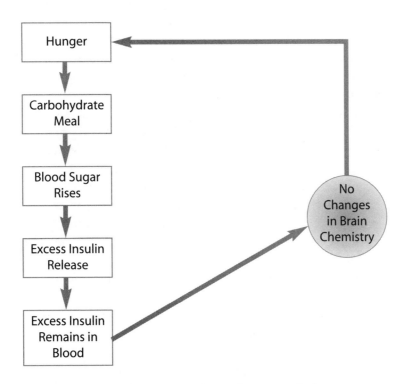

Figure 3.4. Carbohydrate Addict's Metabolism

point the way. Researchers have observed that people in certain isolated villages around the world share an unusual feature. The Hunzas of the Himalayas, the Okinawans of Japan, the people living in the village of Orroli in Sardinia off the coast of Italy, and the Vilcabamba people of South America all boast an average life expectancy of a century, and their residents are astonishingly free of chronic age-related diseases.

Nobody knows for sure what the ideal diet is, but there is good evidence that the Mediterranean diet may come closer than any other. The science behind the Mediterranean diet shows again that insulin regulation may hold the answer to its health benefits.

There are common elements in the diets of most Mediterranean people. As a rule, the diet is low in saturated fats, with added fat mostly in the form of olive oil. It is high in *complex* carbohydrates (low-glycemic index) and high in fiber, mostly from fruit and vegetables. The total fat in the diet is around 30 percent. The ratio of monounsaturated to saturated fats is high (usually 2:1 or more). This is because olive oil (80 percent monounsaturated oleic acid) is the principal fat and is being combined in the diet with large quantities of fresh fruits, vegetables, and minerals. Other components of the diet include cheese, eggs, fish, fowl, garlic, onions, and yogurt. Red meat is consumed only in small quantities to enhance flavor.

While imbibing wine is customary with this diet, widespread usage of hard liquor is not. For millennia, wine has been consumed in moderation, almost always during meals, and as a rule, in the company of friends—the ancient Greek word *symposium* means *drinking in company,* but with the added connotation of intellectual exchange.

In the landmark Seven Countries study, Dr. Ancel Keys and his colleagues showed that the Mediterranean diet group had lower mortality rates from all causes compared with Northern European and American groups. Again, the Mediterranean diet is relatively low in *refined* carbohydrates, which have emerged as the major culprit in the excessive amounts of insulin in obese patients.

The *New England Journal of Medicine* has recently reported that people who ate a Mediterranean-style diet had a 25 percent reduced risk of dying from cancer and heart disease. One of the most interesting aspects of the Mediterranean diet is that it contains many of the healthy fats, including those found in avocados, fish, nuts, and olive oil. In fact, this diet has an even higher fat content than the Heart Association diet. As a reminder, fats do not need insulin regulation. When a person consumes olive oil, for example, insulin is not released. It is only released in the metabolism of sugars and carbohydrates and, to a small extent, proteins. This study, involving 22,043 adults from twenty to eighty-six years of age, reflects many of the findings of the famous Lyons Diet Heart Study in France.

In this trial of people who had previously been diagnosed with a heart attack, those following the Mediterranean-style diet suffered 73 percent fewer heart attacks and 70 percent fewer deaths than those on the Heart Association diet. Indeed, the Mediterranean style of eating makes great heart sense.

Pan-Asian Modified Mediterranean (PAMM) Diet

Dr. Stephen Sinatra has coined the term *PAMM diet,* which combines the healthiest foods found in China, Japan, and Thailand with fresh fish, fruits, olive oil, and vegetable selections from the Mediterranean diet. To this he adds flaxseed; groats; mushrooms; low-glycemic grains, such as spelt; and soy. Dr. Sinatra's top picks, Asian-style, include:

- Broccoli with sesame seeds;

- Green salad with ginger;

- Green tea;

- Omelet with scallions;

- Seaweed and cucumber maki rolls;

- Shiitake mushrooms;

- Tofu (Szechuan style).

On the PAMM diet, Dr. Sinatra recommends that about 25 to 30 percent of your calories come from protein; 30 to 35 percent from healthy fats; and 40 to 45 percent from slow-burning, low-glycemic carbohydrates, including fresh fruits and vegetables and such legumes as chickpeas and lentils. Dr. Sinatra also recommends not using any white flour (bread, bagels, crackers, etc.). He is a strong believer in a gluten-free approach to optimum health. His PAMM diet is very similar to both Dr. Sears's Zone diet and Dr. Arthur Agatston's South Beach diet; all three embrace moderate protein, healthy fat, and low-glycemic carbohydrate consumption to keep insulin production at ideal levels within the body.

The recent emergence of the South Beach diet as an effective means of weight loss and lifestyle adaptation further strengthens our position that excess insulin leads to weight and fat gain, and that moderation is the key to healthy eating. The South Beach diet diverges from the Zone and PAMM diets in that it consists of different phases for weight loss and maintenance. The first phase of the diet emphasizes the ingestion of very low-glycemic carbohydrates, such as lettuce, coupled with lean proteins and some healthy fat. In the second or third stages, as part of a weight-maintenance plan, the dieters can gradually add moderate amounts of carbohydrates, such as bread and alcohol.

Atherosclerosis (heart disease) can be attributed to postprandial (after-eating) inflammation because the amount of insulin (inflammation) released into your body is dependent on what and how much you eat at each meal. Research is now showing why food regimens, such as the Mediterranean diet, those of our Paleolithic ancestors, and the Zone diet, can guide you in making the best dietary and lifestyle choices to prevent atherosclerosis and other chronic diseases.

FOOD IS POWERFUL MEDICINE—A DIETARY FEAST FROM A TO Z

Once food (protein, carbohydrates, and fats) is broken down into its basic components (amino acids, glucose, and fatty acids) and sent to the bloodstream, it has a more powerful impact on your body and your health than any drug your doctor could ever prescribe.

As we have pointed out, Americans are still much more likely to die of lifestyle-related diseases, such as cancer, diabetes, heart disease, and strokes, than people who live in Third World countries; the reason is largely due to what we put on our plates. Numerous studies reveal that people who live in less affluent countries, with diets rich in unprocessed whole grains and plenty of fresh fruits and vegetables, have much lower rates of cancer and heart disease than those in the wealthier, more advanced nations because, as we have learned, these foods generally have a protective effect against our so-called diseases of civilization.

Scientists are increasingly finding health-enhancing chemicals in fruits, vegetables, herbs, and such common spices as garlic and turmeric. These protective compounds are called *phytonutrients,* and many of them are powerful antioxidants. Here is an A-to-Z sampling of some of the best and tastiest out there—a bounty of health for you, ready for the plucking.

APPLES

Key ingredients pectin and quercetin act to:

- Lower cholesterol;
- Protect against cancer;
- Protect against heart disease.

BERRIES

Key ingredients anthocyanin, ellagic acid, and pectin act to:

- Benefit vision;
- Protect against cancer;
- Lower cholesterol.

CARROTS
Key ingredients alpha-carotene, beta-carotene, calcium, and pectate act to:
- Protect against cancer;
- Protect against heart disease;
- Protect against stroke.

DARK-GREEN LEAFY VEGETABLES (such as spinach and kale)
Key ingredients folic acid, lutein, and alpha-lipoic acid act to:
- Prevent macular degeneration;
- Help protect against heart attack;
- Protect against cancer.

ECHINACEA
Key ingredients of complex polysaccharides act as:
- Immune stimulants;
- Anti-inflammatories;
- Antiviral/antibacterial agents.

FRUITS, CITRUS (grapefruits, oranges, lemons, limes, tangerines)
Key ingredients d-limonene, flavonoids, lycopene, and vitamin C act to:
- Decrease cholesterol;
- Protect against cancer;
- Protect against cardiovascular disease.

GARLIC
Key ingredients ajoene, selenium, and sulphur compounds act as natural antibiotics and antifungals, and also act to:
- Prevent blood clots and heart disease;
- Protect against cancer.

HAWTHORN BERRIES (tea)
Key ingredients flavonoids and procyanidins act as anti-inflammatories and also act to:
- Lower blood pressure;
- Protect against heart disease.

Ipecacuanha root

Key ingredient emetia acts as an anti-inflammatory and acts to:

- Ease indigestion;
- Protect against cancer.

Juices from tropical fruits (guavas, kiwi fruit, mangoes, pineapples)

Key ingredients fiber, lycopene, many antioxidants, and vitamins E and C act to:

- Protect against cancer;
- Protect against heart disease;
- Stimulate immune system.

Kava kava

Key ingredient kavalactones acts to:

- Help insomnia;
- Induce relaxation;
- Reduce anxiety.

Legumes (dried beans, lentils, peas)

Key ingredients fiber and folate act to:

- Help control diabetes;
- Lower cholesterol;
- Protect against cardiovascular disease.

Melons (cantaloupes, honeydew, watermelon)

Key ingredients beta-carotene, lycopene, potassium, and vitamin C act to:

- Help lower high blood pressure;
- Protect against cancer;
- Protect against cardiovascular disease.

Nuts and seeds

Key ingredients arginine, B vitamins, fiber, magnesium, selenium, vitamin C, and zinc act to:

- Balance eicosanoid hormones;

- Help with weight loss;
- Increase HDL levels;
- Protect against heart disease.

ONIONS

Key ingredients quercetin and selenium act to:

- Protect against cardiovascular disease;
- Protect against stomach cancer;
- Reduce risk of stroke.

POLYPHENOL TEAS (*Camellia sinensis*) (black tea, green tea, oolong)

Key ingredients catechins and polyphenols act to:

- Lower risk of heart disease;
- Prevent oxidation of LDL cholesterol;
- Protect against cancer.

QUININE (Peruvian bark)

Key ingredients alkaloids and chinchora act as:

- Antimalarials;
- Membrane stabilizers;
- Nighttime muscle-cramp relievers.

RED GRAPES AND WINE

Key ingredients phenolics, quercetin, and resveratrol act to:

- Prevent oxidation of LDL cholesterol;
- Protect against heart disease and blindness;
- Regulate blood flow and circulation.

SOY PRODUCTS AND TOFU

Key ingredients genistein, isoflavones, and phytoestrogens act to:

- Lower blood cholesterol and triglycerides;
- Prevent oxidation of LDL cholesterol and clogging of arteries;
- Protect against cancers (breast, prostate).

Tomatoes (cooked with oil)
Key ingredients chlorogenic acid, lycopene, and p-coumaric acid act to:
- Decrease risk of esophageal cancer;
- Protect against cancer (prostate, cervix);
- Protect against heart disease.

Unusual spices (curry powder, turmeric)
Key ingredients curcuminoids and phenolic compounds act to:
- Benefit digestion and liver function;
- Lower cholesterol and reduce inflammation;
- Protect against cystic fibrosis.

Vegetables, cruciferous (broccoli, Brussels sprouts, cabbage)
Key ingredients fiber, indoles, and sulforaphane act to:
- Lower cholesterol;
- Protect against cancer;
- Protect against macular degeneration.

Walnuts
Key ingredients polyunsaturated fats and some omega-3s (EFAs) act to:
- Prevent heart disease;
- Reduce cholesterol;
- Reduce stroke risk.

Xiao yao wan (bupleurum) (dry root, often taken as a tea [Sho-saiko-to formula])
Key ingredient *Paeonia* acts to:
- Reduce bleeding;
- Reduce menstrual cramps and pelvic pain;
- Reduce PMS symptoms.

Yellow and orange vegetables (red and yellow peppers)
Key ingredients carotenoids and flavonoids act to:
- Protect against cancer;
- Protect against heart disease;
- Stimulate immune function.

ZEAXANTHIN-CONTAINING VEGETABLES (beet, collard, mustard,
Swiss chard, watercress)
Key ingredient zeaxanthin acts to:

- Help vision;
- Lower cholesterol;
- Prevent cancer (especially cancer of the cervix).

Nutrient-Rich Vegetables

At CuisinArt's organic hydroponic farm (*see* Appendix D), all vegetables ripen fully before they are picked, which makes them very nutritious and gives them that flavor of having been picked in the backyard garden. Since it is generally true that once fruits or vegetables reach their fully mature state, they will have synthesized the maximum amount of vitamins and absorbed the maximum amount of minerals possible, by harvesting vegetables in their prime-ripened stage, we can preserve the highest nutritional value of the product until it arrives on your plate.

Studies with tomatoes have shown that the vine-ripened versions have from two to five times as much provitamin A, and more than five times as much vitamin B_6, as immature green ones. You may purchase tomatoes that are red in a supermarket, but they may have been picked green and then gassed with ethylene to turn them red. And the fruit, even if it is red, does not have the same nutrition or flavor as the vine-ripened version. Similarly with sweet bell peppers, the final stage of this ripened fruit is not green, but red, yellow, or orange, depending upon the variety.

SPA-MEDICINE WEIGHT-MANAGEMENT PROGRAMS

Americans spend over $55 billion per year on weight-loss programs, most of which are doomed to fail. To most people, weight loss is about calorie counting, deprivation, and endless rules and restrictions. We now have the science and technology to make weight loss, or maintaining your ideal weight, simple and attainable. By becoming educated about the evolving science of Dr. Sears's OmegaZone Dietary Program, you will lose weight and feel good about yourself without ever feeling deprived.

As discussed earlier, more than twenty years ago many physicians recognized that obesity and high cholesterol were major risk factors for cardiovascular disease, the number-one health problem in America, and encouraged their patients to reduce body fat by eating less fat and more carbohydrates. How wrong we were. Most Americans are still paying the price for this nonfat, high-carbohydrate craze, but you can avoid this mistake with a spa-medicine program, using the OmegaZone Dietary Program.

Myths and Facts about Weight Loss

Myth #1: Eating fat makes you fat.

Fact: Eating fat does not make you fat. It is your body's response to excess carbohydrate in your diet that makes you fat.

Myth #2: It's easy to lose weight by simply restricting calories.

Fact: Losing weight does not necessarily follow eating less.

Myth #3: Diets based on limited choice and caloric restriction work best.

Fact: People get tired of feeling deprived and hungry and these diets usually fail.

Myth #4: Weight loss is all about willpower.

Fact: Weight loss has nothing to do with willpower. You need information, the right information, not willpower.

Myth #5: It is not what you eat, but how much you eat.

Fact: Changing *what* you eat is more important than *how much* you eat. It is important to *decrease* carbohydrate intake and eat the right ratio of protein to carbohydrate at each meal.

Myth #6: All people are created equal; it's simply a question of calories in and calories out.

Fact: Not all people are created equal. Some of us are slow burners. Some of us have an exaggerated insulin response when we eat a carbohydrate load, some of us don't. A weight-loss program must be individualized for your particular needs.

Myth #7: A person's metabolism is not all that important when it comes to losing weight.

Fact: Your metabolism is important and a measurement of your BMR (basal metabolic rate) will show you how important it is. Some of us need hormonal, nutraceutical, detoxification, or pharmacological agents to normalize our body's metabolic rate, and some of us don't.

Myth #8: Counting calories and knowing all the food tables and portion sizes is critical.

Fact: Spa-medicine dietary programs can help you navigate toward your ideal weight with remarkably little effort.

Myth #9: When I feel hungry, I need food.

Fact: Learn to distinguish thirst from hunger. Often a glass of water will satisfy. Try to drink six to eight glasses of water daily.

Myth #10: Exercise is not important for losing weight.

Fact: Exercise is essential, not only for losing weight, but also for maintaining weight.

No matter what diet you choose, aging can be slowed by reducing caloric intake, reducing free-radical damage, lowering insulin levels, and improving hormonal communication throughout the body. Weight management, as opposed to a weight-loss diet, becomes a systematic, lifelong approach to diet and nutrition, where food is used like a drug to prevent chronic disease and aging.

As with any successful weight-loss regimen, your weight should initially drop fairly rapidly within the first few weeks, and you will continue to lose weight until you reach your optimal weight. This may take three to four months, or up to six months or longer for those with more serious weight problems.

You will notice many of your chronic health problems beginning to improve. Your joints will no longer be as stiff. Your blood pressure and blood-sugar levels will even out. For the first time, constipation and irritable bowel syndrome will be gone. Your blood fats will decrease as your energy and sense of well-being increase. Your skin, nails, and hair will improve.

To achieve all this, it is important to learn the essentials of nutritional eating. Here are a few guidelines to get you started.

- **Educate yourself about nutrition and longevity.** Learn how nutrition can help you live better longer. To the best of our knowledge, the most effective program for this is the OmegaZone Dietary Program, which we fully endorse.

- **Become involved in menu planning and cooking.** Shop wisely by reading labels and selecting quality produce. Fully understand the power of foods and learn how best to prepare them.

- **Add variety to your meals.** Eat plenty of colorful fruits, vegetables, and whole-grain cereals. Eat more healthy fish, organic meat, and DHA-fortified eggs. Drink plenty of water. Remember to watch the ratio of protein to carbohydrates eaten at each meal.

- **Eat five times a day.** Always eat breakfast, lunch, and dinner. Add an afternoon and evening health snack. Vegetables and nuts are good choices. A high-protein, low-carbohydrate bar is also convenient. Eating this way, you will never feel deprived.

- **Control your portions.** Use your fist as a measure of your meal because your stomach is about the size your fist. A typical protein serving fits in the palm of your hand and is no thicker than it. You do not have to finish all the food on your plate, so try to stop eating before the full feeling hits.

- **Make mealtime special.** Prepare your meal so that it looks sensual and colorful, and tastes great. Select one or two sites in your home and create an ambiance in which to enjoy your meal. Surround yourself with your loved ones or friends and celebrate each meal.

- **Monitor your weight.** Your weight can serve to alert you to potential health problems and is one of the most important biomarkers you can use on your path to wellness and longevity. Increasing weight is often the first sign of unregulated insulin.

- **Get to know the glycemic index and the glycemic load.** The former measures the rate of entry of various carbohydrates into the bloodstream. The faster the rate of entry, the higher the insulin level. The latter measures the total quantity of carbohydrates.

- **Consider the link between nutraceuticals and longevity.** Research has confirmed the importance of supplementing your diet with specific vitamins and minerals to optimize your well-being and longevity. Supplementing with omega-3 fish oils, for example, is essential to controlling your eicosanoid hormonal balance.

Maintain Your Weight While Eating Out

Studies show that over half of all meals in America are now eaten outside of the home. You can protect yourself from any weight gain associated with this troublesome trend by making an effort to eat in more often, and by following these simple guidelines when dining out.

- **Stop and think before heading out.** Which are the healthier restaurants? Do they have a wide selection from which to choose? Ethnic restaurants, including Chinese, Greek, Indian, Japanese, and Thai, with their emphasis on vegetarian and seafood meals, are often healthier than typical American fare. Avoid fast-food restaurants whenever possible, but when there is no other choice, order broiled fish or chicken and tell them to *hold the bun*. Salads are also a good choice wherever you dine.

- **Stay in control.** Every time you are away from home, remind yourself that you are in charge of what food you select and pay for. Try to eat those foods that are most similar to your diet at home.

- **Skip the bread.** If you must have some bread, dip it in small amounts of olive oil instead of slathering on the butter. Olive oil's monounsaturated fats are good for your arteries and will make you feel full longer.

- **Choose quality protein.** Eat low-fat protein foods, such as fish, chicken, range-fed beef, bison, or turkey. Avoid foods rich in saturated fats and cholesterol, such as fatty cuts of beef and pork, and organ meats (liver, pâté). Avoid sandwich meats.

- **Drink water with wine.** Having water with your wine will keep you fuller and help you drink the wine more slowly. Water also helps prevent dehydration. Whether dining out or at home, drink alcohol in moderation, no more than one to two glasses per day.

- **Plan ahead for holidays.** Holiday food, eaten either at home or in a restaurant, is notorious for adding weight. Stockpile nutrient-rich, low-calorie foods at holiday time and try to cut your appetite by snacking on them before dining out. This is one time to watch not only what you eat, but also how much you eat. Again, watch the alcohol intake.

- **Beware of fruit juices.** Processed juices are concentrated sources of carbohydrates, and most commercial juices are basically flavored sugar water. Enjoy them sparingly—and dilute them—whether dining in or out. It is far better to accompany your meals with bottled water and a twist of lemon or lime. Herbal or green teas are also excellent choices.

- **Avoid sodas.** They are extremely high in sugar and have little or no nutritional value.

- **Hold the pasta.** Be wary of all refined and high-glycemic carbohydrates, such as pasta, rice, potatoes, breads, and sugar. Use carbohydrates as condiments.

- **Order healthy desserts.** A bowl of fresh, mixed berries, fruit with yogurt, or a scoop of sorbet is an excellent choice, rather than black forest cake and other decadent choices.

Final Note

Compared to the Atkins Diet (high protein and fat), the OmegaZone Dietary Program is a moderate carbohydrate, moderate protein, and moderate fat program. Severe ketosis (excess acid in the blood and urine) occurs when people consume too much protein and too few carbohydrates. The body reduces abnormal ketone levels by increased urination, and this water loss (up to four pounds) accounts for much of the initial weight loss seen on the Atkins Diet. Unfortunately, the body eventually adapts to continued ketosis by altering the action of the fat cells.

Within three to six months, the fat cells become fat magnets that are ten times more active in their ability to accumulate fat. Fat loss thus slows and fat begins to accumulate again.

We prefer the science behind the OmegaZone and the long-term weight-loss results we see. Additionally, our colleague, Dr. Blake Tearnan, covers some important issues in Appendix H that will assist you in meeting your weight-loss objectives and achieving your optimum weight. Table 3.7 below provides a guide to desirable weights, taking height and age into consideration.

TABLE 3.7. Desirable Weights

Height without shoes	Weight without shoes (women or men)	
	Age 19 to 34	35 and Up
5'0"	97–128	108–138
5'1"	101–132	111–143
5'2"	104–137	115–148
5'3"	107–141	119–152
5'4"	111–146	122–157
5'5"	114–150	126–162
5'6"	118–155	130–167
5'7"	121–160	134–172
5'8"	125–164	138–178
5'9"	129–169	142–183
5'10"	132–174	146–188
5'11"	136–179	151–194
6'0"	140–184	155–199
6'1"	144–189	159–205
6'2"	148–195	164–210
6'3"	152–200	168–216

Desirable Body Fat Percentages

WOMEN		MEN	
30 years	14 to 21 percent	30 years	9 to 15 percent
30–50 years	15 to 23 percent	30–50 years	11 to 17 percent
50+ years	16 to 25 percent	50+ years	12 to 19 percent

Source: Kelly Brownell: LEARN Program for Weight Control

Chapter 4

Pillar Three —
Exercise

When you gain control of your body,
you will gain control of your life.

—BILL PHILLIPS, *BODY FOR LIFE*

EXERCISE—THE UNIVERSAL LONGEVITY BOOSTER

If we told you there was a simple solution to a broad array of health issues, from cardiovascular disease to depression to bone health, you might say we were dreaming. But it's true. You can sidestep osteoporosis, lift your spirits, and protect your heart all at the same time . . . simply by moving your body for about thirty minutes a day, most days of the week.

Yes, we're talking about exercise—the third pillar of wellness. Its importance as part of a lifelong plan for weight maintenance, disease prevention, and longevity cannot be overstated. There is no other lifestyle change that brings so many immediate and long-lasting benefits to your health and well-being.

Just to get you warmed up, here are thirty reasons to exercise:

1. Burns extra calories and decreases food cravings;

2. Decreases fluid-related symptoms, such as PMS;

3. Decreases frequency and severity of asthma attacks;

4. Decreases tobacco use;

5. Enhances sexual performance;

6. Helps relieve constipation;

7. Improves cerebral circulation;

8. Improves digestive function;

9. Improves immune function;

10. Improves mental alertness and reaction time;

11. Improves posture, coordination, and balance;

12. Improves quality of sleep;

13. Improves self-confidence and self-esteem;

14. Improves vision and reduces risk of glaucoma;

15. Increases lean muscle mass;

16. Increases longevity;

17. Increases maximum oxygen uptake;

18. Increases metabolic rate;

19. Increases strength of ligaments and tendons;

20. Lowers resting heart rate and increases endurance;

21. Preserves muscle mass and strength;

22. Prevents cardiovascular disease;

23. Prevents chronic diseases, such as cancer and diabetes;

24. Prevents lower back pain;

25. Reduces blood pressure;

26. Reduces risk of breast, colon, and prostate cancer;

27. Reduces risk of type-2 diabetes, especially with weight control;

28. Releases growth hormone important for antiaging;

29. Relieves anxiety, depression, and stress;

30. Strengthens bones.

Even modest physical activity can keep you younger. A recent study in the *Journal of the American Medical Association* found that one of the key reasons Americans don't exercise is the common myth that a person needs to do taxing and rigorous workouts to get benefits. The Centers for Disease Control and the American College of Sports Medicine also report that just half an hour a day of moderately intense activity, such as housecleaning, gardening, or walking can provide most of the health benefits of exercise.

More recent good news comes from Dr. Steven Blair and his colleagues at the Institute of Aerobics Research in Dallas, Texas. These researchers studied physical fitness and health in 10,224 men and 3,120 women. Each person underwent a detailed medical exam that included a maximal stress test on a treadmill and then, based on the treadmill test, everyone was grouped into one of five categories of fitness and subsequently followed for an average of eight years.

The categories ranged from very unfit (fitness level 1) to very fit (fitness level 5). Figure 4.1 below depicts the risk ratio (which represents the death rate) for men and women, depending on their level of fitness. The risk for the very fit people in level 5 is given a value of 1; risks for the other levels are given ascending numbers.

There are several striking aspects to this study. First, it is another piece to the puzzle showing that people who exercise and are physically fit live longer. Perhaps the most heartening news is that even modest levels of fitness are associated with greatly reduced risk. Note especially the substantial decline in risk for both men and women by moving from the least fit group (1) to the next group (2). This big risk reduction occurs as they go from being completely sedentary (group 1) to moderately active (group 2), walking for thirty minutes four times a week, for example.

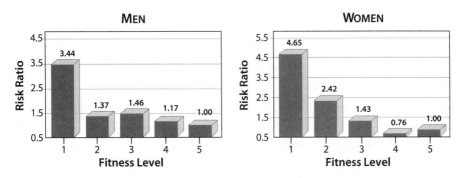

Figure 4.1. Fitness Level and Health—Risk for Death

MYTHS AND FACTS ABOUT EXERCISE

Misguided beliefs about exercise often dampen our enthusiasm for it. Let's get to the root of the most pervasive myths about exercise.

Myth #1: Aerobics is better for shaping your body than weight training.

Fact: To change your physique, you must train with light weights.

Myth #2: Weight training is mostly for young athletes.

Fact: Weight training is even more important as you age to prevent muscle wasting (sarcopenia).

Myth #3: The more you exercise, the better the results.

Fact: Too much exercise prevents you from getting the results you desire.

Myth #4: Women who lift weights get bulky and look masculine.

Fact: Weight training is the only way for women to create a toned look.

Myth #5: I know a lot about exercise and exercise equipment.

Fact: There is a huge difference between knowing what to do and actually doing it.

Myth #6: There is no proof that exercise helps you live longer.

Fact: Studies such as Dr. Steven Blair's at the Institute of Aerobic Research in Dallas show that even moderate exercise can extend longevity.

Myth #7: To burn calories, running is much better than walking.

Fact: Walking burns about the same number of calories as running the same distance and is easier on the joints.

Myth #8: The muscles of an older person are not as responsive to weight lifting as the muscles of a younger person.

Fact: The muscles of older people are just as responsive to weight training as those of younger people.

Myth #9: Advanced age is an irreversible condition that results in many chronic diseases, such as diabetes, heart disease, and hypertension.

Fact: You can adopt an exercise program that maximizes your ability to age much more slowly and prevent many chronic diseases. Your health largely depends on you, no matter what your age.

Myth #10: With resistance exercises (weights), the type you do is far more important than how you do them.

Fact: How you do these exercises is very important. You must perform them passionately to produce the results you want to achieve.

DEVELOP YOUR OWN EXERCISE PRESCRIPTION

Exercise can be as simple as recognizing those things you already love doing—dancing, gardening, walking—and making it a point to do them three to six days a week (*see* Appendix E for calorie values associated with various activities). You can also explore a more structured program that includes both cardiovascular (aerobics) and resistance (weight training) workouts on alternating days. You are the only person who knows how to best fit in your exercise prescription each day—find something you really enjoy and make it part of your everyday life. Begin each session with about ten minutes of warm-up.

Let's take a closer look at each stage and type of exercise.

Warm-Up/Stretching

Beginning a strenuous exercise program with tight, stiff muscles is the most common way to injure yourself. It is important to warm up. Start by doing something that gets your muscles moving, such as walking for five minutes or doing a series of simple stretches.

Yoga is an ideal practice for those interested in high-level wellness. The word *yoga* means union—a discipline that helps unite body, mind, and spirit. Hatha yoga consists of a series of physical postures (asanas) and breathing exercises (pranayamas), which can be easily learned. One of our favorites is the sun salutation, shown in Figure 4.2 on page 78. Regular practice increases balance, flexibility, grace, and strength.

Strength Training

Strength training is essential for preventing osteoporosis and muscle wasting (sarcopenia), especially for those over the age of fifty. We like the Training-for-LIFE Experience by Bill Phillips. It is a simple, practical program that really works. A good friend of Dr. Simpson's, Amy Yarnel, participated in a program of this type and the doctor was astounded by the dramatic effect this training method had on her in a very short time.

Phillips's concepts fit well in a spa-medicine program. He recommends a regimen of thirty-six weight-training exercises. Several of these rotated over the course of a week work all of the major muscle groups in your body, including the abdominals, back, chest, shoulders, biceps, triceps, quadriceps, hamstrings, and calves. With a little practice, you will be able to properly conduct all these exercises.

Phillips's principles for training include instructions to:

- Weight train for no more than forty-five minutes, three times a week;

- Alternate the training of the major muscles of the upper and lower body;

- Perform two exercises for each major muscle group in the upper and lower parts of the body;

- Follow a specific intensity index and push yourself a little harder every week by adding more weights;

- Plan your training by deciding what time you're going to exercise, which exercises you will be doing, how much weight you will be lifting, how many *reps* you are aiming for, and how long it will take you to complete the session;

- Keep a written log of all workouts.

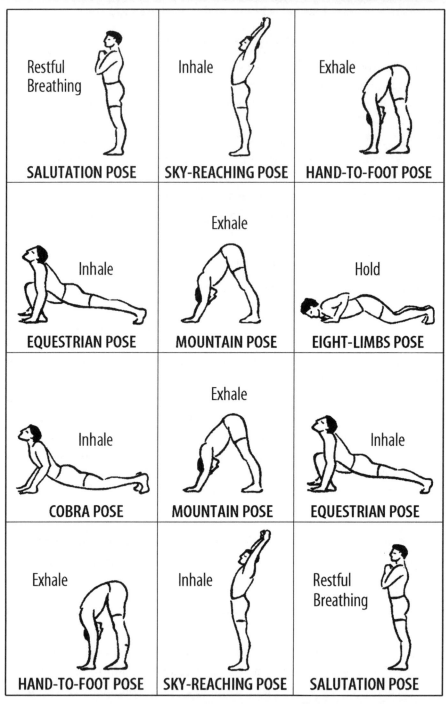

Figure 4.2. Sun Salutation *(Surya Namaskar)*

Spa wellness trainers will familiarize you with these and other exercises. For home study, we recommend Bill Phillips's books, including *Body for Life*.

Aerobic Exercise—Get Moving

An aerobic activity is any exercise in which the body uses a sufficiently large and continuous amount of oxygen to completely burn carbohydrates (glycogen), free fatty acids, and triglycerides. If you persevere, your muscles, lungs, heart, and blood vessels will work harder today than they did last week (but not get pushed into the anaerobic zone, in which muscle glycogen is used for fuel and lactic acid is formed as a byproduct). By performing progressive levels of aerobic exercise, the body gains new capacity, and the conditioning that results is associated with greater life expectancy, lowered risk of heart disease, and many other positive effects.

When planning your aerobic exercise, keep these three variables in mind, and never increase more than one in any given exercise session.

- **Frequency:** The activity should be performed at least three to five times a week.

- **Intensity:** Your heart rate must be elevated to within 60 to 70 percent of the maximum rate. (You can estimate your maximum heart rate by subtracting your age from 220. If you are forty, your maximum heart rate should be 180.)

- **Time:** Your heart rate should remain at this level for at least fifteen minutes. (You can check your heart rate by feeling your pulse at the wrist. Place the index and middle fingers of your left hand on the inside of your right wrist. Count the number of beats that pulse per minute. This is your heart rate.)

Fitness instructors will help you design an exercise prescription during your spa medicine program. Your exercise program is designed to:

- **Enhance vitality** by reversing the usual deterioration that people past age forty-five often experience, such things as metabolic slowdown, glucose intolerance, and declining strength;

- **Postpone or prevent chronic disease,** such as cardiovascular disease, hypertension, osteoporosis, and type-2 diabetes;

- **Prevent a weakening of the body** caused by a change in body composition in favor of fat, at the expense of muscle—some 80 percent of a young adult's normal weight is lean body mass, only 20 percent is fat, and by the time most of us reach age seventy, the ratio is closer to 50:50.

TAKE A WALK FOR GOOD HEALTH

Walking, by itself or in addition to the above, is one of our favorite forms of exercise, for the following reasons:

- Fast walking is an excellent form of cardiovascular exercise.
- Walking for forty-five minutes, three to five times a week, burns almost the same number of calories as running.
- Walking can be done by almost anybody in almost all settings.
- Walking can be done at a variety of paces.
- Walking is easy—no special training is required.
- Walking can be done with friends, music, and at any time.
- Walking is inexpensive—you only need good shoes to protect your feet.

A morning walk before breakfast is a great way to boost your metabolism, burn more fat, and have more energy throughout the day.

HOW MUCH EXERCISE IS TOO MUCH?

- **Breath test:** If you can still talk comfortably while you exercise, you can probably step up the pace. If you cannot, you are training too hard and need to slow down. If you experience dizziness, faintness, loss of muscle control, nausea, severe shortness of breath, any pain or tightness in the chest, stop exercising immediately, and *if the symptoms persist, immediately seek professional help.*
- **Breathing recovery rate:** If you still find yourself short of breath ten minutes after exercising, your exercise is too strenuous.
- **Heart-rate recovery:** Five minutes after exercise, your pulse should be less than 100 beats per minute. If it isn't, you are pushing yourself too hard.
- **Fatigue:** Exercise should be stimulating and invigorating. If you feel worn out and tired most of the time, you are overdoing it and should slow down.

BEFORE YOU EXERCISE

If you have any of the following problems, it is important to obtain a medical clearance before starting an exercise program.

- A history of heart disease, including a heart attack, cardiac arrest, congestive heart failure, myocarditis, valve disease, or any other heart disease that was ever treated by a doctor.

- A history of chest pain diagnosed as angina pectoris.

- Any known cardiac arrhythmias (abnormal heart beats or abnormal heart rhythm).

- A history of strokes.

- Any use of medications for the heart or blood vessels during the last three months, including medicine for chest pain, arrhythmias, congestive heart failure, or hypertension (high blood pressure). The medications include beta blockers (propranolol), digitalis, nitroglycerin, procainamide, and quinidine. If there is a question about any other medicine, check with your doctor.

- Any acute infectious disease (colds, flu, virus, etc.).

- Any musculoskeletal, neuromuscular, or orthopedic disorders that would make walking uncomfortable or dangerous.

- Any renal (kidney), hepatic (liver), or other metabolic problems.

- A resting blood pressure greater than 160 mm Hg systolic or 100 mm Hg diastolic.

- Any previous medical advice not to exercise.

- Any suspicion of yours that exercise may be harmful for you.

This list was adapted from the *LEARN Program for Weight Control,* by Kelly D. Brownell, Ph.D.

EXERCISE AND LONGEVITY—THE INTRIGUING CONNECTION

According to Michael Roizen, M.D., adopting a combination of exercises can reduce your biological age by over eight years. He includes the three types of exercise mentioned earlier—general physical activity, stamina-building activities, and strength and flexibility exercises—and shows how each affects the aging process differently.

First, general physical activity, such as housecleaning, gardening, and walking—virtually anything that uses your muscles—contributes to about 40 percent of the age-reducing effects attributed to exercise. All of these exercises can be performed without even breaking a sweat.

Second, activities that raise your heart rate—aerobic exercises that require stamina, such as biking, jogging, and swimming—contribute to another 40 percent of age-reducing effects.

Third, Dr. Roizen advocates exercises for strength and flexibility. Building and strengthening muscles through weight lifting and stretching contribute the remaining 20 percent. This is, however, the critical 20 percent because these exercises help to prevent muscle wasting, one of the most common, but least recognized, diseases of aging. Without a healthy muscular system, you'll find it challenging to maintain your health and well-being. Strength training is at the core of the Superslow Zone programs. (*See* Resources and Medi-Spa Directory.)

As you will learn, most of the benefits of exercise are due to improved hormonal control and a reduction in inflammation. Advanced age is not an irreversible biological condition of increasing chronic disease. Rather, it is a dynamic state that, in most people, can be changed for the better, regardless of how many years they have neglected their body in the past.

BIOMARKERS OF AGING

Biomarkers, as we said, are predictive biological markers that can give you an idea of how well (or not) you are aging. If you examine the overall population and track any biological function—be it muscular strength or mental function—performance generally declines with age. Each biomarker of aging—a biological process that can be measured and is universal—usually decreases 2 to 6 percent for each decade after age thirty-five.

This decrease is an average measure for the population. By adopting certain lifestyle patterns, such as exercise and optimizing your hormonal status with OmegaZone nutrition and nutritional supplements, you can alter this trajectory for the better. As Roizen points out, "For every seventy-year-old who is debilitated from cardiovascular disease, there's another who's running road races or traveling the globe."

Your body can be rejuvenated. You can regain aerobic stamina, flexibility, muscular strength, and the vigor and vitality you had thought were gone forever. Whether you are in middle age or pushing eighty, the biomarkers of aging can be significantly altered. In the case of many specific physiological functions, they can actually be reversed.

Most of the twenty biomarkers that follow are dependent on exercise. Many of these biomarkers were presented in the excellent book, *Biomarkers,* written by Drs. William Evans and Irwin Rosenberg. You and you alone have the ability to alter each of these biomarkers of aging. This is why, when you take control of your body, you gain control of your life.

TWENTY BIOMARKERS OF VITALITY
THAT YOU CAN CHANGE FOR THE BETTER

Your age in years (chronological age) has little to do with how old you are biologically (biological age) and how old you look and feel. We want you to think about yourself in terms of the following twenty biomarkers of vitality.

Biomarker 1:   Muscle mass

Biomarker 2:   Strength

Biomarker 3:   Resting metabolic rate (RMR)

Biomarker 4:   Body fat percentage and distribution

Biomarker 5:   Antioxidant levels

Biomarker 6   Aerobic capacity

Biomarker 7:   Blood sugar tolerance

Biomarker 8:   Triglycerides/HDL ratio

Biomarker 9:   Cholesterol/HDL ratio

Biomarker 10:   Blood pressure

Biomarker 11:   Vital (lung) capacity

Biomarker 12:   Bone density

Biomarker 13:   Your body's ability to regulate its core temperature

Biomarker 14:   Skin elasticity and thickness

Biomarker 15:   Eicosanoid balance

Biomarker 16:   Static balance

Biomarker 17:   Reaction time

Biomarker 18:   Auditory threshold

Biomarker 19   Visual accommodation

Biomarker 20   Hormone levels

BIOMARKER 1—MUSCLE MASS

Muscle, to a far greater extent than most people realize, is responsible for the vitality of your whole physiological well-being. A strong, toned musculature makes all sorts of wonderful contributions to your overall health. A high ratio of muscle to fat on the body:

- Causes metabolism to rise—meaning you can more easily burn fat and alter your body composition in favor of beneficial muscle tissue;

- Increases your aerobic capacity—and the health of your whole cardiovascular system;

- Triggers muscle to use more insulin—thus greatly reducing your chances of developing high blood pressure, diabetes, and many other age-related diseases;

- Increases growth hormone, an antiaging hormone par excellence;

• Helps maintain high levels of HDL cholesterol, thereby reducing your chance of developing heart disease and other vascular diseases, such as strokes.

An important goal of exercise is to build lean muscle at the expense of fat. Most people carry around too much body fat and too little muscle. Those with a high ratio of muscle to fat on their frame have a higher resting metabolic rate (RMR), and they don't have to worry as much about gaining weight. As we age, we lose about 6.6 pounds of lean-body mass (muscle) each decade. This rate increases over the age of forty-five, until age seventy when many people have 50 percent of their weight as fat.

Two factors are responsible for how much muscle you retain over time. The first is how much you use your muscles. The second is the level of tissue-maintaining anabolic hormones circulating in your blood, the most potent of which are testosterone and growth hormone. We now know that certain nutrients, such as arginine, glutamine, and lysine, can also enhance lean muscle and decrease body fat.

BIOMARKER 2—STRENGTH

Studies have shown that from age twenty to seventy, we lose at least 30 percent of our total number of muscle cells. In addition, the muscle cells that remain begin to atrophy—each cell becomes smaller—and the end result is decreased muscle strength. Gradual muscle loss is the catalyst for a number of age-related diseases, such as osteoporosis and type-2 diabetes. Today we know, however, that this decline in muscle size and strength is not inevitable. With regular exercise, older people can sustain muscle growth and strength similar to younger people. CAT scans and muscle biopsies have proven that muscle mass and strength can be regained, no matter what the age or condition a person is in before starting an exercise program.

BIOMARKER 3—RESTING METABOLIC RATE (RMR)

Researchers believe that older people's reduced muscle mass is almost wholly responsible for the gradual reduction of their resting metabolic rate. A person's RMR drops about 2 percent per decade, starting at age twenty.

Too many calories, coupled with too little exercise, a reduced musculature, and a declining metabolic rate adds up to more and more fat. Unless this cycle is broken, it will only worsen over time. Because of the expense and the cumbersome manner in which RMR readings were previously measured, they were very difficult to do, but new techniques, such as Body-Gem, make it easy.

BIOMARKER 4—BODY FAT PERCENTAGE AND DISTRIBUTION

With advancing age, most of us gain fat even though our body weight hasn't increased that much. The average sixty-five-year-old sedentary female is about 43 percent fat, while the average twenty-five-year-old female is around 25 percent fat. Males remain somewhat leaner at sixty-five; about 38 percent of body weight is fat.

Increasing the proportion of desirable lean-body mass to unwanted fat is a more desirable goal than just losing weight. Concentrate on shedding fat and gaining lean muscle. The body-mass index (BMI) is an effective method for judging optimal weight in relation to your height. The ideal BMI for a certain sex and age yields the lowest risk of chronic disease and premature mortality. If your BMI is 20 percent above the ideal for your age and sex, you may be at risk. Your BMI can be determined by comparing your age, sex, and weight against a standard set of tables. A BMI of less than 23 is optimal.

Body fat distribution is another predictor of disease; in fact, it may be as important a factor in disease prediction as the percentage of total body mass that is fat, which makes it essential to know where fat is stored in your body. Evidence suggests that people who store fat above their hips have a greater risk of developing diabetes, heart disease, and strokes than those who store fat below their hips.

It appears that it is healthier to be shaped more like a pear than an apple. If you have a BMI that's higher than ideal, plus a large bulge of fat around your midriff (a waist circumference greater than 38"), your risk of disease is magnified. Regular exercise plays an important role in maintaining a more youthful looking and, most important, healthier body.

BIOMARKER 5—ANTIOXIDANT LEVELS

Studies have shown that a high dietary intake of carotenoids reduces the risk of various cancers, cardiovascular diseases, and other degenerative diseases.

A new biophotonic scanner uses a sensitive, noninvasive laser technique to quickly measure (in ninety seconds) the antioxidant levels in the skin of a person's palm. This can help in adjusting the supplement intake to ensure optimal antioxidant levels. Antioxidant levels in tissue remain stable over several weeks.

BIOMARKER 6—AEROBIC CAPACITY

Most people's aerobic capacity begins to decline after age twenty. By age sixty-five, aerobic capacity is typically 30 to 40 percent less than in young adults, but the decline is slowed in those older people who exercise. Your peak heartbeat also declines with age—the formula for maximum heart-rate becomes 220 minus your age.

To check your heart rate, a three-minute step test can also be easily performed. A client steps up and down off of a twelve-inch bench at the rate of twenty-four steps per minute, and the result is compared to the norm for men and women of similar age.

Aerobic capacity is the single best test of fitness and functional capacity. In older people, exercise conditions the muscles more than the heart. The more muscles that are demanding oxygen, the greater your utilization of oxygen and your aerobic capacity, which is what helps keep you fit.

BIOMARKER 7—BLOOD SUGAR TOLERANCE

With age, your body loses its ability to effectively handle glucose, and your chance of developing type-2 diabetes increases. By age seventy, some 20 percent of men and 30 percent of women have an abnormal glucose tolerance test (GTT).

Research has shown that your level of activity, body-fat ratio, and the type, amount, and frequency of carbohydrates you eat has more to do with the development of diabetes than your ability to secrete insulin. We believe this creeping blood-sugar intolerance is one of the most devastating age-related changes. Certain (carbohydrate-addicted) individuals are more prone to developing this dysfunction. People at risk should eat a higher protein, healthy fat, lower carbohydrate diet (such as a Zone meal). Along with diet, strength-building exercises are a key to regulating your glucose metabolism.

Insulin control is achieved primarily through balancing protein and carbohydrates at each meal to maintain stable blood sugar levels for four to six hours. (This is staying in the Zone.) A fasting blood-insulin level may be one of the best indicators of a person's overall health. Less than 12 is good and an ideal level is 5.

Chronic elevation of blood sugar results in an increased concentration of glycosylated hemoglobins, a major component of which is hemoglobin AIC (HBAIC). This is the estimate of the degree of high blood sugar over five to eight weeks (normal HBAIC is 3.8 to 6.3 percent). New research indicates that a fasting blood sugar level greater than 70 *milligrams* percent places a person at an increased risk of disease.

BIOMARKER 8—TRIGLYCERIDES/HDL RATIO

We believe the triglyceride/HDL ratio is a more important biomarker than the familiar cholesterol/HDL ratio because research has shown that this ratio is a better predictor of future heart disease than total cholesterol or even LDL cholesterol.

The TG/HDL ratio is an indirect marker of both your insulin level and your eicosanoid hormones, and an ideal ratio is 2. If your ratio is 4 or more, you are on a path to chronic disease, and future cardiovascular vulnerability. The fastest way to lower the TG/HDL ratio is to follow a spa-medicine program that includes the OmegaZone Dietary Program coupled with omega-3 EFA supplements.

BIOMARKER 9—CHOLESTEROL/HDL RATIO

Divide your total cholesterol by your HDL cholesterol to assess your particular measure of this biomarker. The goal for women and men over age fifty is a ratio of 4.5 or lower. Advancing age does not appear to have much effect on the total cholesterol/HDL ratio. (In fact, a low HDL is a greater heart-disease risk for women than a high LDL.) It's the harmful LDL and VLDL (very low-density lipoprotein) form of cholesterol that rises with age. LDL should not exceed 60 to 70 percent of the total cholesterol. Dietary changes can help lower LDLs. Actions that are helpful for raising the good HDL cholesterol include detoxifying the liver, exercising, going off birth control pills, lowering body fat, quitting smoking, and reducing alcohol intake.

Note: Medical conditions, such as diabetes, kidney, liver, or thyroid disease can increase LDL. Also some medications—anabolic steroids, diuretics, and others—may increase LDL levels.

BIOMARKER 10—BLOOD PRESSURE

Unlike people living in the United States, most populations around the world show no increase in blood pressure with age. Numerous medical doctors believe that normal systolic blood pressure is less than 135, while a normal diastolic blood pressure is less than 85, but recent research indicates that a normal blood pressure is 110/70.

To get an accurate measurement of blood pressure, it is best to get a minimum of three readings at different times. African-Americans have a higher genetic risk for hypertension and consistently run higher readings after the age of twenty.

There are several ways to reduce high blood pressure. Since more than 30 percent of the population is salt sensitive, those people need to watch their salt intake and not let it exceed 2,000–3,000 milligrams of sodium per day. Exercise is also a potent tool to help control blood pressure. In fact, people who are fit have a 34 percent lower risk of developing hypertension. Reducing insulin and inflammation by restricting carbohydrate intake is the major key to controlling blood pressure. For further information on how to achieve blood pressure control using diet, lifestyle, and targeted nutritional supplements, read *Lower Your Blood Pressure in Eight Weeks,* by Dr. Stephen Sinatra.

BIOMARKER 11—VITAL (LUNG) CAPACITY

To test your lung function, all you need is a candle and box of matches. Light the candle and try blowing it out; repeat, moving the candle farther away each time, until you are unable to blow it out. (If you can blow out a candle from 3 feet away, you most likely have adequate lung capacity.) This is a rough measurement of your vital capacity, which many antiaging doctors consider one of the strongest predictors of longevity. Again, exercising regularly can help you increase your lung capacity. Smoking is one of the lifestyle factors that will seriously decrease your vital capacity.

BIOMARKER 12—BONE DENSITY

Age-related declines in mineral content can leave older people with weaker, less dense, more brittle bones. A combination of poor dietary habits, hormonal changes, deficient calcium absorption, smoking, and a sedentary lifestyle are the primary risk factors. When this bone loss reaches the point where there's a substantial increase in the risk of fracture, it's called osteoporosis.

Research has shown that, on average, an individual loses approximately 1 percent of bone mass a year (the rate is slower in men than in women). Taking calcium, magnesium, and other bone-building nutrients, and doing regular weight-bearing exercise, such as walking, running, and cycling can effectively reduce the rate of bone loss and help prevent osteoporosis. Exercise also helps to increase the body's absorption of calcium.

BIOMARKER 13—YOUR BODY'S ABILITY TO REGULATE ITS CORE BODY TEMPERATURE

Our bodies adjust our internal temperature to stay within a degree of 98.6°F or 37.5°C. This vital ability to regulate temperature diminishes with age, which makes both hot and cold weather pose an increased risk as people age. Older people also have a reduced sensation of thirst, and it takes a warmer internal temperature to make an older person sweat. In addition, reduced cardiac output means more heat remains trapped inside the body, and this is detrimental because it can interfere with cell function. Reduced kidney function can also complicate dehydration and thermoregulatory problems as we age.

Again, exercise can help. Staying in shape no matter what your age enables you to retain healthy amounts of water, sweat more when you work out in the heat, and lose fewer electrolytes.

BIOMARKER 14—SKIN ELASTICITY AND THICKNESS

A simple test for this biomarker is to pinch the skin on the back of your hand between your thumb and forefinger for five seconds. How long does it take to flatten back out completely?

Age:	20–30	40–50	60–70
Time:	0–1 sec.	2–5 sec.	10–50 sec.

Through its effects on growth hormone and insulin, exercise can greatly increase the elasticity of your skin. You can also quickly hydrate and improve your skin's elasticity simply by drinking six to eight glasses of pure filtered water each day.

BIOMARKER 15—EICOSANOID BALANCE

As we saw in the nutrition chapter, a balance of good and bad eicosanoids is a key facet of healthy aging. Certain fish oils are high in omega-3 fats, important because they modulate the balance of good and bad eicosanoids. Bad eicosanoids are derived from long-chain omega-6 fatty acids called arachidonic acid (AA). Enhanced production of good eicosanoids requires EPA (eicosapentaenoic acid) and DHA (docosahexaenoic acid) found in fish oil because they inhibit the production of AA.

An exciting, recently developed biomarker is a blood test that measures your ratio of AA to EPA, which is the best way to measure the ratio of bad to good eicosanoids throughout your body. Ask your local physician about this SIP (silent inflammation profile) test, which is becoming more available from several labs in the United States, or visit the website www.zonecafe.com.

BIOMARKER 16—STATIC BALANCE

Stand on a flat surface. Keeping your eyes closed, lift your left foot (if you are right-handed) about six inches off the ground while bending your left knee at about a 45-degree angle. Have someone time you (and catch you if necessary) to see how long you can do this without opening your eyes.

Age:	20–30	40–50	60–70
Time:	28 sec.	18 sec.	4 sec.

Exercise increases balance, bone strength, coordination, posture, and the strength of ligaments and tendons. Tai chi and yoga are especially effective for maintaining good balance and aging gracefully.

BIOMARKER 17—REACTION TIME

With your arm outstretched and your hand positioned vertically, have a friend suspend an eighteen-inch ruler just above your thumb and middle fingers. Then, have your friend let go of the ruler without warning, as you move to catch it between your fingers as quickly as possible. Exercise improves mental alertness and reaction time.

BIOMARKER 18—AUDITORY THRESHOLD

The upper limit of normal hearing is 25 decibels. A young adult's hearing acuity is better than an older adult's (assuming the younger person hasn't spent his or her life in front of an amplifier at a rock concert). Thus, 40 decibels is the usual screening level used for people sixty-five years and older. Failure at any frequency above this level necessitates referral to a physician. There is evidence that exercise helps hearing.

BIOMARKER 19—VISUAL ACCOMMODATION

Slowly bring a newspaper to your eyes until the regular-sized letters start to blur. Measure the distance between the eyes and the paper with a ruler (the closer to your face you can read the newspaper, the better the accommodation). Exercise is known to improve vision and reduce the risk of glaucoma. *Save Your Sight,* by Drs. Marc and Michael Rose, offers natural ways to prevent and improve visual accommodation.

BIOMARKER 20—HORMONE LEVELS

The hypothalamus, located in the brain, controls the release of hormones from various glands in the body. As you age, the hypothalamus loses its ability to regulate and produce hormones, such as estrogen, progesterone, testosterone, DHEA, pregnenolone, and human growth hormone. These hormones are the real juice of life, and after ages thirty to thirty-five, many of these hormones begin to decline.

We are often astounded at how revitalized men and women feel as quickly as six to eight weeks after beginning bio-identical hormone replacement (*see* Chapter 9). Hormones can be readily measured in blood or saliva. One of the few ways of increasing growth hormone—the key hormone in antiaging—is with exercise.

WE'LL HELP YOU GET MOVING

One of the advantages of a spa-medicine program is having access to scientifically accurate new technology, which can help you customize your exercise and nutrition program.

At rest, your body burns between 1,400 and 1,900 calories a day. This is your resting metabolic rate (RMR). The higher your RMR, the faster you will burn calories and the more quickly and easily you will lose weight. We have found that clients often need to be detoxified before they are able to increase their RMR and lose weight. Zone medi-spas use far-infrared saunas to help detox clients so they can achieve weight loss when other methods have failed. Zone medi-spas also utilize the Superslow Zone—just two twenty-minute training sessions a week produce incredible results. (*See* Resources and Medi-Spa Directory.)

Your resting metabolic rate is approximately 1 calorie per kilogram per hour. If you weigh 132 pounds (60 kg), you will burn 60 calories an hour, or 1,440 calories a day. Gender, percentage of body fat, and other factors also affect RMR, as will the fact that some people are slow burners and others are fast burners. Since a low RMR may be responsible for difficulty losing weight, actual measurements of the RMR are important.

Ideally, you should expend 3,500 calories of energy a week in exercise above and beyond your RMR. Appendix E gives the different amount of calories expended by the various activities during a typical spa medicine program.

Your first goal is to discover ways of boosting your overall activity level. With every movement you improve your physical fitness. Keep busy with housework, gardening, and mowing the lawn, not to mention fun things like dancing and sex—they are all activities that burn extra calories. The point is to get your muscles moving. The more active you are, the younger you feel.

Think about your daily routine. What can you do to create more activity in your routine? Personal trainers and health guides in a spa will explore your activities of daily living in addition to helping you customize an exercise program tailored to your needs. Remember, a well-rounded exercise program combined with good nutrition is a juggernaut against the aging process.

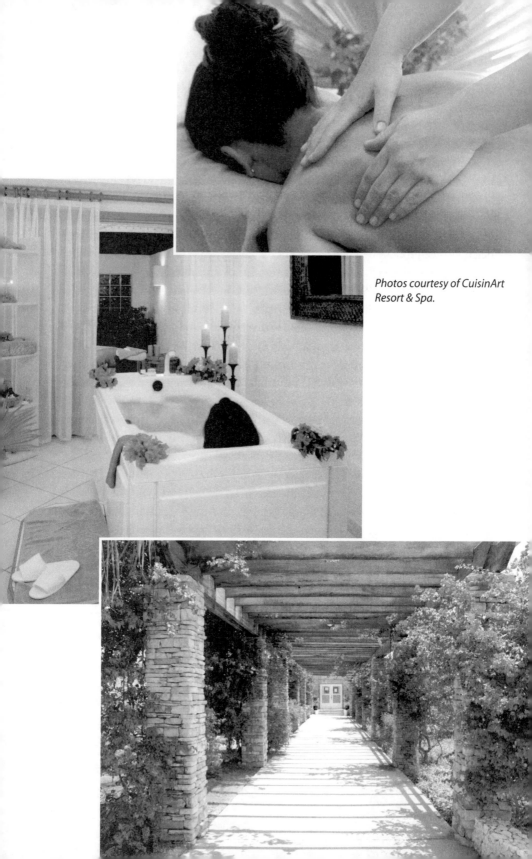

Chapter 5

Pillar Four —
Mind-Body Health

*Living and perceiving only through the head is why life gets so
confusing, stressful, and dry. Without enough heart, you feel like you're
living just to survive. Through the heart you access more of your real
spirit and learn to become who you really are.*

—DOC LEW CHILDRE, *FREEZE FRAME*

INTRODUCTION TO MIND-BODY MEDICINE

The research that really began modern mind-body medicine took place in 1974
at the Rochester School of Medicine and Dentistry, when psychologist Robert
Ader showed that the immune systems of white rats had learned specific condi-
tioned responses. Until this time, learning was thought to take place only in the
brain and nervous system.

Ader gave the rats a nausea-producing drug called cyclophosphamide to condition them to associate saccharin water with nausea and avoid it—classic Pavlov-
ian conditioning. The problem was that many of the rats, although young and
healthy, were getting sick and dying. Ader discovered that, in addition to causing nausea, cyclophosphamide was also lowering the number of T cells (immune-
system cells that help the body fight infection) in the immune system.

Eventually, just giving the rats saccharin water alone (without cyclophosphamide) was all that it took to decrease T cells. Classical conditioning had triggered a learned association between the taste of saccharin water and the suppression of T cells—which, in turn, made the rats more susceptible to disease and
death. Until this experiment, the medical profession had believed that the central
nervous system and the immune system were completely separate entities.

This research has been replicated many times since then, and the findings
have given birth to a new field called *psychoneuroimmunology* (PNI). An explosion
in PNI research has shown how the mind, beliefs, and emotions can profoundly
affect physical well-being and the course of health. One of the most thought-

provoking researchers on the scene today is Candace Pert, Ph.D., author of *Molecules of Emotion: Why You Feel the Way You Feel*. Pert played a key role in the discovery of opioid (synthetic opiumlike narcotic) receptors in 1972, and her ongoing research into neuropeptides (compounds of two or more amino acids in nerve tissue) has kept her at the forefront of mind-body–medicine research. In a nutshell, she is convinced that these tiny chemical messengers, which are found throughout the body, communicate in a way that gives each body part a voice. She also believes that peptides are responsible for emotions ranging from anger to sadness, as well as deeper states of consciousness, such as bliss and wonder.

As researchers learn more about the hormones and neurotransmitters that the brain uses to communicate with the rest of the body, we are gaining a much deeper understanding of the stress response. The scientific evidence of the mind's influence on the body comes from four major areas:

1. **Physiological research** investigates the many connections between the brain and the different body systems.

2. **Epidemiological research** (the study of causes and distribution of diseases) shows the correlation between psychological factors and illnesses in the population.

3. **Clinical research** explores how we can alleviate, prevent, or treat mind-body diseases once they appear.

4. **Longevity research** suggests that, besides influencing lifestyle choices, the worldview of a person acts directly on her or his health, either helping or hurting the individual. A person's worldview may, in fact, be one of the most important factors in well-being and longevity.

STRESS

Hans Selye, M.D., is credited with originating the concept of stress and first recognizing its vital role in our health. As a young medical student in Prague in 1925, what impressed Selye during hospital rounds was that no matter which specific disease a patient had—heart, kidney, liver, or lung—the patients all looked and felt ill. He identified these symptoms as part of a *general* disease condition. Then, in 1936, while doing research at the Banting and Best Institute in Montreal (where insulin was discovered), he thought he had discovered a new hormone while looking at the organs of dissected rats. Being a true scientist, he injected saline only to the control subjects and then restudied the animals. He noticed similar internal effects—stomach ulcers, enlarged lymph nodes, atrophy of the thymus gland—in both groups. What struck Selye even more was that simply immobilizing the rat, without injecting anything, also produced the same result. Selye recognized that this general response to any stressor was very simi-lar to what he had observed as a medical student in Prague. In 1938, the journal *Nature* published an article about this work, "A Syndrome Produced by Diverse Nocuous Agents," and the concept of stress in the twentieth century was born.

In the mid-1800s, the eminent French physiologist Claude Bernard had already recognized that the role of the *milieu interieur* (inner state) was essential to understanding health and disease. In the early 1900s, the famed Harvard phys-iologist, Walter Cannon, author of *Wisdom of the Body,* described the fight-or-flight response—the internal response of the body to a threat or perceived threat. The body releases stress hormones, collectively called *catecholamines* (ephinephrine and norepinephrine, for example), which begin a cascade of events that prepare a person or animal to run or fight.

This was all well and good for a caveman facing a saber-toothed tiger, but most of the threats (stressors) we face in modern life are more likely to be psy-chological and cannot be handled by fighting or fleeing. At McGill University in the 1950s, Selye demonstrated that the body reacts to modern-day stressors as though it were still facing the same physical threat as our early ancestors.

It is important to recognize that there are two forms of stress—short term (acute) and long term (chronic)—and that each has very different health conse-quences (*see* Figure 5.1 on page 96). Initial reactions to stress are largely governed by the *autonomic nervous system* (ANS), that part of the nervous system over which we usually have no direct voluntary control. It has two branches—the *sympathetic nervous system* (SNS) that causes the arousal response described above, and the *parasympathetic nervous system* (PNS), which has the opposite effect of calming and relaxing the body. Most stress-management techniques, including meditation and biofeedback, aim to induce a positive parasympathetic state by reducing the responses from the overtaxed SNS.

When your body responds to a near miss on the freeway—acute stress—it is instantly flooded with hormones that temporarily increase your breathing, blood pressure, heart rate, and muscle tension. Your stomach and intestines become less active, and blood sugar rises to provide a burst of energy. After a short while, as the emergency passes, these symptoms usually abate.

If you are under chronic stress, however—for example, constant deadlines, a rocky marriage, an unfulfilling job—your body secretes excess cortisol, a hor-mone that will harm your nervous and immune systems over time. There is grow-ing evidence that the overproduction of this and related stress hormones plays a major role in a wide variety of illnesses. Cortisol is the most deleterious hor-mone our bodies produce; too much of it will damage the brain and accelerate the aging process.

When it comes to mind-body health, we would like to explore three basic questions throughout the rest of this chapter, namely:

- What psychological events have the greatest effects on health?
- How precisely do these events affect the body physiologically?
- How can we best intervene to enhance well-being?

The first thing to realize is that stress is *not what happens* to someone—those outside forces are the stressors (*see* Figure 5.2 on page 97)—but rather how a person *reacts to what happens*. Research at the Institute for Heart Math confirms this and indicates that the amount of stress you feel is based on your perception of an event, person, or place, far more than on the impetus of stress itself. In other words, when you feel stress, you perceive a threat to your physical or mental well-being that you may or may not be able to respond to adequately.

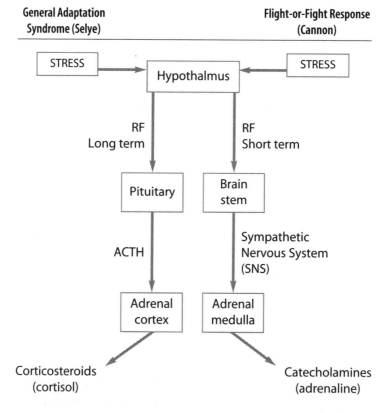

Figure 5.1. Neuroendocrine Mechanisms in Stress Responses

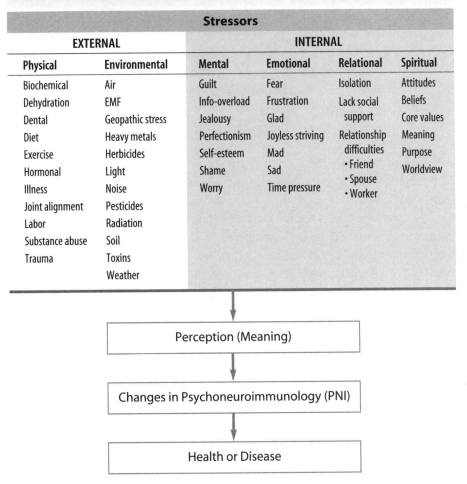

Stressors					
EXTERNAL		**INTERNAL**			
Physical	**Environmental**	**Mental**	**Emotional**	**Relational**	**Spiritual**
Biochemical	Air	Guilt	Fear	Isolation	Attitudes
Dehydration	EMF	Info-overload	Frustration	Lack social	Beliefs
Dental	Geopathic stress	Jealousy	Glad	support	Core values
Diet	Heavy metals	Perfectionism	Joyless striving	Relationship	Meaning
Exercise	Herbicides	Self-esteem	Mad	difficulties	Purpose
Hormonal	Light	Shame	Sad	• Friend	Worldview
Illness	Noise	Worry	Time pressure	• Spouse	
Joint alignment	Pesticides			• Worker	
Labor	Radiation				
Substance abuse	Soil				
Trauma	Toxins				
	Weather				

Perception (Meaning)

Changes in Psychoneuroimmunology (PNI)

Health or Disease

Figure 5.2. Effects of External and Internal Stressors

HEART RATE VARIABILITY (HRV)

The emerging science of heart rate variability offers a window into the heart and its relationship with the nervous system, the head, and emotional well-being. The medical community is beginning to recognize that a supercharged sympathetic nervous system (SNS) can set you up for cardiac problems, such as congestive heart failure, and even sudden death. Other conditions that can contribute to chronic SNS-activation include anxiety, depression, diabetes, hypertension, insulin resistance, obesity, and sleep apnea. Behaviors and lifestyles, including abuse of stimulants, chronic stress, hostility, sedentary lifestyle, sleep deprivation, smoking, social isolation, and unhealthy diets, are also contributors.

Other indicators of abnormal functioning of the autonomic nervous system (ANS) include a resting heart rate greater than ninety beats per minute, an inability to achieve 85 percent of the age-predicted maximal heart rate on a treadmill (for those not taking cardiac drugs), along with an abnormal heart-rate recovery rate, and a failure to decrease the heart rate by twelve beats per minute during the first minute after peak exercise.

Dr. Sinatra predicts that a hyperactive sympathetic nervous system (SNS), the branch of the ANS that causes the arousal response, will soon be recognized as an independent risk factor for acute cardiac disease. Any method, including the mind-body approaches discussed here, that improves the function of the ANS, while reducing SNS activity, can greatly improve and nurture your cardiovascular system.

The fight-or-flight response is elicited in acute stress, resulting in increased sympathetic nerve activity and the release of the hormone epinephrine (adrenaline). These physiological changes are, as we said, of short duration. Chronic stress elicits what is known as long-term general-adaptation syndrome which can lead to exhaustion. This weakened state involves the pituitary-induced release of corticosteroid hormones, including harmful cortisol.

THE MIND'S ROLE IN HEALTH

A June 1985 editorial in the *New England Journal of Medicine* (*NEJM*), concerning the effects of social and psychological factors on the course of cancer, stated that, "Most reports of such a connection are anecdotal; it is time to acknowledge that our belief in disease as a direct reflection of mental state is largely folklore."

In 1991, just six years later, the *NEJM* published a landmark study that showed a *direct* link between mental state and disease. Today, the influence of the mind's role in health is undisputed as more and more PNI research proves what Peter and the Apostles knew 2,000 years ago:

"How is it that you have continued this deed in your heart? You have not lied to men but to God. . . . When Ananias heard these words, he fell down and died." This is from Acts of the Apostles 5: 4–5, and is, perhaps, the earliest recorded example of the profound effect that a state of mind can have on the heart.

The case of the famous Scottish anatomist, John Hunter, is a more recent example of how anger can be the Achilles heel of the heart. In a lecture to his colleagues, Hunter professed, "My life lies in the hands of any rascal who can annoy me." Truer words were never said. Hunter died suddenly following an argument with one of his peers.

TYPE A—HOSTILITY AND THE HEART

Heart disease now accounts for slightly more than 50 percent of all deaths reported in the United States. In the 1960s, while working at the Harold Brunn Institute for Cardiovascular Research at San Francisco's Mt. Zion Hospital, Drs. Meyer Friedman and Ray Rosenman identified a cluster of behaviors—constant hurriedness, free-floating hostility, and intense competitiveness—that seemed to be present in most of their patients with heart disease. They coined the term *type A* to describe these people. Other individuals, whom they called type-B people, did not have these qualities.

Over the years, researchers have recognized that hurriedness and competitiveness are not as toxic as hostility. People who are prone to hostility show longer increases in blood pressure and stress hormones than others. Check to see how

Heartbreak and Heart Disease

Dr. Sinatra wrote *Heartbreak and Heart Disease* in 1998, after ten years of psychotherapy training on how emotionality and spirituality can affect the heart. Dr. Sinatra wrote that, of all the emotions, heartbreak was one of the most devastating to the heart; it could, over time, lead to heart disease, and the best treatment for it, he said, is emotional release. This all began in 1984, after he had conducted a weekend seminar on stress and tension that was attended by forty people. Following it, he published a paper discussing what he had learned there about biological hormones in relation to suppressed feelings. In this workshop of both men and women, stress hormones were collected via twenty-four-hour urine measurements, and he found that the women, who were able to cry, hug one another, network with one another, and be open about their feelings of heartbreak, had very low levels of stress hormones in their urine. These women, who were more able to express their feelings, had no heart disease. For the men though, he found that those who would not communicate their feelings were particularly vulnerable to heart disease. The men who were withdrawn and did not cry, who buried their feelings of heartbreak and lived in a state of denial, had astronomically high levels of stress hormones in their urine, and 80 percent of them had advanced heart disease. This was the first time Dr. Sinatra reported that men who do not cry, or who hold on to their feelings, were much more vulnerable to heart attacks. That workshop so opened his eyes, in fact, that he decided to become a psychotherapist and entered two long psychotherapy programs dealing with behavior, emotionality, and the heart.

The essence of heartbreak is complicated, its roots often stemming from childhood, with issues of unconditional love at the heart of the matter. For more on this complex, invigorating subject, please refer to Dr. Sinatra's book *Heartbreak and Heart Disease*.

hostile you tend to be by taking the following quiz, Test Your Hostility Level, by
Redford B. Williams, M.D., of Duke University Medical Center.

TEST YOUR HOSTILITY LEVEL	Yes	No
In the express checkout line at the supermarket, do you often count the items in the baskets of the people ahead of you to be sure they aren't over the limit?		
When an elevator doesn't come as quickly as you think it should, do your thoughts quickly focus on the inconsiderate behavior of the person on another floor who's holding it up?		
Do you frequently check up on family members or coworkers to make sure they haven't made a mistake in some task?		
When you are held up in a slow line in traffic, the bank, or the supermarket, do you quickly sense your heart pounding and your breath quickening?		
When little things go wrong, do you often feel like lashing out at the world?		
When someone criticizes you, do you quickly begin to feel annoyed?		
If an elevator stops too long on a floor above you, are you likely to pound on the door?		
If people mistreat you, do you look for an opportunity to pay them back, just for the principle of the thing?		
Do you frequently find yourself muttering at the television during a news broadcast?		

If you answered YES to three or more questions, your hostility level is probably high. If this is the case, it would be a good idea to begin practicing the relaxation response, the freeze-frame technique, or one of the other mind-body therapies discussed on the following pages.

TYPE B PERSONALITY

In contrast to type-A individuals, those classified as type B do not experience the same sense of time urgency and show little hostility to others. They tend to play for fun and relaxation, not to exhibit their superiority at any cost. They can relax without guilt, just as they can work without agitation.

TYPE C—THE CANCER PERSONALITY

While at the University of California School of Medicine at San Francisco, psychologist Lydia Temoshok extensively researched cancer progression and PNI. She hypothesized that cancer patients tend to be uncomplaining, cooperative, and resistant to expressing emotions, particularly anger and hostility. This fits with the general impression that cancer patients tend to be nice people. She termed this personality type C, for cancer prone.

Researchers have shown that humor, positive emotions, and social support can, on the other hand, boost immune function and protect against developing cancer. In 1989, David Spiegel, M.D., conducted studies at Stanford University, which showed that women with breast cancer who received supportive group therapy survived twice as long as those who did not. Not only does an unhealthy lifestyle increase cancer risk, but it is now clear that your attitude, emotions, and social environment can increase your risk as well.

Hope is a component of optimism. British psychiatrist Dr. Steven Greer, M.D., links hope to a quality called *a fighting spirit*. Research in the 1980s on women with breast cancer found that 80 percent of those who had a fighting spirit were still alive after ten years, while only 17 percent of those who felt helpless had survived.

LEARNED HELPLESSNESS AND SELF-EFFICACY

When Martin Seligman, Ph.D., and his colleagues at the University of Pennsylvania exposed animals to painful electric shocks they were unable to escape, the animals learned to be passive. When given subsequent shocks they could easily avoid, the animals lay down and didn't even try to escape.

Many people with chronic illness fall into a similar pattern of learned helplessness. Those who score high for learned helplessness have lower self-esteem, more anxiety and depression, and greater day-to-day problems with their disease.

Self-efficacy, the power of a person to be effective and produce a desired effect in themselves, was popularized by Albert Bandura at Stanford University. It is an assessment of competence, a belief that certain actions can be performed and specific tasks can be completed, and is the opposite of learned helplessness. It influences the choices we make, the effort we put forth, and how long we persist in the face of obstacles. It is related to confidence—the belief that you have the ability to meet the threat or challenge facing you. Self-efficacy is a trait we see in healthy individuals able to cope with the most demanding situations.

EMOTIONAL LONGEVITY

Successful aging can be defined as experiencing minimal disease or disability, maintaining a high level of mental and physical functioning, and being engaged in life right up to the end of life.

Dr. Robert Sapolsky, writing in *Why Zebras Don't Get Ulcers,* shows that up to 15 percent of the people who get ulcers are not infected with *Helicobactor pylori* (*H. pylori*) bacteria. Furthermore, although most people who have ulcers also have *H. pylori,* only about 10 percent of those infected with *H. pylori* actually get an ulcer. According to Sapolsky, in the presence of major life stressors, the addition of a small amount of bacteria inevitably leads to an ulcer. Likewise, in the presence of lots of bacteria, it takes only a small amount of stress to cause an ulcer.

The point is, successful aging depends on both biological and nonbiological dimensions. It turns out that what determines the wide differences in longevity are several new dimensions in health, as described by Norman Anderson, Ph.D., a professor at Harvard University's School of Public Health. They are:

• Emotions;

• Environment and relationships;

• Faith and meaning;

• Personal achievement and equality;

• Thoughts and actions.

How do you score on the Emotional Longevity Screening Questionnaire below? It is important to remember that our biological status is only one of several broad categories of factors that influence our health and longevity.

Emotions are somewhat unique in that they act as a kind of well-being thermometer. They are unique in being the one pathway that all the dimensions of health share.

EMOTIONAL LONGEVITY SCREENING QUESTIONNAIRE	Yes	No
1. I have feelings of stress.		
2. I have feelings of fear/anxiety.		
3. I have feelings of anger.		
4. I have feelings of grief (broken heart).		
5. I have feelings of cynicism.		
6. I have feelings of being unable to love.		

	Yes	No
7. I have feelings of guilt.		
8. I have feelings of a sense of inadequacy.		
9. I have feelings of no will to live.		
10. I have feelings of depression.		
11. I have feelings of being helpless and hopeless.		
12. I have feelings of hostility.		
13. I have feelings of sadness.		
14. I have feelings that my life has no purpose.		
15. I have feelings that I don't belong.		
16. I have a feeling of purpose in my work and life.		
17. I feel good about my education and earnings.		
18. I have feelings of love for my family.		
19. I have feelings of joy with my many friends.		
20. I have feelings of gratitude.		
21. I have feelings of love for my significant other.		
22. I feel a strong spiritual orientation in my life.		
23. I feel I have achieved a good socioeconomic position.		
24. I feel I am in control of my life.		
25. I have feelings of joy.		
26. I have a sense of optimism.		
27. I feel that my life is an open book.		
28. I feel that my life is meaningful.		
29. I have feelings of peace.		
30. I have feelings of a divine presence.		

Score:

For questions 1–15, add the number of NO answers. For questions 16–30, add the number of YES answers. Then combine the two for a total.

0–15   Poor emotional longevity

15–20   Good emotional longevity

21 or more   Great emotional longevity

COPING AND COHERENCE

In determining health or disease, individual differences in the way people cope with stressful events may be more important than the stressors themselves. Just as negative psychological traits can intensify the effects of stressors, positive ways of coping can buffer their effects.

Psychologist Suzanne Kobasa at the City University of New York has measured a style of coping she terms *hardiness,* which can protect against illness. She studied a group of business executives and found that certain personality traits were present in the healthiest leaders of companies. One trait was seeing life's demands as a challenge rather than as a threat. Another was commitment to something meaningful, such as their work, family, and so on. The final trait was a sense of being in control, similar to Bandura's self-efficacy.

The late Aaron Antonovsky, who lived and worked in Israel, studied individuals who had survived the Holocaust, and confirmed that a person's attitude toward life had a significant impact on his or her well-being. People who score high on a sense-of-coherence test feel that their circumstances make sense—they have enough meaning to justify the effort and investment of energy that any inherent problems demand. People with a strong sense of coherence can choose the most appropriate strategy to deal with the stress of a particular situation.

Several studies have shown that well-educated people are healthier, even after accounting for income differences. In the integral health model (*see* Appendix A), we believe that when an individual integrates the various structures of consciousness outlined, her or his resulting worldview will, in turn, enhance a personal sense of well-being. Such an individual combines Kobasa's hardiness, Bandura's self-efficacy, and Antonovsky's sense of coherence.

The awareness of twentieth-century medicine owed much to a concept known as the medical model. The underlying assumption was that each disease has a single cause that can be identified by objective testing, and the result is that the solution is in the hands of doctors and hospitals (and drugs and surgery) and does not depend on the actions of the person with the disease. This model, which virtually ignores the person's thoughts and emotions, may work up to a point for acute conditions, such as pneumonia or bone fracture (though even there a person's attitude influences recovery), but it is extremely limited when applied to chronic illness, such as arthritis, cancer, heart disease, and the many other diseases of civilization now prevalent in the world.

We believe that medicine in the twenty-first century will follow a much more complete, integrated approach and will recognize how imperative a person's worldview is to well-being. The limited scope of the current medical establishment makes it ill-suited to deliver this new model of integral health. In the decades ahead, as the full benefits of this new, complete medicine are recognized, we anticipate an explosion in spa medicine.

THE RELAXATION RESPONSE

Dr. Herbert Benson was fascinated by the fact that people had higher blood pressure during times of stress. After finishing his cardiology training at Harvard in the 1970s, he focused his attention on the link between mind and body, looking for a way to treat stress-induced high blood pressure.

Initially, Benson studied biofeedback on monkeys and then worked on people, practicing meditation with psychologist Robert Keith Wallace. They found dramatic physiological changes as the study's participants shifted from everyday thinking into meditation. They recorded significant chemical and hormonal changes, as well as changes in blood pressure, brain-wave function, breathing, and heart rates.

Before this, there had only been two conditions known to decrease metabolism below the resting state: sleep and hibernation, and it took several hours or days to do so, but meditators were able to produce these changes in three to five minutes. Interestingly, to conduct his experiments, Benson was using the same lab as Walter Cannon, who had developed the concept of the fight-or-flight response in the early 1900s. It all fit together with the research of Walter R. Hess, who won the Nobel Prize in 1949 for his work in the 1930s and 1940s that showed, by stimulating certain areas of the brain in lab animals, he could produce a response exactly opposite to the fight-or-flight response—a response he called a "protective mechanism against overstress."

Benson showed that this protective mechanism was what he had found in the meditators, and he coined the term *the relaxation response* to describe this basic physiological response in human beings. More recently, he cited evidence that religion and/or faith in God lowers mortality rates and improves health by reducing anger, anxiety, depression, and blood pressure. He writes that "Faith quiets the mind like no other form of belief." Prayer creates peace and positive images that foster healing.

He and his colleagues spent several years researching secular and religious literature from around the world to analyze what the key ingredients were that turned off a person's inner dialogue and elicited the relaxation response. They turned out to include four simple elements:

- A quiet environment without interruptions;
- A mental device (mnemonic), such as a rhyme or mantra;
- A passive, accepting attitude;
- An upright yet relaxed position.

A wide array of techniques can elicit the relaxation response, which is technically considered a set of integrated responses that lower the arousal of the sympathetic nervous system (SNS). The resulting relaxed state is characterized by:

- Changes in the EEG, indicating relaxation;
- Enhancement of some immune functions;
- Redistribution of blood flow;
- Reduction in blood pressure;
- Reduction in heart rate;
- Reduction in oxygen consumption;
- Reduction in respiratory rate;
- Reduction in tissue sensitivity to stress hormones.

And this relaxed state can be elicited by:

- Autogenic training;
- Breathing;
- Complete absorption in a pleasant experience;
- Freeze-frame;
- Guided imagery;
- Meditation;
- Progressive muscle relaxation;
- Repetitive exercise, such as tai chi;
- Self-hypnosis;
- Walking.

To achieve the relaxation response, you can repeat a simple, neutral word, such as *one,* for several minutes. Benson and his colleagues noted even more profound physiological changes when people incorporated what he terms *the faith factor* into repeating a simple prayer or statement reflecting their spiritual roots or beliefs. For example, you could use the words *shalom* or *om.* Or the phrase "The Lord is my shepherd" or "Hail Mary, full of grace." After you have chosen your phrase, close your eyes, and breathe in through your nose. Say your word or phrase silently as you exhale. When stray thoughts come by, gently release them and continue your mantra. Use this technique for ten to fifteen minutes, once or twice a day, as needed.

Most medi-spas offer a number of relaxation methods in order for a guest to choose whichever ones he or she feels most comfortable with. One of our favorites is the freeze-frame technique, popularized by Doc Lew Childre from the Heart Math Institute in Boulder Creek, California. Learning how to freeze-frame means understanding how to choose your perceptions of reality so they are the healthiest and most productive possible (*see* Figure 5.3 on page 108). As you know, the amount of stress you feel is based on your perception (worldview) of events and not on the stressful events themselves (stressors).

How to Freeze-Frame

1. Recognize the stressful feeling.

2. Make a sincere effort to shift your focus to the area around your heart. Pretend you're breathing through your heart to help focus your energy in this area. Keep your focus there for ten seconds or more.

3. Recall a positive fun feeling or time you've had in life, when you felt really happy and loved, and attempt to reexperience it.

4. Now, using your intuition, common sense, and sincerity, ask your heart what would be a more beneficial response to the stressful situation you started with. If you choose one that will minimize future stress, it will be the most heart healthy.

5. Listen to what your heart says in answer to your question.

Freeze-frame aids you in becoming more sensitive to your heart's directive, which is using the power to really change from the inside out. The best way to begin to practice freeze-frame is with those little things that come up, such as traffic jams, things that bug you, problems at work, and so on.

It's important to use a freeze-frame technique that really gets to the emotionality of your heart. For example, Dr. Sinatra's wife, Jan, will visualize her smiling grandchildren when she is under severe stress and tension. Just the image of her grandchildren and the love and affection she has for them instantly brings her back to feelings of joy, which neutralize the toxic emotional reactions. Try to find something that truly works for you and practice it—it could be a lifesaver.

Self-Hypnosis with Suggested Deep Relaxation

To induce self-hypnosis, sit comfortably and, from a prerecorded tape, receive instructions that should ultimately calm and relax you. Once you are in this state

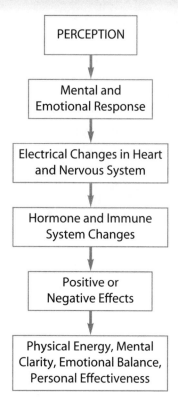

Figure 5.3. Perception Changes Health

of increased suggestibility, where brain waves become slower, and blood pressure, breathing rate, and heart rate all decrease, hypnotic suggestions of your choice are presented to you.

Guided Imagery

A twenty-minute relaxation exercise helps you focus attention and center your mind. Imagery is often used in conjunction with hypnosis. Hypnosis is the induction of a particular state of mind, while imagery is an activity. You either focus on a predetermined image to help control a particular problem (active imagery) or you allow your mind to present images to you that give insight into a problem (receptive imagery). Vivid imagery of either type appears to send a message from your brain, via the limbic system (your emotional center), to the endocrine glands and the autonomic nervous system (ANS). The more fully you imagine, the better the results. Imagery is valuable in mind-body medicine and healing because it can bring about physiological changes, provide psychological insight, and enhance emotional awareness. Think of your emotions as the means by which thought creates change in the body.

Autogenic Training

Autogenic training, another useful technique to induce the relaxation response, was developed in the 1940s by Johannes Schultz in Germany. It includes actively focusing on feelings of warmth and heaviness in the limbs, with a passive focus on breathing to let it happen.

Progressive Muscle Relaxation

Described by Edmund Jacobson in the 1920s, a quiet place and a passive attitude are essential to this technique. You are taught to detect even the slightest muscle contraction as you scan your body from head to toe and achieve a deep degree of muscle relaxation.

Bioenergetics

Bioenergetics is a form of psychotherapy that originated in the 1950s from Wilhelm Reich's vegetative therapy, which, in turn, stemmed from his belief that emotions were trapped in the body. Alexander Lowen, a student of Reich's, coined the term *bioenergetics*—body-oriented psychotherapy. Freeing up emotions, using emotional release and techniques to open up the breathing, is a way of discharging chronically repressed, pent-up tensions and spasticities from the body, important because unreleased emotions can have a deleterious effect on health and wellness. Bioenergetic therapists frequently use emotional release as a form of discharging negative elements from the body, and they will encourage the expression of anger, sadness, or even rage. Hitting, crying, and kicking are various techniques to help rid the body of chronic spasticities that limit a person's joy and the feeling of being fully alive.

Bioenergetic therapist training is a long and arduous process requiring careful scrutiny by peers. As this type of therapy also investigates sensitive issues of sensuality and sexuality in determining the overall health of the person, bioenergetic therapists must be well grounded. And for certification, they must have gone through extensive therapy themselves, in order to make them well suited and well trained to help people overcome deep-seated emotions that can be thoroughly toxic to the body.

Keep in mind that, for optimum mind-body health, physical, environmental, *and* psychological factors all play an important role in managing the stress in your life. Table 5.1 is a summary of some recommended solutions involving all three components.

TABLE 5.1. Summary of Stress Solutions

Physical	Environmental	Psychological
Nutrition	Full-spectrum light	Worldview
Exercise	Water purifier	Meditation
Massage	Air filter	Counseling/bioenergetics
Breathing	Cleansed food	Social support
Bodywork	Natural-care products	Freeze-frame

One-Pointed Meditation and Mindfulness Meditation

There are two major types of meditation. *One-pointed* meditation, mentioned earlier, employs a mental device—a phrase or a sound—to produce the relaxation response and is called Samahdhi practice.

The other form of meditation is known as *Vipassana,* or mindfulness meditation. In the practice of mindfulness meditation, the goal is to completely empty your mind of everything except the present. Massachusetts psychologist and author Jon Kabat-Zinn writes:

> When thoughts or feelings come up in your mind, you don't ignore them or suppress them, nor do you analyze or judge their content. Rather, you simply note any thoughts as they occur as best you can and observe them intentionally but nonjudgmentally, moment by moment, as events in the field of your awareness.
>
> By observing your thoughts and emotions as if you had taken a step back from them, you can see much more clearly what is actually on your mind. The key to mindfulness is not so much what you choose to focus on, but the quality of the awareness that you bring to each moment. It is very important that it be nonjudgmental—more of a silent witnessing or a dispassionate observing, than a running commentary on your inner experience.

Kabat-Zinn points out that by fully accepting what each moment offers, you open yourself to experiencing life much more completely. Acceptance offers a way to navigate life's inevitable ups and downs—what Zorba the Greek called "the full catastrophe" of living with grace, humor, and some understanding of a larger reality or what we call wisdom. Calmness, equanimity, increased awareness, insight, and even profound peace and joy can be experienced with practice.

In addition to having fewer symptoms, people on this path have a willingness to look at stressful events as challenges rather than as threats, and they experience a greater sense of control and meaning in their life. Mindfulness practice may also benefit health by increasing your sense of connection to other people and the environment. Many report feeling they are part of the greater flow of life, a feeling many describe as a sense of oneness with the world, of feeling complete and part of a larger whole.

Mindfulness meditation and an understanding of our psychohistorical development over time are the essence of eternity medicine, which we will introduce later (*see* Afterword).

MEANING MEDICINE

As you can see, the amount of stress you feel is based more on your *perception* of a person, situation, or event than on the event (stressor) itself (*see* Figure 5.4 below).

Our thoughts result not only from the brain's adaptation and evolution over the last few million years, but also from *the meaning we attach to our sensory impressions of the world.* Everything we have ever known, or felt, or will feel is ultimately a linguistic invention. How we come to order our thoughts (worldview) is thus critical to our psychological health and well-being.

As we shall see, until a larger reality—what might be called the wisdom self—is discovered, a person's life experience will continue to be derived from, and limited to, the personal, conditional thought system (ego-self). A larger consciousness, or wisdom self, is characterized by such positive emotions as humor, joy, love, and wonder.

We have long been interested in what allows individuals to go beyond obvious healthy lifestyle choices to a deeper sense of well-being. Our shared belief is that a sense of the spiritual and an integral worldview are the common sources of inner health and wholeness.

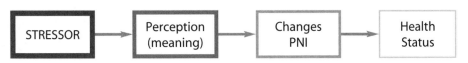

Figure 5.4. The Relationship Between Stress, Meaning, and Health

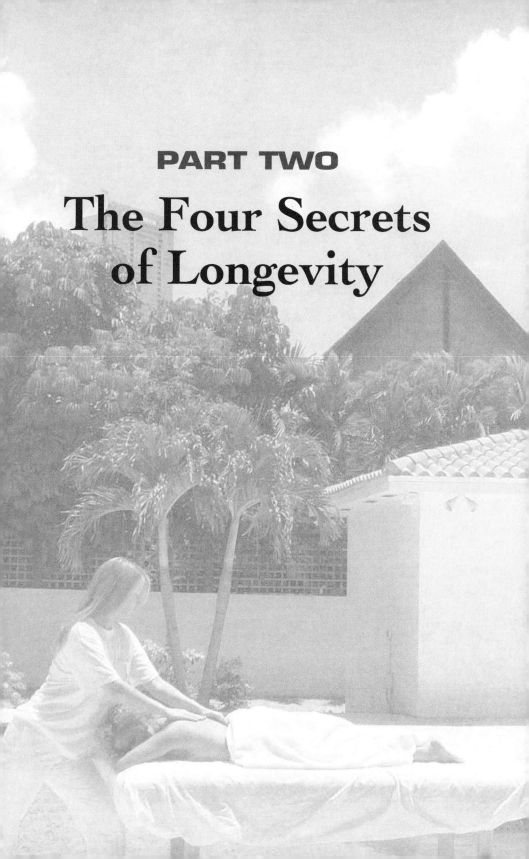

PART TWO
The Four Secrets of Longevity

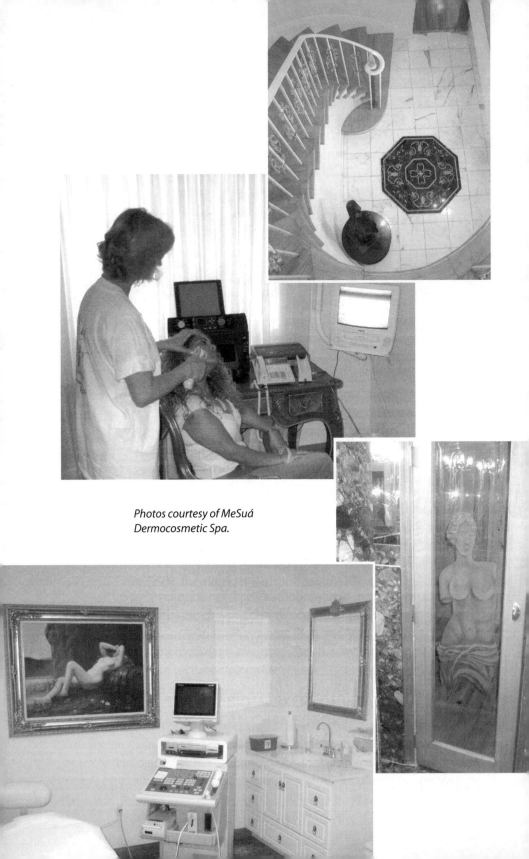

Photos courtesy of MeSuá Dermocosmetic Spa.

Chapter 6

Why We Age

When you have eliminated the impossible,
whatever remains, however improbable, must be the truth.

—Sir Arthur Conan Doyle (1859–1930)

EIGHT THEORIES OF AGING

Scientific research has led to the formulation of a number of aging theories, but truthfully, aging most likely results from a combination of theories, such as the eight discussed in this chapter. Similarly, the four secrets of longevity are an amalgam of these same theories and can, in combination with the four pillars of wellness, illuminate your gateway to the ageless zone.

1. THE DNA/GENETIC THEORY

Some scientists regard this as a planned obsolescence theory because it focuses on the programming encoded in our DNA, the blueprint each of us has received from our parents. We are born with a unique code and a predetermined tendency for certain ways of functioning, physically and mentally, that under this theory regulate our rate of aging. But the timing of this type of genetic clock can be greatly influenced. For example, DNA is easily oxidized, and free-radical damage can result from diet, lifestyle, pollution, radiation, toxins, or other outside influences, which means that each of us has the ability to either accelerate or slow down the damage caused by oxidized DNA.

The telomerase theory of aging is one of the most recent regarding gene damage. First discovered by scientists at the Geron Corporation in California, it is now understood that telomeres (the sequences of the nucleic acids in DNA that extend from the ends of chromosomes) shorten every time a cell divides. The shortening of these telomeres is believed to lead to cellular damage because the cell is not able to duplicate itself correctly. Each time it divides, it duplicates itself a little less precisely than the time before, and each subsequent reproduction makes the cell weaker and weaker until, eventually, there is cellular dysfunction leading to aging and, ultimately, death.

Further recent research by Don Kleinsek, Ph.D., one of very few genealogists looking for the genes involved with aging, indicates that telomeres can be repaired by the introduction of the relevant hormone. If this theory holds up, it means that once we know what each telomere is responsible for, it *may* be possible to precisely introduce the necessary hormone or nutrient to aid genetic repair, as well as maintain balance in the body.

Another key element in rebuilding the disappearing telomeres is the enzyme telomerase, currently found only in germ and cancer cells. Telomerase appears to repair and replace telomeres, which helps to regulate the clock that controls the life span of dividing cells (*see* The Hayflick Limit Theory of Aging on page 118).

2. THE NEUROENDOCRINE THEORY

First proposed by Professor Vladimir Dilman and Ward Dean, M.D., this theory focuses on the neuroendocrine system and elaborates on its wear and tear. It is a system with a complicated network of biochemicals, which control the release of hormones that are governed by the hypothalamus, a walnut-sized gland located in the brain.

The hypothalamus also governs the various chain reactions that instruct other organs and glands to release their hormones. The hypothalamus responds to the body's hormone levels, acting as a guide and feedback system controlling the body's overall hormonal activity.

As we grow older, however, the regulatory ability of the hypothalamus loses its precision, and the receptors for individual hormones in the body become less responsive to them. Accordingly, as we age, the secretion of many hormones around the body declines, and their effectiveness is also reduced due to the diminished sensitivity of their receptors.

These are some of the reasons why some doctors recommend drugs that act as receptor *resensitizers*. One such drug improves insulin sensitivity (metformin), and another improves noradrenaline sensitivity (modafinil).

One theory for why the hypothalamus loses its ability to regulate is that it becomes damaged by the hormone cortisol, which is produced by the adrenal glands located on the kidneys. Cortisol is now considered to be a *dark* hormone produced when the body undergoes prolonged stress. It is known to be one of the few hormones that increases with age and, over time, is responsible for a vicious cycle of continued hypothalamic damage, leading to an ever-increasing degree of cortisol production, and then even more hypothalamic damage—a real catch-22 situation.

As the hypothalamus loses its ability to control the system, the resulting damage could lead to hormonal imbalance. If this is the case, spa-medicine programs that decrease stress, and therefore decrease cortisol levels, are important for restoring hormonal balance.

3. THE FREE-RADICAL THEORY

This now-familiar theory of aging was developed by Denham Harman, M.D., at the University of Nebraska in 1956. The term *free radical* denotes any molecule that has a free, unpaired electron, which makes it react with healthy paired molecules in a destructive way.

Because the free-radical molecule has an additional electron, it creates an extra negative charge. This unbalanced energy incites the free radical to bind itself to another balanced molecule as it tries to steal an electron. If it succeeds, the balanced molecule becomes unbalanced and is now turned into an unpaired free radical, itself looking to annex an electron.

It is known that chemical toxins, diet, drugs (including alcohol and tobacco), heavy metals, lifestyle, radiation, and strenuous exercise, and so on, all accelerate the body's production of free radicals.

Moreover, there are additional, *natural* free radicals in the body, a result of energy output, particularly from the mitochondria (the cell's engine). The simple acts of breathing, eating, and drinking form free radicals as the body yields the universal energy molecule adenosine triphosphate (ATP). And oxygen is a particularly potent free-radical producer. What a paradox that oxygen—vital for life— generates life-shortening free radicals.

Free radicals attack the structure of cell membranes, which then create metabolic waste products. These toxic accumulations, in turn, interfere with cell communication; disturb DNA, protein synthesis, and RNA; lower energy levels; and generally impede vital chemical processes.

There is a solution to this problem, however, as free radicals can be transformed by free-radical scavengers, otherwise known as antioxidants. Specific antioxidants will bind to particular free radicals and help to stabilize them.

Free radicals come in a hierarchy according to their potential for damage, with the hydroxyl-radical and the superoxide-radical at the top of the list. In order to successfully combat the damage of dangerous free radicals, therefore, it is necessary to take a variety of antioxidants—you can thus help to eliminate many of them. Included in this broad cross-section of antioxidants are alpha-lipoic acid, beta-carotene, coenzyme Q_{10}, grapeseed extract, and the important vitamins C and E. All these substances will be discussed in full in Chapter 8.

4. THE MEMBRANE THEORY OF AGING

The membrane theory of aging was first described by Professor Imre Zs-Nagy of Debrechen University, Hungary. According to this theory, age-related changes and inflammation in the cell impair its ability to transfer chemicals, electrical processes, and heat.

As we grow older, the cell membrane becomes less lipid (less watery and more solid). This impedes its efficiency in conducting normal cell function and leads, in particular, to a toxic accumulation. As we grow older, this cellular toxin, lipofuscin, develops deposits in the brain, heart, lungs, and skin. Indeed, some of the age pigments in the skin, commonly called liver or age spots, are composed of lipofuscin. It is known that lipofuscin levels are much higher in people with Alzheimer's disease than in healthy people.

The cell's declining efficiency also means that the essential, regular transfer of sodium and potassium between cells is impaired, thus reducing communication. It is also believed that transfer of electricity and heat between cells is also impaired.

Professor Zs-Nagy researched substances that could help remove lipofuscin deposits and improve cellular membranes and communication, and developed the drug centrophenoxine (Lucidril), perhaps the most efficient drug currently available. Other, nondrug substances that have shown an ability to remove lipofuscin include DMAE and the amino acids acetyl-L-carnitine and carnosine.

5. THE HAYFLICK LIMIT THEORY OF AGING

Named after its discoverer, Dr. Leonard Hayflick, this theory of aging suggests that the human cell has a limited number of times it can divide. Part of this theory may be affected by cell-waste accumulation.

Working with Dr. James Moorehead in 1961, Dr. Hayflick theorized that the human cells' ability to divide is limited to approximately fifty times, after which they simply stop dividing (and hence die). As cells split to help repair and regenerate themselves, it is possible that the DNA/genetic theory of aging plays a role here. Maybe each time a cell divides, it loses some blueprint information, until eventually (after fifty-odd times of dividing), there is simply not enough DNA information left to complete any sort of division.

Dr. Hayflick showed that nutrition has an effect on cells, with overfed cells dividing much faster than underfed cells. And studies by him and others have shown that caloric restriction in animals significantly increases their life span and that, in essence, animals that are fed less live longer. Is this because they are subject to less free-radical activity and therefore less cellular damage? Or is it that inflammation caused by insulin and glucose damage is less prevalent in them than in overfed animals?

Whatever the reason, the Hayflick Limit Theory indicates that we need to slow down the rate of cell division if we want to live long lives. Cell division can be slowed down by expanding your lifestyle to include the four pillars of wellness and the four secrets of longevity.

6. THE MITOCHONDRIAL DECLINE THEORY

The mitochondria are the power-producing structures found in every cell of every organ. Their primary job is to create adenosine triphosphate (ATP), which they accomplish with the help of nutrients, such as acetyl-L-carnitine, coenzyme Q_{10}, NADH, and some of the B vitamins. ATP is literally the life-giving chemical because every movement, thought, and action we make is generated from it. Yet very little ATP can be stored in the body, and it cannot by itself be introduced into the body, as a supplement would be. It is estimated that a 180-pound man needs to create, on average, 80–90 pounds of ATP daily. Under strenuous exercise, the body's use of ATP can rise to as much as 1.1 pounds per minute, but its reserves of ATP are generally no more than 3–5 *ounces* so, under those same strenuous exercise conditions, this works out to approximately eight seconds' worth of ATP available. Given this factor, it becomes apparent that the mitochondria have to be very efficient and healthy in order to produce a continuous supply of the essential ATP that makes possible the necessary repair and regenerative processes. Chemically speaking, under normal conditions the mitochondria are fiery furnaces and are themselves subject to a lot of free-radical damage. They also lack most of the defenses common to other parts of the body, so as we age, the mitochondria are continually damaged by free radicals and become less efficient, fewer in number, and tired. Some eventually die, which results in a decline of crucial ATP production.

Since organs cannot borrow energy from one another, the efficiency of each organ's mitochondria is essential to that particular organ's repair processes and functions. If a particular organ's mitochondria fail, then so does that organ (which of course can lead to death). Unlike nuclear DNA (the DNA in the nucleus of a cell, as opposed to the DNA in the mitochondria outside the nucleus), mitochondrial DNA does not have natural regenerative mechanisms, which makes enhancement and protection of the mitochondria an essential part of preventing and slowing aging. This protection can come from a broad spectrum of antioxidants, such as coenzyme Q_{10}, alpha-lipoic acid, and vitamin C, as well as such substances as pregnenolone and D-ribose (a five-sided sugar). In addition, acetyl-L-carnitine and hydergine may be particularly useful—experiments have shown that both substances greatly improve the mitochondrial condition of aged animals.

7. THE CROSS-LINKING THEORY OF AGING

Proposed by J. Bjorksten, this theory, also referred to as the glycosylation theory of aging, holds that it is the binding of glucose (simple sugars) to protein, a process that occurs in the presence of oxygen, which causes various problems associated with aging. Once this binding (cross-linking) has occurred, the protein becomes impaired and is unable to perform as efficiently. Living a longer life is going to lead to the increased possibility of oxygen meeting glucose and protein and causing known cross-linking disorders, including cataracts and tough, leathery, yellow skin. To witness cross-linking in action, simply cut an apple in half and watch the oxygen in the air react with the glucose in the apple, first turning it yellow and brown, and then, eventually, tough. Diabetes is often viewed as a form of accelerated aging and the imbalance of insulin and glucose leads to numerous health complications. In fact, people with diabetes have two to three times the numbers of cross-linked proteins and glucose as their healthy counterparts.

The cross-linking of proteins and glucose may also be responsible for cardiac enlargement and the hardening of collagen, which may result in an increased susceptibility to cardiac arrest. Cross-linked proteins and glucose have also been implicated in kidney disorders, skin aging, and Syndrome X (metabolic syndrome).

It is also theorized that sugars binding to DNA may cause damage that leads to malformed cells and thus cancer. The contemporary diet is, of course, a very sweet one—we are bombarded with simple sugars in everything, from soft drinks to processed foods. An obvious way to reduce the risk of cross-linking is to reduce sugar (and all refined carbohydrates) in your diet. In addition, there are an increasing number of supplements that show great promise in the battle to prevent, slow, and even break existing cross-links.

8. THE WORLDVIEW–WELL-BEING THEORY

Dr. Simpson believes that an integral worldview (*see* Appendix A) is the key ingredient for inner health, wholeness, and longevity. The psychohistorical development of consciousness is central to this theory. Once we assimilate the entirety of our human existence into our awareness, we develop a sense of coherence—we see the world as comprehensible, manageable, and meaningful. This integral worldview, besides helping individuals make healthy lifestyle choices, also has a direct effect on a person's well-being and longevity. This probably works in tandem with several of the above mechanisms of aging. For more information on this ordering of consciousness (integral worldview), visit the website www. eternitymedicine.com.

Whatever aging theory we consider, the final result is a monumental cellular deficiency primarily resulting from inflammation and toxic overload.

THE RATE OF AGING

Women outlive men by ten years, partly because women are routinely screened for breast and uterine cancer, whereas men will usually see a physician only after becoming ill. Another reason may be that, up to this point, most hormone replacement therapy has been directed toward women, even though men have the same symptoms as menopausal women and have similar hormonal levels, low testosterone, and elevated FSH and LH levels.

For most of us, the aging process begins around age thirty, and after age forty, all of us are slowing down. The medical term is *catabolic,* or breaking down. Prior to age thirty, most individuals are in an anabolic state—they are building new body tissue. One of the goals of *Spa Medicine* is to help you reverse the catabolic state and move you once again toward an anabolic state in order to help you *live better longer.*

Obviously, the earlier you start, the simpler it is and the more benefits you will receive; however, it is never too late. People who start a program in their sixties and seventies can still realize significant benefits.

We now know that the major diseases of aging, such as cancer, diabetes, heart disease, and osteoporosis, are largely preventable. Thanks to recent scientific progress, we have the tools to decrease genetic damage, enhance immune function, improve the circulation to the brain and heart, and generally augment a person's vitality.

We encourage all clients visiting medi-spas to first complete their wellness program, since detoxifying the body, nutrition, exercise, and mind-body practices are all vital for longevity. In a medi-spa longevity program, we focus on practical methods to enhance your life span—we are not only looking to increase the number of your years but also to improve the quality of those extra years. The program is individualized for each participant—different nutraceuticals, enzymes, cosmeceuticals, hormones, pharmaceuticals, and cell therapy may be included as part of your longevity program.

The ultimate goal of the longevity program is to square the normal aging curve (*see* Figure 6.1 on page 122). As you can see, you can intervene at any time and shift the curve to the right with a medi-spa program (MSP).

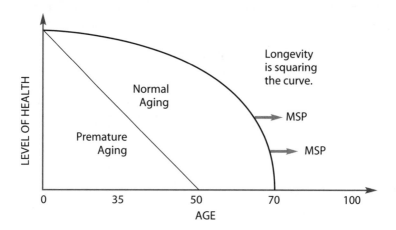

Figure 6.1. Live Better Longer with a Medi-Spa Program (MSP)

Chapter 7

Secret One —
Reduce Inflammation

Instead of different treatments for heart disease,
Alzheimer's, and colon cancer, there might be a single
inflammation-reducing remedy that would prevent all three.

—*TIME* (COVER STORY) FEBRUARY 23, 2004

INFLAMMATION

Most of us have some idea what inflammation is. If a wound gets hot, turns red, hurts, and swells, we recognize that inflammation is at work. In this instance, inflammation is a beneficial process, serving to immobilize the area of injury as the rest of the immune system mobilizes to heal.

Regardless of the source of assault on our bodies, inflammation is the first-alert mechanism that calls into action the cells responsible for surveillance and protection, heralding them to go to work and limit the damage. These cells attack and destroy the invaders, then clean up the damaged cells, repairing and clearing as they go, until a healthy state is restored. As such, inflammation is your body's first line of defense against injury or infection.

SILENT INFLAMMATION

Unlike the above example, researchers now recognize another kind of inflammation: silent inflammation, or SI. This type of internal inflammation has an insidious nature and is the culprit behind the many chronic diseases that are primarily caused by poor lifestyle habits and environmental pollutants. The chronic and continuous low-level demand that silent inflammation places on the body's defense systems results in an immune-system breakdown. In SI there is no regulated progression of a healthy inflammatory response, no planned sequence from the first alarm to the formation of the last new cell. Many of these reactions become intermingled and hamper one another.

The body tissues themselves may lose their ability to recognize cells that are "self" from those that are not, and the body may mistakenly identify its own cells as foreign invaders. This internal programming error then continues to trigger and retrigger immune responses, setting the stage for autoimmune diseases, such as lupus, multiple sclerosis, and scleroderma. The result is chaos, and what is even more disturbing is that this process may be happening year after year without our even being aware of it.

We now know that inflammation plays a central role in the chronic illness that remains our number-one killer: coronary artery disease. In fact, elevated markers of silent inflammation, such as homocysteine, CRP, and Lp(a), have been found to be more predictive of heart disease than such traditional risk factors as elevated cholesterol levels (50 percent of those hospitalized for heart disease have normal cholesterol levels).

A landmark study showed that people with high levels of C-reactive protein (CRP), one of the cardinal markers of inflammation, were over four times more likely to have heart attacks than those with low CRP levels. Researchers then began to link C-reactive protein, along with other markers of inflammation, to a wide range of chronic diseases, including Alzheimer's disease, arthritis, Parkinson's disease, and even cancer. Chronic silent inflammation is now accepted as a warning that something is drastically out of balance in a person's overall health.

Although chronic inflammation can cause a variety of disorders, many of us (and unfortunately this includes many physicians) do not know the warning signs of this kind of inflammation or the best ways to treat it. This knowledge is critical because, if a person has one inflammatory condition, the odds that he or she will develop another condition increase dramatically. Researchers have discovered, for example, that a woman with rheumatoid arthritis has a 100 percent increased risk of experiencing a myocardial infarction. And other recent research has demonstrated that higher CRP levels are also associated with age-related macular degeneration, so the same individual can have more than one condition caused by SI. For all these reasons, slowing down this chronic inflammation syndrome is vital to successful age management, so it is crucial that everyone becomes aware of it, understands its causes, and takes measures to stop it.

CAUSES OF INFLAMMATION

There are many factors that trigger inflammation. They are found in both our internal and external environments and include excessive levels of the hormone insulin, emotional stress, environmental toxins (heavy metals), free-radical damage, nanobacteria and other bacterial infections, obesity, overconsumption of hydrogenated oils, periodontal disease, radiation exposure, smoking, spirochetes, such as the *Borrelia* that causes Lyme disease, viral infections, such as cytomegalovirus (CMV), and some pharmacological drugs. Let's take a closer look at a few of these examples.

Insulin

The most powerful drug you can consume is the food you eat each day. Depending on the ratio of macronutrients (carbohydrates, fats, proteins) you take in at each meal, your daily diet will either keep you in an optimum zone for good health, or it won't. The Zone is a physiological state in which the hormones (especially insulin) influenced by the diet are kept in ranges consistent with optimal health. A perfect Zone meal is composed of macronutrients proportioned in ideal balance, as follows:

- Carbohydrates: 40 percent
- Fat: 30 percent
- Protein: 30 percent

Combining macronutrients according to the ratio listed above will keep you in the Zone. The goal is to keep insulin levels less than 12 µU/ml, although an ideal level is 5 µU/ml. We now know that the Zone diet helps keep eicosanoids (hormonelike substances), insulin, and weight at ideal levels, which, in turn, lowers silent inflammation levels. And remember that the health consequences of failing to keep insulin levels in range can be heart disease, insulin resistance, obesity, type-2 diabetes, and many other unwanted health complications.

Controlling Insulin

Insulin control is achieved through balancing the ratio of protein and carbohydrates at each meal to maintain stable blood-sugar levels for four to six hours. We agree with our colleague Dr. Barry Sears who states, "Hormonally, you are only as good as your last meal, and you will be only as good as your next meal." This means, for optimal health, you have a dietary choice to make every four to six hours. Accordingly, the following is advised.

- Try to eat a Zone meal within one hour of waking.
- Every time you eat, aim to balance protein, carbohydrates, and fat.
- Try to eat five times a day—three meals and two light snacks.
- Eat more vegetables and fruit; eat less bread, pasta, potatoes, and rice.
- Eat a serving of slow-cooked oatmeal topped with seasonal fruit twice a week for fiber, gamma linolenic acid (GLA), and phytonutrients.

- Always supplement your diet with fish oil and other nutraceuticals.

- Use monounsaturated oils (such as olive oil) whenever possible on vegetables and salads.

- Choose low-glycemic carbohydrates whenever possible.

In addition to excess insulin, heart disease and aging are accelerated by increased blood sugar, elevated cortisol levels, and free radicals. And all these contributing factors can be modified by the Zone diet, which works to establish hormonal equilibrium in the body.

The essential fatty acids, omega-6 and omega-3, are also key dietary components. As mentioned in Chapter 3, when these two types of essential fatty acids are metabolized they produce eicosanoid hormones, which can have dramatically different physiological reactions. Eicosanoids have been labeled either good or bad, depending on how they affect the body. Good eicosanoids, produced from omega-3 fatty acids, are anti-inflammatory by nature, while bad eicosanoids cause inflammation. The metabolism of essential fatty acids is ultimately controlled by one particular enzyme in the body, delta-5-desaturase, which produces arachidonic acid (AA), a long-chain omega-6 fatty acid that is the precursor of the proinflammatory (bad) eicosanoids. (*See* Figure 7.1 below.)

Two dietary constituents profoundly affect the activity of the enzyme delta-5-desaturase—the levels of long-chain omega-3-fatty acids, eicosapentaenoic acid (EPA), and the levels of insulin. The AA/EPA balance, as measured in the blood, represents the balance of bad and good eicosanoids throughout the body (an ideal AA/EPA ratio is 1.5).

If you eat an imbalance of (too many) carbohydrates, refined sugars, and proteins, you will provoke a greater insulin response. Too much insulin in the body exacerbates AA production, which causes sticky platelets (platelet aggregation) and sets the stage for chronic, silent inflammation while promoting blood clotting at the same time. But high levels of EPA (as found in wild salmon, for example) will counteract the negative effects of AA production and keep inflammation at bay.

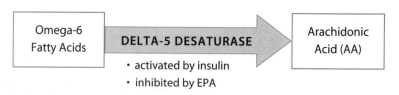

Figure 7.1. The Role of Delta-5 Desaturase in AA Synthesis

Heavy Metals

There are numerous published papers describing adverse clinical effects with aluminum, cadmium, copper, iron, lead, and mercury. According to data from the U.S. Toxics Release Inventory, in the year 2000, industry in the United States released 4.3 million pounds of mercury and mercury compounds into the environment, and generated 4.9 million pounds of mercury compounds in toxic waste. This toxic metal burden increases low-grade inflammation at the cellular level, which interferes with mitochondrial function and energy production, and therefore has a very negative effect on the endocrine (glandular), immune, and metabolic systems.

The cardiovascular, immune, and nervous systems are extraordinarily sensitive to mercury. In one small study of thirteen people with heart disease, investigators found mercury concentrations in excess of 22,000 times normal. Researchers speculated that toxic mercury levels adversely affected mitochondrial activity, which led to the heart problems.

And how do we become mercury toxic in the first place? Quite simply by breathing bad air and eating bad fish. Most mercury vapors come from the industrialization of coal, and they are inhaled into the lungs and then transmitted to tissues. Another important factor is the precipitation of mercury vapors in the water supply through rainfall. The mercury goes into lakes, ponds, and streams, where algae and bacteria—your main entrée if you're a fish—take it in. First small (bait) fish ingest this algae-laden methylmercury, then the bigger fish eat these smaller fish, and on up the food chain, until it reaches us. And the larger the fish, the greater amount of time it's had to accumulate more mercury from its diet of smaller fish, so when we dine on a large mercury-overloaded fish, we are getting a large dose of toxic metal.

A study of the association between fish intake and myocardial infarction, using hair analysis and urinary excretion to measure mercury levels in 1,833 men, showed that those men with the highest hair-mercury levels had twice as many heart attacks and almost three times as many cardiac arrests as the men with lower hair-mercury content. Mercury increases LDL, and high levels of LDL prime the pump for further inflammation.

Although somewhat controversial, many believe that dental fillings are another source of unwanted mercury toxins in the body. If you have any signs and symptoms of mercury overload, such as cardiac problems of unknown origin, confusion, fatigue headaches, insomnia, joint pain, tremors, weakness, or weight loss, to mention a few, you should seriously consider having your old cracked fillings removed by a dentist.

The easiest way to diagnose heavy metal toxicity, as mentioned before, is to ingest a dose of oral DMSA (dimercaptosuccinic acid) and collect the urine for the next twenty-four hours. A proficient lab to have mercury levels checked is Doctor's Data (*see* Resources and Med-Spa Directory). In our respective practices, we commonly perform this test on patients with cardiac disease, fibromyalgia, emotional and neurological problems, and unexplained fatigue.

Free Radicals

Free radicals are highly reactive, imbalanced molecules that steal electrons from cells to neutralize their charge. Free radicals interfere with enzymatic reactions and cause significant metabolic stress, damaging cells and DNA. Simply eating, drinking, and breathing will generate free radicals as byproducts of energy (ATP) production, and alcohol, drugs, poor diets, and radiation, among other causes, accelerate the production of free radicals in the body. Their danger is that they fan the fires of inflammation and attack cell membranes, ultimately disrupting cellular communication. When free-radical damage disturbs the integrity of your cell membranes, they leak, and excessive waste builds up inside the cells.

One of the primary ways we can protect ourselves from free-radical damage is to take oral antioxidants. Because cell membranes are composed mostly of fat, fat-soluble antioxidants, such as alpha-lipoic acid, coenzyme Q_{10}, and vitamin E, can best penetrate into the cell. Antioxidants slow the aging process by promoting cellular repair, inhibiting inflammation, and preventing production of the inflammatory substances that accelerate aging.

Cardiologists frequently cite the process of lipid peroxidation as a focal point for the origin of atherosclerosis (hardening of the arteries). Many antioxidants, particularly coenzyme Q_{10} and quercetin (found in onions), actively block the oxidation of LDL that contributes to silent inflammation.

Nanobacteria

Although oxidized LDL cholesterol creates plaque that helps set the stage for atherosclerosis, there are other causes of cardiovascular disease. Controversial nanobacteria are increasingly considered an important explanation for this disease.

Nanobacteria, formally known as *Nanobacterium sanguineum,* are so minute that they eluded researchers for decades. They're one-one thousandth the size of normal bacteria, and until recently, nobody believed that anything so small could even be alive. It turns out, however, that nanobacteria are not only very vital and thriving, but they may be causing damage to our health in more ways than we can imagine.

One of our missions has been to explain how and why heart disease occurs in people who don't exhibit the traditional risk factors. If we can identify the cause, then we can help prevent thousands of unexplained deaths each year. There have been numerous hypotheses, but so many never pan out. Take *Chlamydia pneumoniae,* the pathogen that causes acute respiratory disease, for example. In news reports from just a few years ago, authorities proclaimed that infection with this bacterium probably accounted for much of the unexplained plaque in people. They hoped that doctors could treat the *C. pneumoniae* and thereby eradicate the plaque. Well, further research uncovered that *C. pneumoniae* was only found in a small percentage of all plaque and was certainly not pervasive enough to be a major cause for it.

An Apt Analogy

To help illuminate what the discovery of nanobacteria could ultimately mean for our health, let's take a look at *H. pylori* and ulcers. It was only after years of having patients undergo gastric surgery that doctors learned that the real culprit in many ulcers was a bacterium known as *Helicobacter pylori.* Surgeons were putting their patients with ulcers through major surgery, cutting their vagus nerve (the extensive cranial nerve that extends to the abdomen) and revamping part of their small intestine when, in most cases, the only treatment needed was antibiotics.

In the same way, in another alarmingly common procedure, cardiac surgeons have been cutting and pasting blood vessels to bypass plaque-filled arteries. We may learn, instead, that a course of the right antibiotic is all that's needed for severely calcified arteries.

Scientists from the Hungarian Academy of Sciences have reported finding nanobacteria in more than 60 percent of carotid-artery-clogging plaques studied. The Hungarians also validated previous research reports of how truly minuscule these bacteria are, and how easily they can enter the body via blood exchange and blood products. Their protective calcified apatite coat makes nanobacteria highly resistant to heat, radiation, and all antibiotics except tetracycline. Nanobacteria have been implicated in nephrolithiasis, polycystic kidney disease, and renal stone formation.

More research will determine whether nanobacteria are the real culprits behind coronary arteriosclerosis. For now it is prudent to keep in mind that microbes could play a substantial factor in causing the silent inflammation that can culminate in cardiovascular disease. We'll now discuss some of the research that looks at other viruses and spirochetes as potential causes of inflammation, as well as the relationship between periodontal disease and the heart.

Spirochetes

In 1982, Willy Burgdorfer discovered the cause of Lyme disease when he isolated spirochetes of the genus *Borrelia* from the mid-gut of ixodes ticks. Some researchers believe that as many as 60 million people in the United States are infected with *Borrelia*, but that Lyme disease occurs in them only when their immune systems become overloaded. Dr. Simpson estimates that at least 30 percent of his patients with Lyme disease are also mercury toxic, and he believes that this mercury toxicity severely compromises their immune systems and leaves them vulnerable to the *Borrelia* spirochetes.

Lyme disease has been reported in forty-seven states and on four continents, and ticks are not the only sources. Blood transfusions, fleas, mosquitoes, sexual intercourse, and unpasteurized cow's and goat's milk have also transmitted the disease. People with Lyme disease are often simultaneously infected with other viruses and bacteria.

The spirochetes responsible for Lyme disease do best in an anaerobic (low-oxygen) environment and cannot tolerate large quantities of oxygen. They can change their shape and chemical structure, and are more evolved than bacteria in many ways. Furthermore, these spirochetes can turn off several surface proteins, which have the effect of keeping the immune system from being able to detect them. This stealth-type camouflage of theirs prevents antibodies from attaching to them, and prevents the enzymes in the blood from finding and destroying them. In this way, the spirochete can penetrate any tissue in our bodies, including our blood vessels, brain, heart, and mouth.

Viruses

Many researchers now believe that coronary artery disease (CAD) is largely an inflammatory process characterized by decades of cyclic irritation, injury, healing, and reinjury to the inside of blood vessels.

Organisms like cytomegalovirus (CMV) and other viruses have been implicated in contributing to inflammation and the subsequent elevation of C-reactive protein (CRP). This elevated CRP can lead to a fivefold increase in risk for heart disease. Dr. Hannah Valentine, a cardiologist at Stanford University Medical Center, found that people with CMV who were given heart transplants developed atherosclerosis, as did rats under identical circumstances. However, if the rats were given an antiviral drug to kill CMV, they did not develop atherosclerosis.

Iron is required for the growth and reproduction of many infectious viral organisms. Research has shown that the tendency of menstruating women to have lower iron levels than men may be the reason for their longer average life span. Since natural substances like lactoferrin, malic acid, and pectin can safely chelate iron out of the system, we recommend nutraceuticals containing these components as part of your longevity program.

Periodontal Disease

There is a significant relationship between periodontal (gum) disease and chronic inflammation. Multiple microbes, including bacteria, spirochetes, and viruses, can grow in and around the teeth and periodontal sections of the mouth and cause a decline in the immune system, making the area susceptible to chronic low-grade inflammation and subsequent increases in CRP levels. In one study of fifty people referred for angiography and assessed for periodontal disease, there was a significant relationship between the extent of coronary atherosclerosis and periodontal disease.

Cardiologists are especially aware of the link between gum disease, halitosis, oral hygiene, missing teeth, and a strong probability of subsequent cardiovascular disease. Practicing good oral hygiene and taking antioxidants, such as coenzyme Q_{10}, essential fatty acids, and magnesium, can help support gum health, thereby reducing chronic inflammation.

Toxic Blood Syndrome

Toxic blood syndrome is blood that has been compromised by heavy metals, infections, and other toxins. Ninety-five percent of chronically sick people have excess blood coagulation, which hampers blood flow, and many of these have toxic blood syndrome, characterized by such markers for inflammation as elevated levels of C-reactive protein, ferritin, fibrinogen, homocysteine, Lp(a), and oxidized LDL. (Inflammation is now considered the primary culprit responsible for vascular disease.) In a study, elevated levels of C-reactive protein (CRP) were the most significant of twelve predictors of future cardiac events in 28,263 healthy postmenopausal women, and was the strongest risk factor associated with an acute coronary event, such as plaque rupture or myocardial infarction. In acute myocardial infarctions, those with higher C-reactive protein levels have a higher death rate than those with lower CRP levels.

Homocysteine

A higher level of homocysteine is not only a risk factor for cardiovascular disease, it has also been implicated in Alzheimer's disease, cancer, low birth weight, neural tube defects, and osteoporosis. Homocysteine is directly toxic to blood vessels in the brain and heart. Elevated levels wreak oxidative stress, cause DNA damage to the nerves, endothelial dysfunction, and even a weakening of the mitochondrial membrane.

High levels of homocysteine have been shown to double the incidence of Alzheimer's disease. In one study of 1,092 people who were initially dementia-free, over an eight-year follow-up, 111 developed dementia and 83 developed full-blown Alzheimer's disease. Those with high homocysteine levels had double the Alzheimer's risk of those with lower homocysteine levels, and as the homocysteine levels went up, so did the risk levels.

One of the most important factors in lowering homocysteine is the use of the B vitamins, including B_6, B_{12}, betaine hydrochloride (trimethylglycine), calcium folinate, folic acid, and pyridoxal phosphate. Beets, broccoli, garlic, and SAMe are also effective in reversing toxic homocysteine back into harmless methionine. A large percentage of people, however, particularly those of European and French Canadian decent, cannot adequately metabolize synthetic folic acid. For these people, homocysteine levels will persist despite the use of B vitamin components.

What are acceptable levels of homocysteine? A homocysteine level less than 7 is ideal. Levels over 10 are unacceptable, especially in those with presenile dementia or arteriosclerotic cardiovascular disease. And high homocysteine levels are especially treacherous in the company of elevated lipoprotein(a) (Lp[a]) because together they can induce clots. On an anecdotal note, Dr. Sinatra has seen elevated homocysteine in the company of high Lp(a) in many of his patients who have heart disease, and he treats it aggressively in them, as well as in those at risk for developing it.

Lipoprotein(a)

Lipoprotein(a) is a cholesterol particle that is highly inflammatory and thrombotic. In a ten-year follow-up of myocardial infarctions in 5,200 participants, those with the highest Lp(a) levels had a 70 percent increase in myocardial infarctions. For the cardiologist, Lp(a) is a difficult risk factor to neutralize because the statin drugs are known to increase Lp(a), so it is important for physicians to track Lp(a) levels whenever they are treating high cholesterol with any statin drugs.

We have found that the toxic effects of Lp(a) can often be neutralized by using targeted nutraceuticals. The liver-supporting nutrients are especially helpful, along with coenzyme Q_{10}, Policosanol, and the omega-3 essential fatty acids, such as fish oils, in combination with niacin.

Fibrinogen

High fibrinogen is a phenomenon increasingly observed in postmenopausal women and smokers, and levels greater than 360 milligrams have been associated with coronary calcification. This coagulation protein has been successfully neutralized with bromelain, fish oils, garlic, and natural Cox-2 inhibitors, such as ginger and green teas, as well as enzymes (to be discussed later in this chapter).

Ferritin

Serum ferritin (high levels of stored iron) is also associated with increased risk for myocardial infarctions. The high levels of iron that can oxidize LDL cholesterol may reflect iron overload or hereditary high iron levels. If you have this condition, it is important to cut iron consumption to a minimum and use high-dose vitamin C with caution, as megadoses greater than 500 milligrams daily may lead you to absorb too much iron from your diet.

Toxic Blood and Plaque

In summary, it's important to assess all these toxic-blood components, particularly when treating an individual with a family history of early-onset, or what we call premature, cardiovascular disease. We know that homocysteine and Lp(a) can be genetic, and in assessing arteriosclerosis we need to go beyond cholesterol and triglyceride monitoring and look at these toxic blood components that are becoming increasingly implicated in the formation of plaque.

Younger plaque is soft and covered by a thinner fibrous cap, loaded with cholesterol. It is quite volatile and often goes unnoticed on angiograms. To some extent, many of us have atherosclerosis—the real question is, "Do you have an unstable plaque?" Inside these young fatty plaques, macrophages (the scavenger white blood cells of the immune system) can become engorged and incompetent to do the job they are designed to do. Instead, they evolve into angry foam cells, releasing proinflammatory toxic substances that may result in further instability to the plaque.

It used to be thought that cholesterol was the major marker for atherosclerosis. This is no longer the case. Proinflammatory messengers, referred to as cytokines and leukotrienes, are now recognized as behind-the-scene culprits. When inflammation is present, specific cytokine messengers are put into service to instruct the liver to increase intermediary inflammatory substances, such as CRP, that are released into the blood and serve as indicators of underlying chronic inflammation. By interrupting and arresting inflammation (*see* Table 7.1 on page 134), we can help to prevent atherosclerosis, hypertension, heart disease, stroke, and even sudden death. Let us look at what we can do to lower inflammatory mediators and minimize silent inflammation in the body.

TEN WAYS TO REDUCE INFLAMMATION

Inflammation can be kept in check using the following methods.

1. Detoxification

The chemical cocktail of stress, pesticides, industrial wastes, poor diet, heavy metals, chronic infections, and drugs greatly contribute to the silent inflamma-

TABLE 7.1. Sinatra Smart Zone for Optimum Health

The smart zone is what Dr. Sinatra considers a safe zone in terms of preventing cardiac problems, and below are the tests for it that you should include in your blood workups. Each test is followed by Dr. Sinatra's suggested optimum health ranges, which are consistent with better-than-normal lab results. The recommendations on the right are ways you can improve your scores if they're not in the healthy range. To use this table, make a note of any lab results that are outside the smart-zone levels in your tests, then choose treatment from the list of recommendations on the right.

Blood Tests	Sinatra-Smart Zone Levels	Recommendations to Maintain Optimum Health
Albumin	4.2–5.0 G/dL	If less than 4.2, immune-system support is needed; reduce allergies; promote personal hygiene.
CoQ$_{10}$	1.0–1.8 ug/ml	30–60 mg Q-Gel daily (see note below for therapeutic levels).
C-reactive protein	<.80 mg/dL	Statin drugs (10–20 mg Pravachol or 20–40 mg Zocor); exercise; baby aspirin; 2 grams omega-3 fish oils; 400 IU vitamin E daily.
Fasting blood sugar	<100 mg/dL	Weight loss; exercise; restrict carbohydrates, especially high-glycemic carbohydrates, such as sugars; use lower glycemic carbohydrates, such as broccoli, chick peas, or lentils, that lower insulin levels; 100–300 mg alpha-lipoic acid; 60–90 mg Q-Gel; 200 IU vitamin E.
Fasting insulin	<12 microunits/L	Same recommendations as fasting blood sugar.
Ferritin	Females: 40–80ng/mL Males: 20–50ng/mL	If greater than than 100 ng/mL, check for hemochromatosis (check iron and iron-binding capacity). If total iron, total iron-binding capacity, and ferritin are all elevated, assess for genetic hemochromatosis (excess iron). If positive for hemochromatosis, you may need to donate blood 1–3 times a year. Check drinking water for high iron content. Do not take more than 500 mg vitamin C a day.
Fibrinogen	180–350 mg/dL	If greater than 350, take 500–1,000 mg of garlic daily; 1–2 grams Norwegian fish oil; 500–1,000 mg bromelain once a day; 6–9 Wobenzyme* tablets daily in divided doses; drink ginger and/or green tea.
Folate	>10 ng/mL	800 mcg folic acid daily.
Hemoglobin A1C	<6% of total HGB	Reduce weight; exercise; 100–300 mg alpha-lipoic acid daily; consider metformin if lifestyle changes do not improve percentages.
HDL	Females: 40–120 mg/dL Males: 35–120 mg/dL	Assess for insulin resistance if HDL is low; reduce weight, exercise; use less high-glycemic carbohydrates; 500–1,000 mg niacin or 750–1,500 mg niaspan; 1,000 mg pantethine; 1000–1,500 mg guggulipid; 500–1,000 mg L-carnitine.
Homocysteine	<10 umol/L	800 mcg folic acid; 40 mg B$_6$; 200 mcg B$_{12}$; 250–1,000 mcg trimethylglycine; eat more beets and broccoli.
LDL	60–150 mg/dL	*See* Total cholesterol. If LDL is greater than 130 in presence of documented coronary artery disease, statin therapy is indicated (10–20 mg Pravachol or 20–40 mg Zocor daily).

Blood Tests	Sinatra-Smart Zone Levels	Recommendations to Maintain Optimum Health
LP(a)	<30 ng/dL	250 mg niacin 3–4 times a day (may cause flushing) or 750–1,500 mg niaspan daily (niaspan is a long-acting niacin for which a prescription is needed); 500–1,000 mg Vitamin C; 1–2 grams Norwegian fish oil; avoid all trans fatty acids; females: consider natural estrogen; males: avoid soy; and consider testosterone.
Total cholesterol	125–225 ml/dL	Lose weight; exercise; increase fiber; flax**; oatmeal; oats; soy products; 200 mcg chromium; 30–60 mg Q-Gel; 50–100 mg tocotrienol formula; 400–800 mg garlic, 500–1,500 mg plant sterols (phytosterols) daily; probiotics.
DHEA (female)	Age 30–39: 60–400 mcg/dL 40–49: 70–350 mcg/dL 50–59: 40–180 mcg/dL > 60: 20–150 mcg/dL	For men under age fifty, low levels of DHEA are definitely a risk factor for heart disease and may suggest vital exhuastion. Women with low DHEA levels are also at risk. Women can take 10–20 mg.
DHEA (male)	Age 31–50: 60–450 mcg/dL 51–60: 80–400 mcg/dL 61–83: 200–280 mcg/dL	Men can take 20–25 mg as a soluble wafer. Your doctor can use a compounding pharmacy to formulate.
Triglycerides	50–180 ml/dL	Weight reduction; exercise; restrict carbohydrates; at least 2 grams fish oil daily.

Optional tests for newer inflammatory markers:
  Interleukin-6
  Oxidized LDL
  Tissue necrosis
  Factor alpha
		If interleukin-6, tissue necrosis factor alpha, and oxidized LDL are elevated, a more complicated inflammatory process is indicated, especially if fibrinogen and CRP levels are significantly increased. If such is the case, then treatments to target inflammation reduction must be initiated. Recommended statin therapy in combination with 2 g Norwegian fish oil; 6–9 Wobenzyme tablets daily in divided doses on empty stomach. Also strongly recommendeded is an exercise program. Make sure your healthcare professional follows up with subsequent inflammatory assessments to track your progress.

		Unless otherwise specified, the above are recommended daily doses.

NOTE: These suggested therapeutic CoQ$_{10}$ levels are for the following medical conditions:

2.0–2.5 ug/mL	If you have high blood pressure, mitral valve prolapse (MVP), arrhythmia, diabetes, or periodontal disease.
2.5–3.5 ug/mL	If you have mild to moderate congestive heart failure, angina, or chronic fatigue syndrome.
>3.5 ug/mL	If you have severe congestive heart failure.

* Wobenzyme is a commercially prepared combination of enzymes that reduce inflammation; it is a favorite among Olympic athletes to reduce muscle soreness.

** 2 Tbsp crushed flaxseeds a day in a healthy shake with 8 oz. soy milk, or sprinkle them on cereals or salads.

Published in *The Sinatra Health Report,* May 2003

tion in our bodies as we age. As the toxic load increases, so does the incidence of chronic disease (*see* Figure 7.2 below).

We believe that regular detoxification should become part of a healthy lifestyle. Although you should always avoid obvious toxins whenever possible, it is extremely difficult to avoid many toxins that are present everywhere in the environment today. That is why each of us should incorporate certain daily detoxification strategies to help flush out the toxins that are circulating in the blood or are lodged in soft tissues and vital organs.

Remember, these strategies should include diets, such as the OmegaZone diet, bathing, infrared saunas, massages, and liver and colon cleansing on a regular basis. Also, a detoxifying nutraceutical formula can provide additional protection from the various toxins. A detox formula should include liver-supporting nutrients, such as artichokes, L-carnitine, and milk thistle. Alpha-lipoic acid and other sulphur-containing nutraceuticals will help chelate heavy metals, and indole-3-carbinol will help rid the body of xenoestrogens.

2. Diet and Weight Loss

Over 65 percent of the American population is now overweight. Researchers speculate that tobacco will soon be replaced by obesity as the major risk factor today. Recent research suggests that fat cells have become the home for inflammatory cytokines. In fact, accumulated fat around the waist acts just like an extra endocrine gland, probably one of the major reasons that obese people tend to get more cancer, type-2 diabetes, and heart disease, as well as other inflammatory disorders.

The obesity and diabetes epidemics are linked to metabolic syndrome (an

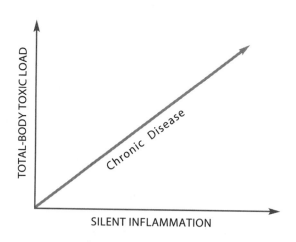

Figure 7.2. Silent Inflammation and Chronic Disease

altered metabolic rate due to chronically high insulin levels) with its deadly quartet of elevated blood pressure, elevated triglycerides and decreased HDL, high insulin levels, and weight gain (apple shape).

Metabolic syndrome also puts people at increased risk for cardiovascular problems. In fact, the most important finding in treating hypertension in the last decade has been an understanding of metabolic syndrome and its relationship to insulin resistance, a condition that can be reversed only through diet and exercise. Hippocrates, considered the father of medicine, knew best, ages ago, when he proclaimed, "Let food be your medicine."

For a diet to become a lifestyle, it must be convenient and not too complex. Most people become overwhelmed trying to decide what they should and should not eat based on the latest medical news. Designing a Zone meal is simple and involves dividing a plate into three sections. First, fill one-third of it with a protein (a typical portion fits in the palm of your hand), and fill up the other two-thirds of the plate with low-glycemic vegetables (broccoli, cauliflower, dark leafy greens, and others that won't raise your blood sugar rapidly), and fruit. Finally, eat a heart-healthy fat, as found in almonds or avocados, or add a dash of olive oil to your salad or greens. This is the way we have been genetically designed to eat.

Dr. Sinatra prefers a Pan-Asian Modified Mediterranean (PAMM) way of eating, using the Zone principles, because cultural societies following traditional Asian and Mediterranean diets have the lowest rates of cancer and heart disease in the world. For more information, please visit these websites: www.zonecafe.com and www.drsinatra.com.

3. Nutraceuticals

Nutraceuticals are components of foods or dietary supplements that support healing. They include antioxidants, coenzyme Q_{10}, enzymes, fish oils, garlic, green tea, L-carnitine, minerals, and vitamins. At the microscopic level, many of these nutraceuticals can penetrate into the cells and help eradicate free-radical damage, while decreasing inflammation at the same time.

Carotenoid and flavonoid nutraceuticals can have a positive impact on the body. For example, antioxidant flavonoids, especially quercetin, were studied in the European Zutphen Elderly Study. As reported in the *Lancet*, researchers looked at mortality in older men and found that a higher death rate was associated with a lower flavonoid intake. The flavonoids consumed by the male subjects came primarily from black tea, green apples, and onions. Their results confirmed that all-cause mortality was reduced in those men consuming greater than 30 milligrams of flavonoids per day.

The cardiovascular benefits of similar oligomeric proanthocyanidins (OPCs, which add the bright colors to many fruits and vegetables, belong in the flavonoid class of nutrients) have also been noteworthy. OPCs inhibit free radicals, the oxidation of LDL, and sticky blood platelets (platelet aggregation). They improve the elasticity and integrity of blood vessels, and have a role in lowering blood pressure. In animal research, OPCs have also demonstrated a cholesterol lowering effect.

The French Paradox is a term that describes the discrepancy between the traditional high-fat French diet and their comparatively low incidence of heart disease. It has been suggested that their consumption of red wine is what offsets their high-fat diet. Researchers postulate that red wine has high concentrations of OPCs quercetin and resveratrol, as well as other flavonoids, and it is these grape skins that are responsible for this victory over heart disease.

Magnesium

Magnesium is a mineral with favorable cardiovascular benefits. It acts like a calcium channel blocker to prevent spasms in the walls of blood vessels. Magnesium has a profoundly positive influence on blood vessels and makes blood platelets less sticky. In fact, a magnesium deficiency has been observed in those with insulin resistance and diabetes. Taking 400–800 milligrams of magnesium is recommended for anyone with Raynaud's disease or for anyone who wants to block coronary artery spasms or lower blood pressure.

In one study, magnesium decreased many symptoms associated with mitral valve prolapse, including anxiety, chest pain, palpitations, shortness of breath, and weakness. (Coenzyme Q_{10} also has known cardiac benefits and was instrumental in helping to improve the quality of life for the people in this study.)

Coenzyme Q_{10}

Coenzyme Q_{10} has a crucial role in cellular energy production and is critical in the proper functioning of the mitochondria, which it contributes to by recycling ATP (adenosine triphosphate) as well as being a cofactor in its production. People with cardiomyopathy, hypertensive cardiovascular disease, mitral valve prolapse, and especially those with statin-induced diastolic dysfunction have shown improvement when they took coenzyme Q_{10}.

Coenzyme Q_{10} can also help treat angina, arrhythmias, congestive heart failure, and toxin-induced cardiotoxicity. And pretreatment with coenzyme Q_{10} for weeks before an elective coronary artery bypass graft (CABG) has been shown to help with speedier postoperative recuperation.

Since its discovery in 1972, there have been multiple controlled trials on the use of coenzyme Q_{10}, with more than forty showing some benefit and only four showing none. One yearlong, double-blind study of 641 recipients showed a 20 percent reduction in hospitalizations for the coenzyme Q_{10} group compared to those taking the placebo, and the coenzyme Q_{10} group had a better quality of life, as well as lower medical bills.

Another topic of special emphasis in relation to coenzyme Q_{10} is statins. The number of these drugs prescribed every year is astounding and may have a link to the increased number of cases of cardiomyopathies. Statin drugs can cause profound deficiencies in coenzyme Q_{10} so it should be supplemented by anyone receiving a statin drug, such as 3-hydroxy-3 methylglutaryl coenzyme A-reductase inhibitors. Coenzyme Q_{10} treatment has been helpful in counteracting diffuse muscular pain, a noted side effect of statin therapy.

The body's own production of coenzyme Q_{10} drops off with aging, and while its side effects—abdominal discomfort, excess energy or anxiety, and nausea—are rare, it is contraindicated for healthy pregnant or lactating women because the unborn and newborn produce sufficient quantities of the compound on their own.

Metabolic Cardiology

Metabolic cardiology is going to be one of the next great emerging subspecialties in cardiology, arising from a new emphasis on the relationship between ATP and energy in the heart. Coenzyme Q_{10}, L-carnitine, and D-ribose will be the most significant players. By supporting cellular function, such as ATP production, coenzyme Q_{10} and other similar agents defend heart cells from the ravages of aging, toxins, and the myriad other conditions that wear down mitochondrial function and cause cardiovascular disease.

The synergism of coenzyme Q_{10} and L-carnitine, for example, has been known for approximately fifteen years in such conditions as ischemia, reperfusion injury of the heart, fatty infiltration of the liver induced by alcohol, and hyperbaric oxygen toxicity in experimental animals. In acute or chronic ischemia, coenzyme Q_{10} and L-carnitine offer significant clinical advantages with absolutely no risk to the patient. These nutrients support cardiovascular function and preserve the inner mitochondrial membrane. They may even support vulnerable cells, particularly older heart cells, and prolong life.

Recently, another new emerging compound has been gaining increasing support among metabolic cardiologists. D-ribose is a biochemical, five-sided sugar that has been extensively investigated. Investigators believe that under certain cardiac conditions, when the heart is deprived of oxygen, there is a profound depression of energy compounds, such as ATP. A drop in ATP means a subsequent decrease in myocardial function, causing the heart to struggle as a pump. Researchers are now learning that D-ribose plummets during ischemic episodes, such as angina and myocardial infarction, and that it takes considerable time to recover and regenerate ATP compounds. Supplementing with D-ribose helps to replenish the severely depleted ATP levels.

Taking D-ribose (15 grams daily) can protect cardiac cells from ischemic episodes and, for anyone with angina, it can increase the amount of time you can exercise before the onset of angina symptoms. The combined antioxidant, membrane-stabilizing, and metabolic activities of coenzyme Q_{10}, L-carnitine, and D-ribose will play a significant role in myocardial ischemia.

As new research unfolds, these nutraceuticals provide an exciting platform in cardiovascular disease to improve the quality of life for people with heart problems. Metabolic cardiologists will upgrade the level of care for their patients as they gain further insight into this new great emerging field in cardiovascular medicine.

4. Enzymes

Within a single cell there are roughly 100,000 genes, the majority of which have enzymes, the workhorses of the living cell, in them. All enzymes are proteins, and all are composed of long chains of amino acids. Also recognized as the life force of the body, enzymes are involved in nearly every one of its metabolic processes. As we age, or develop a disease, our bodies have fewer and fewer enzyme stores at their disposal (a sixty-year-old has 50 percent fewer enzymes than a thirty-year-old, for example).

Enzymes function as catalysts and make things work faster. They have the ability to initiate, accelerate, and terminate biochemical reactions in the body. Enzymes increase the activity of the cells that are important to a healthy immune system, and they are integral in maintaining balance in the body. Provided there are sufficient enzymes, cases of acute inflammation can heal in a few days. With chronic silent inflammation, however, the continued shortage of enzymes leads to an eventual breakdown of the reactions needed to remove diseased tissue from the body and return it to normal health. Enzymes are important biological response modifiers and play a vital role in controlling inflammation and promoting health.

Cancer and Enzyme Therapy

It is well known that people with cancer also have excess blood coagulation or toxic blood. Wobenzym therapy, used exclusively by Olympic athletes over the years to reduce inflammation in tendons, muscles, and joints, will often help normalize the blood of cancer patients, in addition to improving blood flow and preventing fibrosis (the formation of abnormal tissue).

Rheumatoid Arthritis and Enzyme Therapy

One in seven Americans has some form of arthritis, and most forms involve inflammation. One of the more common and disabling types is rheumatoid arthritis, considered an autoimmune disease, where the body attacks itself. Many people have benefited by taking up to twenty enzyme tablets a day.

Multiple Sclerosis and Enzyme Therapy

Multiple sclerosis (MS), an inflammatory disease of the central nervous system, is another prototypical autoimmune disorder that conventional medical practitioners have had little success in treating. A number of causes of demyelination (degradation of the fatlike myelin coverings of nerves) have been suggested, including chronic viral infections, Lyme disease, mercury toxicity, selenium deficiency, and an imbalance of saturated and unsaturated fatty acids in the diet. In Salzburg, Austria, Dr. C. Neuhofer has been able to limit the progress of her own MS, as well as the many patients she has treated, using enzyme therapy.

In addition to Wobenzym, newer enzyme preparations, such as Nattokinase, have been gaining popularity for reducing inflammatory mediators, such as C-reactive protein and Lp(a). In the future, enzymes such as Nattokinase and Wobenzym, as well as fish oil, will be utilized in reducing the total inflammatory load in the body.

5. Omega-3 Fatty Acids

Leading medical institutions worldwide have confirmed that daily supplementation with high-grade fish oil, rich in omega-3 essential fatty acids, is your most powerful weapon for controlling inflammation.

There is overwhelming evidence in the cardiovascular literature that omega-3 essential fatty acids are appropriate in the treatment and prevention of cardiovascular disease, and the *Lancet* recently published another, very important, study of 11,000 Italian participants with myocardial infarction. Over a three-year period, the group given fish oil had a 45 percent lower incidence of sudden cardiac death and a 20 percent reduction in all causes of death. Those receiving fish oil also had reduced blood pressure, suppressed platelet activity, lowered triglyceride levels, and a marked lessening of cardiac arrhythmias. Perhaps the most noteworthy benefit of fish oil is its favorable impact on heart rate variability (HRV). Omega-3 essential fatty acids also reduce plaque rupture by literally getting inside plaque to stabilize it and render it less vulnerable to rupture. Eating healthy fish or taking fish-oil supplements is an absolute must, especially for those most at risk for cardiovascular disease. In fact, just two fish meals per month will reduce an individual's risk of sudden cardiac death by 50 percent.

Unfortunately, because most fish have become contaminated with toxins, such as dioxins, mercury, and PCBs, consuming fatty coldwater fish as your primary source of omega-3s is now being questioned. There is, however, a solution to this dilemma—the OmegaRx brand of fish oils formulated by Dr. Barry Sears's lab. These pharmaceutical-grade fish oils have been concentrated and purified to the highest standards possible. They are toxin-free and can be ingested without any fear of toxins or contaminants found in the fish we eat, or in the standard omega-3 supplements. For these reasons, we can heartily recommend them. OmegaRx fish oil supplements are available through the website www.zonecafe.com.

The certification process for OmegaRx measures the levels of contaminants in parts per billion. OmegaRx is found to be at least 100 times purer than the typical health-food-grade fish oils. It sets the standard for fish-oil purity and goes beyond the same quality control standards established for the oils that were used in recent clinical trials.

If you make no other changes in your diet to enhance insulin control and reduce inflammatory mediators, consider supplementing with OmegaRx to help maintain brain, cardiovascular, and immune function. Dr. Sears's recommended daily maintenance dosage is four OmegaRx capsules or 1 teaspoon of OmegaRx liquid. The half-life of fish oil is two days so you only need to take it once a day.

6. Control of Chronic Infections without Antibiotics

Current research from the National Institutes of Health (NIH) and elsewhere shows that while chronic infections are really never eradicated, they can be controlled as long as a person remains on an antimicrobial program. The disadvantages of living on antibiotics, however, do not make this an attractive or plausible way to live.

Research has shown that some people who have taken tetracycline for acne for years have less atherosclerosis. This makes sense when we recognize that many people have chronic infections, such as CMV and nanobacteria, that contribute to the silent inflammation and the elevated CRP levels we see. It is our opinion that if we boost the body's natural immunity with select nutraceuticals, and we practice good oral hygiene, we can thwart many of these chronic infections. And, unlike antibiotics, these formulas can be taken for an entire lifetime without any substantial risk.

We have already discussed how infections cause Lyme disease, and how useful Wobenzym and other enzymes are in the treatment of these chronic infections. After studies done in Florida at Hemex Laboratories (www.hemex.com), researchers are now convinced that the presence of any form of infection is associated with inflammation and severely toxic blood. Therefore, to help get adequate blood flow to the infected tissues to completely eradicate these stubborn infections, we believe it is essential to take targeted nutraceuticals.

Garlic is also important because most infections cannot grow well in its presence. Malic acid helps bind iron so that many harmful organisms requiring iron for their reproductive cycle are kept from replicating. We have found that TOA-free cat's claw (Samento) is very helpful for Lyme disease. Samento (*Uncaria tomentosa*) is extremely potent and able to significantly strengthen the immune system. It also has powerful anti-inflammatory, antioxidant, and antitumor properties. Research shows that Samento eliminates dependence on steroids and inhalers, reduces hepatitis-C and HIV levels, drops CRP levels, and lowers some tumor markers, such as PSA. For more information, contact Nutramedix at 800-730-3130 or visit their websites: www.nutramedix.com or www.samento.com.ec.

Other nutraceuticals, such as elements of colostrum, grapefruit seed extract, rice bran, rhodiola rosea (found in northern Alpine regions), and many different mushrooms, including shiitake and reishi, also have powerful effects in fighting chronic infections and inflammation.

7. Pharmacology

While many physicians are unaware of the important role of eicosanoids, the pharmaceutical industry is very cognizant of these powerful hormones because many of the more popular drugs used today alter eicosanoid levels. Most of these drugs inhibit the enzymes that synthesize eicosanoids and have little effect on the balance of good and bad eicosanoids.

As an example, the cyclooxygenase enzymes (Cox-1 and Cox-2) are responsible for the synthesis of prostaglandins and thromboxanes, but they can be blocked by aspirin, Cox-2 inhibitors, and nonsteroidal anti-inflammatory drugs (NSAIDs). Furthermore, corticosteroids inhibit all types of eicosanoid synthesis. Although blocking the synthesis of bad eicosanoids may reduce inflammation, the anti-inflammatory and other beneficial properties of good eicosanoids are obstructed in the process, and the undesirable side effects of corticosteroids make their long-term use inadvisable.

Recent research indicates that the cardiovascular benefits of statin drugs (originally used to decrease cholesterol levels) may be primarily due to their anti-inflammatory actions that reduce C-reactive protein levels. (As mentioned earlier, C-reactive protein is associated with generalized inflammation and is considered a significant biomarker for the development of heart disease.) New research suggests that although statin therapy may be helpful in reducing inflammation, it also increases insulin levels and insulin resistance, which could pose a future risk for diabetes, heart disease, and obesity.

Our position on statins was summarized in a recent editorial in *The Southern Medical Journal*. Although there is little doubt that statin therapy can significantly reduce the incidence of coronary problems, especially for those who are at the greatest risk of developing coronary artery disease, overutilization of statins in anyone who does not have overt coronary artery disease or silent inflammation should be avoided.

Electron beam computerized tomography (EBCT) has demonstrated an association between high coronary calcium burden (indicated by a score greater than 1,000) and cardiac events, which suggests that statin therapy may prove beneficial for high-risk coronary people and for those with diabetes, high cholesterol, and high inflammation. It is not, however, considered smart medicine for otherwise healthy people to overuse these potent drugs, with their known and unknown side effects. We also do not know the long-term effect of statin therapy, especially since there are no studies for anyone taking statins longer than ten years. Cancer and heart problems that are associated with the statin drugs may cause us to rethink our posturing on statin therapies in the future. For now, we implore physicians to selectively use statin therapy to address the health needs of each patient and to avoid prescribing them simply to treat high cholesterol numbers alone.

8. Exercise and Stress Management

There is no doubt that exercise should be an indispensable part of any person's total health program, not only because of its many benefits, but also because of the sense of well-being that exercise provides.

The benefits are mostly a consequence of the hormonal and weight-loss changes that various types of exercise induce. The real key is that the more intense the exercise, the more the hormonal responses are affected. Moderate-to-higher–intensity aerobic exercises reduce insulin (and therefore inflammation), and increase glucagon levels—exactly as a Zone-favorable diet does. However, high-intensity exercises, such as boxing, marathon running, wrestling, and other professional and Olympic sports, can cause enormous oxidative stress and subsequent antioxidant insufficiency. The most common antioxidants that are depleted with regular intense exercise include coenzyme Q_{10}, magnesium, and vitamin E. In premenopausal female athletes, severe iron deficiencies may also be noted.

High-intensity exercise can enhance the oxidation of LDL, and emotional stress can cause inflammation just as easily as oxidized LDL. The medical community now recognizes that a supercharged sympathetic nervous system (SNS) can set you up for cardiac events and sudden death. Heart rate variability, an assessment of sympathetic and parasympathetic nervous system balance or imbalance, can now be performed in an office setting. Anger, hostility, and the inability to express feelings are also serious cardiovascular risk factors. In addition to exercise, various mind-body approaches listed in this book can be very effective in altering SNS response and inflammation.

9. Chelation

Chelation therapy has already helped more than a million people improve, and current research suggests this might be due to the way it helps the endothelium, the layer of cells lining our blood vessels, by increasing the production of nitric oxide, an essential substance of great importance that transports oxygen to the tissues of our bodies. (Over 90,000 scientific papers have been published on the role of nitric oxide in the body.) The epithelium functions much more efficiently when chelation lowers the levels of heavy metals and inflammation.

Chelating agents may be administered orally or intravenously and will remove lead and toxic metals from your body in a safe, economic way. Dr. Gary Gordon of Prescott, Arizona, provides over 500 published extracts that demonstrate the powerful detoxification results achieved through chelation with oral EDTA. There is good evidence that the antioxidant and anticoagulant benefits of this therapy may also enhance longevity.

The chelation of heavy metals in the body also reduces iron. Since iron is an important source of food for various microbes, limiting its supply will limit microbe survival and ultimately decrease inflammation.

10. Bio-identical Hormone Replacement

As we age, all our hormones decrease. By the time most of us reach our fifties, our hormone levels are about half what they were in our thirties. The goal of bio-identical hormone replacement therapy (HRT) is to restore our hormones to the levels of a young thirty-five-year-old. Optimum hormone levels are essential for minimizing the development of diseases caused by inflammation. (*See* Chapter 9 on bio-identical hormone therapy.)

SUMMARY

Everywhere we turn we are facing evidence that inflammation plays a larger role in chronic disease than we physicians ever thought. To some degree, silent inflammation is insidiously eroding all of our vital organs, including our brain. Although this chapter focused primarily on inflammation in the heart, it could just as well have focused on inflammation in the brain, the skin, or any other vital organ. The various causes of inflammation and treatments to reduce inflammation in these organs are similar to those of the heart.

In treating inflammation, we urge physicians to keep an open mind while using conventional treatment and to investigate alternatives that can improve the quality of life for their patients. Choosing from the best conventional and complementary options is the only logical and ethical thing to do to help douse the inflammatory inferno in our hearts and other vital organs.

Chapter 8

Secret Two —
Nutraceuticals

Nutraceuticals can be broadly defined as components of foods or dietary supplements that have a medicinal or therapeutic effect. In general, nutraceuticals are taken in amounts higher than what can be obtained from a regular diet.

—Arthur Roberts, M.D.

Our bodies require oxygen for metabolism. Without oxygen we cannot produce energy, but a downside of this energy production is its generation of free radicals and inflammation, so one of the main keys to achieving good health is to maintain the right balance of free radicals and antioxidants.

Nutraceuticals are components of foods or dietary supplements that support healing. They include antioxidants, amino acids, enzymes, fish oils, herbs, minerals, and vitamins. Many of these nutrients and antioxidants can penetrate into cells and prevent free-radical damage while simultaneously decreasing inflammation in the body.

TEN PRINCIPLES OF CELLULAR HEALTH AND NUTRACEUTICALS

The following principles are modified from Dr. Matthias Rath's original ideas detailed in *The Heart*.

1. Health and disease are determined by the vitality of the 60 trillion cells that make up our bodies and the various organs comprising them.

2. Nearly all diseases develop within organs at the cellular level. Inflammation is a major cause of most chronic disease.

3. Essential nutrients are needed for the thousands of biochemical reactions in each cell and to minimize the effects of inflammation.

4. The primary cause of cellular malfunction is a deficiency of vitamins, minerals, hormones, and other nutrients required for cell fuel.

5. Stress and aging (both mental and physical) will change the demand for nutrients required by the various cells of organs.

6. Nutrients are also required in different amounts, as determined by an individual's genetic predisposition.

7. Cardiovascular and neurological complications are the most prevalent of all ailments because those cells consume vitamins and other essential nutrients at a higher rate than the cells of other organs.

8. Medi-spas, which integrate the best of both conventional and alternative treatments while focusing on the individuality of each client, are the ideal sites to optimize cellular health.

9. Dietary supplementation with enzymes, hormones, vitamins, and other nutrients is a key process in the prevention and treatment of cardiovascular conditions and other chronic diseases associated with aging.

10. Core nutraceuticals, containing antioxidants, enzymes, minerals, omega-3 fatty acids, and vitamins, should be consumed daily by all individuals. In addition, target nutraceuticals aimed at specific problems should also be taken to help support cell function while correcting cell malfunction in any diseased organs.

THE EMERGENCE OF NUTRACEUTICALS

In the United States, the profit motive often dictates the direction of scientific research. Unlike drugs, nutraceuticals are most often derived from natural products that in most instances cannot be patented. This greatly reduces the financial incentive for a drug company to proceed with years of research and marketing. Most nutraceutical research today is carried out abroad, led by Germany, where about 70 percent of physicians prescribe from about 600 different botanical medicines. Today drugs are a multibillion dollar industry; however, the pendulum is beginning to swing the other way.

The rediscovery of botanical medicine and the emergence of nutraceuticals are helping to redefine health care in the United States and other countries. More and more consumers have noticed their benefits are largely free of the side effects associated with many types of drugs.

Over the past twenty-five years, in our own practices in cardiology, internal medicine, and plastic surgery, we have seen countless patients benefit from taking nutraceuticals. For a majority of nonacute health conditions, we prescribe nutraceuticals and lifestyle changes as first-line therapies, looking to drugs only if these approaches are not effective.

We would like to introduce you first to new research on antioxidants and then cite the brain as a specific example of how targeted nutraceuticals can improve your health and longevity.

I. ANTIOXIDANTS LEAD THE WAY TO A NEW UNDERSTANDING

We now stand at the threshold of a new understanding of how antioxidants can affect the quality and length of human life, thanks largely to such people as Professor Lester Packer, Ph.D., author of *The Antioxidant Miracle*. He and others have made startling new discoveries on how antioxidants can prevent and treat many chronic and degenerative diseases, including arthritis, cancer, cataracts, and heart disease.

Dr. Packer's conclusions concerning the antioxidant effects that increase longevity include:

- Improving concentration and reversing age-related memory loss;
- Protecting against prostate and other cancers;
- Rejuvenating an aging immune system;
- Relieving arthritis and other inflammatory conditions;
- Reversing age spots and protecting against skin cancer;
- Supporting cardiovascular function;
- Turning off *bad* genes.

Antioxidant supplements are readily available, and you are probably taking them, but you may not be taking them correctly. Recently, scientists discovered a dynamic interplay among certain key antioxidants, a relationship Dr. Packer calls *the antioxidant network* because they work in concert to greatly enhance one another's power. What makes network antioxidants special is that they can extend their antioxidant power by recycling or regenerating one another after they have quenched dangerous free radicals. As Dr. Packer states, "The primary job of the antioxidant network is to prevent antioxidants from being lost through oxidation. As one network antioxidant saves the other, the cycle continues, ensuring the body will maintain the right antioxidant balance."

Although there are hundreds of antioxidants, Dr. Packer has identified these five as foundation network antioxidants:

1. Alpha-lipoic acid
2. Coenzyme Q_{10}
3. Glutathione
4. Vitamin C
5. Vitamin E

It is interesting to note that all these foundation antioxidants support the inner mitrochondrial membrane. Whenever we protect the mitochondria (the cell's engine), we stabilize the integrity of the cell and probably extend its life. Dr. Sinatra feels that one of the major causes of congestive heart failure in older people is mitochondrial dysfunction of heart cells leading to impaired contraction in the heart. As an antidote to this, he has been recommending coenzyme Q_{10} to his patients for more than twenty years.

Oxidation—A Paradox of Life and Death

As stated previously, the body requires oxygen for metabolism, to produce energy and sustain life. Unfortunately, free radicals, those molecular snipers that roam the body in search of electrons that will neutralize their charge, are byproducts of oxidative processes and cause cellular damage. An essential means of cultivating good health involves balancing antioxidants and free radicals, and this is what your body's antioxidant defense system does.

Dr. Bruce Ames, a well-known antioxidant scientist, estimates that each human cell gets about 10,000 oxidative *hits* daily to its DNA. If you multiply this by the trillions of cells in the body, you can see how it can add up to a big problem. Free radicals not quickly reined in can cause a great deal of trouble and this is why supplements with antioxidants are indispensable for longevity. When your antioxidant defenses are overwhelmed by a firestorm of free radicals, the condition known as oxidative stress exists. In order to sustain optimum health, you must have enough antioxidants available to handle the free-radical oxidative stress that occurs to a greater or lesser degree every second of your life.

To better understand the process of oxidation, think about the leftovers you wrap up after a meal. One of the reasons wrapping helps is that it keeps oxygen from attacking the leftovers. Although food chemists had long recognized that certain vitamins were good food preservatives and began to call them antioxidants, it did not initially occur to anyone that the same process occurring to the leftover food was occurring in our own bodies.

As we age, the levels of antioxidants fall and the network antioxidants (*see* Table 8.1 on page 151) become overwhelmed by the gradually increasing toxic load on the body. Interestingly, humans and elephants have the highest concentration of antioxidants and the longest life spans, while rats and other rodents have the lowest levels and the shortest life spans.

The Antioxidant Network

The following is a summary of the beneficial effects of the five network antioxidants from *The Antioxidant Miracle,* by Dr. Packer, modified with our comments and suggestions.

TABLE 8.1. Network Antioxidants

FAT-SOLUBLE ANTIOXIDANTS *(Protect fatty part of cell membranes)*	WATER-SOLUBLE ANTIOXIDANTS *(Protect watery part of cell membranes)*
Vitamin E	Vitamin C
Coenzyme Q_{10}	Glutathione
Alpha-lipoic acid*	Alpha-lipoic acid*

*Alpha-lipoic acid is unique and can function in both zones, regenerating fat- and water-soluble antioxidants.

Source: The Antioxidant Miracle

1. Alpha-Lipoic Acid

- Protects against three common age-associated diseases: cataracts, heart disease, and strokes.
- Strengthens memory and prevents brain aging.
- Helps to reduce blood sugar.
- Boosts the entire antioxidant network by helping to recycle oxidized vitamins C and E and coenzyme Q_{10}.
- Can prevent and relieve the complications of diabetes.
- Turns off *bad* genes that accelerate aging, cancer, and polyneuropathy (inflammation of all the nerves of the body).
- Can reverse mushroom poisoning of the liver.
- Has been useful in treating liver disease, such as hepatitis C.
- Reduces advanced glycolation end products (AGES) and helps skin.
- Strengthens the immune system.
- Prevents replication of HIV in cultured human cells.
- Protects against radiation poisoning.

A Note for Smokers

Smoking probably shortens your life by about eight years. Obviously, the best advice is to quit. It might be possible to reduce the diseases associated with cigarette smoke by bolstering network antioxidants, especially lipoic acid. Gamma tocopherol (vitamin E) also appears to be protective for smokers, and since smoking causes a drastic reduction in vitamin C, it should be supplemented as well. We don't, however, recommend beta-carotene in doses greater than 10,000 units for smokers, as high doses of it may enhance lung cancer in them.

RDA: Not established

Recommended amount: 50–100 milligrams

Sources: Synthesized by body but levels fall off with age. Present in small amounts in animal products, especially red meat.

2. Vitamin E

- Reverses the age-related slump in immune function.
- Protects your brain from aging.
- Protects your lungs from automobile emissions.
- Reduces risk of gastrointestinal cancer in both men and women.
- Reduces your risk of strokes and heart disease.
- Protects your skin from UV rays and ozone.
- Relieves arthritis and other inflammatory diseases.
- Reduces risk of prostate cancer in men.
- Reduces risk of breast cancer in women.
- Helps save your vision by preventing cataracts.

RDA: 30 IU daily

Recommended amount: 100–200 IU mixed tocopherols and tocotrienols

Sources: Barley, extra virgin olive oil, leafy vegetables, nuts, rice bran oil, wheat germ.

A Note for Living Better Longer

In studies on human cells, scientists have evidence that vitamin E can prevent aging at the cellular level, where aging begins. Long before we see the more visible signs of gray hair and wrinkles, subtle changes are occurring in our cells. One of the telltale signs of aging is the accumulation of the pigment lipofuscin, especially in the brain and heart. Vitamin E has been shown to prevent cells from accumulating this aging substance in cultured human cells.

3. Vitamin C

- Protects you from heart disease.
- Reduces risk of cancer.
- Protects sperm from free-radical damage.
- Regenerates used-up vitamin E.

- Boosts the immune system.
- Reduces the length and severity of colds.
- Keeps skin young and supple, particularly the fat-soluble form of ascorbyl palmitate.
- Vitamins C and E prevent the oxidation of harmful LDL lipoproteins.
- Protects against cataracts.

RDA: 60 milligrams (100 milligrams for smokers)

Recommended amount: 200–400 milligrams

Sources: Abundant in many fruits and vegetables, including broccoli, cabbage, citrus fruit, cranberries, potatoes, red peppers, and tomatoes.

An Evolutionary Note

Humans (as well as bats and guinea pigs) are one of the few animals that don't produce vitamin C. Some scientists believe that the loss of the necessary enzyme about 45,000 years ago was an evolutionary error. The average foraging gorilla will consume about 5,000 milligrams of vitamin C per day. If a rat were a 170-pound man, it would make about 5,000 milligrams per day, an amount that some believe is closer to an optimal dose for humans. The stress of today's living requires taking more than the woefully inadequate RDA of vitamin C. Smokers, older people, anyone with diabetes, and women on oral contraceptives, all require at least 200 milligrams of vitamin C per day.

4. Coenzyme Q_{10}

- Regenerates vitamin E in the antioxidant network.
- Can prevent and help reverse some heart diseases.
- Can help manage type-2 diabetes.
- Can help improve Parkinson's disease.
- May help prevent Alzheimer's disease.
- May help treat breast cancer.
- Can help treat gum disease.
- Can reduce fatigue.
- Can improve male fertility.

RDA: Not established

Recommended amount: 30–100 milligrams (150–250 milligrams if taking a statin drug)

Sources: Synthesized by the body; also found in seafood and organ meats.

An Historical Note

Coenzyme Q_{10} was discovered by Professor Fred Crane at the University of Wisconsin in 1957. Renowned scientist Karl Folkers, who was the first researcher to identify the structures of vitamin B_6 and B_{12}, isolated coenzyme Q_{10} from beef hearts in 1958 while working at Merck, Sharpe and Dohme. Although recognizing its importance, Merck sold the technology to the Japanese in 1965. Dr. Folkers continued his research at the University of Texas and was the first to suggest that the age-related decline in coenzyme Q_{10} was a contributing factor in many age-related diseases, including heart disease, cancer, and Alzheimer's disease. He reasoned that since high-energy bonds are so important to the function of virtually every cell in the body, it is impossible for any body system to run well if it is not getting adequate fuel. Since coenzyme Q_{10} helps support the formation of adenosine triphosphate (ATP)—the essence of the body's energy—coenzyme Q_{10} will help rescue almost any tissue in need. Cardiologists such as Stephen Sinatra, M.D., have used coenzyme Q_{10} in thousands of patients for more than twenty years, with great success.

The L-Carnitine Connection to Coenzyme Q_{10}

A vital sidekick to coenzyme Q_{10} is L-carnitine, an amino acid found primarily in meat, most often lamb. Because it has a special relationship with coenzyme Q_{10}, we highly recommend this multitalented nutraceutical in doses of 75–150 milligrams per day. Together, coenzyme Q_{10} and L-carnitine act synergistically to burn fats inside the mitochondria, the furnaces of the cells, and this helps the body's energy network function at a highly favorable level, especially in the heart, which derives more than 60 percent of its energy from burning fat.

5. Glutathione

- Important for longevity.
- Recycles vitamin C.
- Can be boosted by lipoic acid.
- Detoxifies drugs and toxins.

- Important for healthy liver function.

- Boosts immunity.

- Helps store and transport amino acids.

- Can help turn off the inflammatory response.

- Forms glutathione peroxidase, the body's most important defense against arteriosclerosis.

- Can be synthesized from the metabolism of N-acetylcysteine (NAC), which is the breakdown product of glutathione. (Oral forms of glutathione are not well absorbed.)

RDA: Not established

Recommended amount: 50 milligrams alpha-lipoic acid daily (as above) and 50 milligrams NAC.

Sources: Abundant in fruits, vegetables, especially avocados, and freshly cooked meats.

A Note on the Master Antioxidant

Glutathione is the cell's primary antioxidant and is found in the watery portion of the cell. Glutathione is produced in the cells from three amino acids—cysteine, glutamic acid, and glycine. Glutathione is the only network antioxidant most experts do *not* recommend supplementing with, due to the fact that it is broken down and no one knows how much glutathione actually passes through the intestinal wall into the cells. Alpha-lipoic acid and NAC will boost glutathione levels in target tissues where it is needed. The B vitamins and such minerals as calcium, magnesium, and selenium also boost antioxidant levels when consumed daily. Adding antioxidants to your wellness and longevity program can help you "To die as young as possible as old as possible," as the Greeks used to say.

The easiest way to take nutraceuticals is in packet form. As part of the Zone Foundation Program, we recommend a multivitamin/mineral combination with added enzymes, omega-3 fatty acids, and an antioxidant cocktail (*see* Table 8.2 on page 156). Although an extra evening dose is a suggested way to take supplements, we understand that people often dislike taking multiple numbers of tablets and capsules. They also want to avoid the extra cost, so a minimum of one packet a day to start is strongly recommended. You can order the Zone Foundation Program at www.zonecafe.com.

TABLE 8.2. Basic Antioxidant Cocktail			
Mixed carotenoids	5,000 IU	Vitamin B_{12}	300 mcg
Vitamin E	200 IU mixed tocopherols and tocotrienols	Vitamin B_6	2 mg
		L-carnitine	75 mg
Coenzyme Q_{10}	30 mg	Magnesium	200 mg
Alpha-lipoic acid	50 mg	Calcium	500 mg
Vitamin C	200 mg	Selenium	100 mcg
Folic acid	800 mcg	Zinc	15 mg

II. BRAIN HEALTH

Many express surprise when they meet someone in their seventies, eighties, or beyond, who is sharp as a tack. While the brain is especially susceptible to the damaging effects of free-radical stress, it is also one of the body's most plastic structures—that is, it is able to respond to targeted nutritional supplements as well as mental stimulation for a lifetime. When it comes to your brain, it's a clear case of use it or lose it. In this section, we'll briefly touch upon the most important nutraceuticals for optimal brain health.

Together with heart disease, memory loss is one of the biggest concerns of our aging population. The most beneficial aspects of aging are wisdom and experience, but the downside of aging is that things we used to take for granted now seem to be changing in a manner that often makes us feel old. Sometimes mental acuity, brain processing, and short-term recall of faces, information, names, numbers, and words are not as quick as they used to be, and some of us accept this age-related memory and cognitive decline as inevitable and natural. This is not necessarily so, and it certainly is not necessarily an early symptom of dementia or Alzheimer's disease. It may be due to age-related factors, but it can also be caused by depression, various medications, or such medical conditions as a low thyroid, a deficiency of vitamin B_{12}, or elevated homocysteine levels.

The first thing to do, even if you have not noticed any symptoms of brain-drain, is check your brain-processing functions to determine what your current level of brain capacity is. You can do this online with an easy, simple brain test called BrainCHECK (www.brain.com).

Our brains are unlike any of our other organs because each tiny region has a very specialized function that is not duplicated anywhere else. That means, if we sustain an injury to a very small area of our brain, we can end up with damage that can severely compromise our ability to function. Even with all our high-tech super computers, the brain is still the most efficient and complicated computer of all. It has yet to be duplicated and it can't be transplanted. Therefore, we must do everything possible to prevent it from becoming damaged.

In order to do that, we must first have a basic understanding of how the brain and nerve cells function. An individual brain cell, or nerve cell, is called a neuron. It has a body in it that receives information from other neurons and, in turn, produces a response that is sent out to other nerve cells or muscles to trigger a body function, such as a thought, movement, vision, smell, taste, tears, and perspiration. Neurons receive information through thousands of little biochemical processes, with the roots (dendrites) attached to the cell body. Information is sent out from the neurons by a long extension of each cell called the axon (only one axon to a neuron), and it is best visualized as a copper wire with insulation, called *myelin,* wrapped around it. Myelin is essential for most nerve cells to conduct electricity normally. The axon then makes contact with another cell, of one type or another, through a junction box called a synapse. It communicates with the next cell down the line by releasing a chemical messenger into the synapse that, in turn, activates that cell. These chemical messengers are called neurotransmitters. One nerve cell can be connected to thousands of other nerve cells through the dendrites (treelike structures in the nerve cells).

The brain has certain basic needs in order to function. First, it needs fuel and that is glucose. The brain cannot survive long without glucose, and glucose deprivation in such conditions as hypoglycemia (low blood sugar) can cause significant brain damage after only a short period of time. Second, it needs to burn the glucose fuel, and for this it needs oxygen, which is carried to it through the cerebral blood vessels—the carotid and vertebral arteries. For our brain to work, our heart must pump blood to it, and to do that, our arteries must be open so the blood can reach the brain. If either of these systems (blood or oxygen) malfunctions, the brain can be permanently damaged in as short a time as five minutes. Third, it needs amino acids, electrolytes, fatty acids, hormones, minerals, and vitamins in order to manufacture neurotransmitters, stabilize electrical connections, maintain metabolic functions and myelin, and strengthen cell walls. Since many of these brain nutrients decline as we age, we need supplementation to replace them. On this subject, the coauthors of *The Better Brain Book,* neurologist David Perlmutter and Carol Colman, discuss the inflammatory and toxic environment of the aging brain.

In order to prevent memory and cognitive loss, it would help to first know what causes it. There are many theories, the most popular of which has to do with oxidative free-radical damage to cells and cell membranes. Oxidation of fatty acids in the walls of nerve cells and damage to the mitochondria (the powerhouse of the cell) tend to cause an accumulation of damaged materials, a loss of dendrites, sick and dying cells, and ultimately cell death. Depending on which regions are damaged, this could manifest as Alzheimer's disease or Parkinson's disease. Other theories involve programmed cell death, or the formation of neurotoxins from ingested materials in food, water, and the atmosphere. And, if not recognized, deficiencies of one or more brain nutrients can also result in memory loss and eventual cell death, plus any accumulation of tiny small infarcts (strokes) will eventually result in decreased memory and ability to think clearly.

Still another school of thought is that memory loss and Alzheimer's disease are due to lifestyle. In his book *Brain Longevity,* Dharma Singh Khalsa, M.D., says that chronic stress causes continued excessive concentrations of cortisol in the body, and this is toxic to brain cells. We agree that reducing your stress and maintaining a balanced and happy spirit are critical to preserve a well-functioning mind, and we believe that, by lowering stress-induced cortisol levels, you can help slow down brain aging, especially Alzheimer's disease.

This prevalent disease has been estimated at 50 percent in individuals eighty-five years or older—the most rapidly growing segment of our population. Whatever the ultimate causes of Alzheimer's disease may be, symptoms of the disease arise when neurons that are damaged or destroyed by free radicals (generated by inflammation) fail to function.

The Importance of Enhancing Brain Function as We Age

The question arises as to when you should start taking compounds to help preserve and heighten cognitive skills. The answer is the earlier the better. Our philosophy is preventive medicine. Once you have been diagnosed with dementia, there is very little, if anything, you can do to effectively slow or reverse the process. So do whatever you can, as early as possible, to enhance, maintain, and retain your brain—without cognitive function, the quality of life descends to a much lower level.

We know there is no fountain of youth, but there are new and emerging compounds that may possibly slow, or even reverse, the memory impairment that can eventually progress to Alzheimer's disease or dementia. Our first priority is to preserve and maintain your self-image and your quality of life for as long as possible. Effective Alzheimer's therapy needs to:

1. Reduce inflammation;

2. Limit the damage of free radicals;

3. Enhance neural function.

1. Reducing Inflammation

Fish oil. Manipulation of dietary fat is a proven method of reducing inflammation. Dietary changes designed to decrease arachidonic acid (by eating less meat and eggs) and increase omega-3 levels have been effective strategies for curtailing inflammatory conditions, including arthritis, multiple sclerosis, and psoriasis. The best source of omega-3s is pharmaceutical grade (purified of toxins) fish oil, the potency of which is determined by its DHA content. Borage seed oil and black currant oil are other sources of activated omega-6 fatty acids, and their potency is determined by the GLA content. Magnesium, vitamin B_3, vitamin B_6, and zinc intensify the anti-inflammatory effects of both essential fatty acids.

Recommended dose: 4 capsules OmegaRx daily
1,600 milligrams EPA (eicosapentaenoic acid)
800 milligrams DHA (docosahexaenoic acid)

For more information about fish oil supplements, visit www.zonecafe.com.

Polyphenols. These are potent free-radical fighters that can help prevent inflammation. They are present in small amounts in most fruits and vegetables, and are abundant in grape seeds and pine bark (Pycnogenol). Polyphenols are excellent for the health of the brain as they can readily cross the blood-brain barrier to nurture brain tissues and diminish inflammation.

Excellent dietary sources include berries, dark vegetables, green tea, red wine, soybeans, and such herbs as bilberry, ginkgo biloba, and milk thistle.

Recommended dose: 120 milligrams Pycnogenol
120 milligrams grapeseed extract

2. Limiting Free-Radical Activity

Alpha-lipoic acid. Lipoic acid is an extremely powerful antioxidant as it is both fat and water soluble, and may therefore freely enter all parts of the cells. It is rapidly absorbed and readily enters the brain to protect neurons from free-radical damage. Further antioxidant protection is derived from its ability to recycle vitamins C and E and regenerate glutathione, one of the brain's most important antioxidants. Lipoic acid also acts as a potent metal chelator and decreases inflammation in the brain.

Recommended dose: 50–100 milligrams a day

Ginkgo biloba. This ancient herb can increase blood flow, decrease clumping of blood, decrease free radicals, and increase glucose to reduce bouts of dizziness, depression, and memory loss. In a study published in *The Journal of the American*

Medical Asociation, the authors concluded that ginkgo biloba was safe and appeared to be capable of stabilizing and improving (for six months to a year) the cognitive performance and social functioning of people with dementia.

Recommended dose: 60 milligrams two to four times a day
Note: Do not use aspirin with ginkgo biloba.

N-acetyl-cysteine (NAC). Glutathione production may be complemented with the oral administration of NAC. This precursor of glutathione has the unique ability to reduce nitric oxide and, in turn, lower free-radical activity, thereby creating a less-hostile environment for delicate brain tissue.

Recommended dose: 1,000 milligrams a day

Vitamin D. This vitamin has strong antioxidant capabilities and is highly fat soluble making it an ideal candidate to act as a bodyguard for the brain. In fact, vitamin D has been shown to be more potent against free radicals than fat-soluble vitamin E. In a Japanese study, 80 percent of the test subjects with Alzheimer's disease were deficient in vitamin D.

Recommended dose: 800 IU a day

Vitamin E. This fat-soluble vitamin is important for balancing free radicals. Because the brain is more than 60 percent fat, which makes it highly susceptible to free-radical assault, fat solubility is a critical antioxidant feature for preserving brain integrity. In a landmark study in the *New England Journal of Medicine,* one test group was given vitamin E, while another was prescribed the drug selegiline; those supplemented with vitamin E excelled in all areas measured, including longevity and cognitive function.

Recommended dose: 400–800 IU a day

3. Enhancing Neural Function

Coenzyme Q_{10}. Although a deficiency of coenzyme Q_{10} is usually associated with heart disease, there is growing evidence of the adverse effects that an insufficient supply of coenzyme Q_{10} can have on the brain. Since most of our cellular energy is derived from the mitochondria, the structures in the cells that manufacture and drive this energy are essential for normal brain function. When this energy powerhouse is malfunctioning, it can result in many of the diseases of aging, including diseases of the brain, and this is where coenzyme Q_{10} comes in. It will help to restore the fuel that allows brain mitochondria to function normally.

Recommended dose: In a recent study of patients with Parkinson's disease, 1,200 milligrams of coenzyme Q_{10}, given daily, significantly improved the quality of life. For healthy people, 30–100 milligrams are recommended.

Chlorophyll. Products such as barley, oat grass, and wheat powders are high in chlorophyll.

Recommended dose: Wheat grass juice or barley grass juice once or twice a day. The juice bar at your local whole-foods market is a great place to start.

III. CARNOSINE

I Can See Clearly Now: Carnosine and Cataracts

We are pleased to present this very recent and exciting report from Marios Kyriazis, M.D., a Russian physician and researcher who has been working on carnosine for the past decade. We present it here because it relates to brain health and nutraceuticals.

Although carnosine (also known as L-carnosine and not to be confused with carnitine) has been known for about a century, its antiaging properties have been extensively studied only during the past few years. There have been over 780 published studies on carnosine, mainly by Russian and Japanese researchers, and more widespread interest in this natural nontoxic product has recently been fueled by Australian and British discoveries about its antiaging actions.

High concentrations of carnosine are present in long-lived cells, such as neurons—nerve cells. A high concentration of carnosine in muscles correlates with a person's having a maximum life span, a fact that makes it a promising biomarker of aging. It is high in active muscles and low in cases of muscular disease, such as muscular dystrophy.

In studies of animals with cataracts, the concentration of carnosine in the lens was low—the lower the concentration of carnosine, the more severe the cataract. Rabbits fed a high cholesterol diet were found to be protected against arteriosclerosis and cataracts when also given carnosine supplements, and in another experiment, dogs given carnosine supplements were protected against cataracts. Recent Russian studies on humans given a particular form of carnosine show that it can indeed reverse the effects of age-related cataracts.

Carnosine is widely believed to be an antioxidant that stabilizes and protects the cell membrane. Specifically, as a water-soluble free-radical scavenger, it prevents damaging fat buildup within the cell membrane. Many antioxidants are aimed at preventing free radicals from entering the tissues but have no effect after this first line of defense is broken. Carnosine is not only effective in prevention, but is also active after free radicals begin to form other dangerous compounds. So it protects the tissues from these damaging *second-wave* chemicals. For example, malondialdehyde (MDA), a harmful end product of a free-radical reaction, is blocked by carnosine. Uncontrolled MDA can cause damage to fats, enzymes, and

DNA, and plays a part in the process of arteriosclerosis, joint inflammation, cataract formation, and aging in general.

Other Benefits of Carnosine

- Carnosine plays a part in neurotransmission, it is a heavy metal binder (chelates metals), and it modulates the activities of enzymes.

- It has wound-healing properties and gives protection against radiation damage.

- It is an immune booster.

- It reduces inflammation and gastric ulcers (particularly when the ulcer is related to stress).

- It impedes the damaging process of glycosylation.

Use with People

After dozens of reports about carnosine's antiaging actions in laboratory experiments on animals, the next logical step was to start using it with people. In the past, carnosine supplements have been used by bodybuilders, athletes, and others, but that use has been confined mainly to reducing muscular fatigue; it has not, heretofore, been used to increase longevity. During a preliminary experiment designed specifically for antiaging, Dr. Marios Kyriazis used L-carnosine supplements (50 milligrams daily) on twenty healthy volunteers, aged forty to seventy-five years, for a period of one to four months. No harmful side effects were reported. Five users noticed significant improvement in their facial appearance (firmer facial muscles), muscular stamina, and general well-being. Five others reported possible benefits, such as better sleep patterns, improved clarity of thought, and increased libido. The rest did not report any noticeable effects, which is not surprising because carnosine is not expected to show any significant noticeable benefits in a short time.

Eyedrops for Cataracts?

Recently the Russians have developed a unique form of carnosine called *n-alpha acetylcarnosine* (NAC). A 1 percent solution of this form was placed into eyedrops and dropped twice daily into each eye of forty-nine people with cataracts.

After six months, results showed that 41.5 percent of the eyes had significant improvement; 27 percent had a general improvement; and the remainder had a gradual improvement. After twelve months of treatment, 88.9 percent of the people studied showed significant improvement, and follow-up studies at twenty-four months showed that these beneficial effects had been sustained. Most important, no serious side effects were noted during the entire period. The main complaint was an initial sensation of heat, which disappeared with continued treatment. This revelation has led to the first reliable nonsurgical treatment for age-related cataracts and indicates that this particular form of carnosine, NAC, is breaking existing cross-links between sugar and protein, as well as inhibiting them.

Cataracts account for about 42 percent of all blindness, and there are 28,000 new cataract cases reported every day. In people over sixty-five years of age, cataract surgery is the most commonly performed surgical procedure, with huge economic implications.

We have, over the past several years, tested a unique NAC form of carnosine. The original company has a proprietary method of producing a very potent and pure form of carnosine, which is highly resistant to carnosinase, the enzyme that breaks L-carnosine down to histamine. We believe that NAC (1 percent) eyedrops twice a day will eradicate most cataracts without the need for surgery. You can obtain NAC and other useful antiaging products from www.eternitymedicine.com.

Targeted Nutraceuticals

If you want to prevent or help support weakened organs and systems within the body, we recommend stepping up your program with targeted nutraceuticals. They very effectively support bone tissue, the brain, cholesterol management, the heart, the immune system, the joints, the libido, the liver, the prostate, and vision. For further information, visit www.zonecafe.com.

We have been involved with the production and distribution of nutraceuticals for more than twenty years and strongly encourage all our clients to take a multivitamin and mineral formula each day. Our Zone Foundation Program includes antioxidants, bone support, mitochondrial support, and omega EFAs to help decrease inflammation. For information about this program, visit our website www.zonecafe.com.

As you've learned, most chronic disease develops at the cellular level and inflammation is perhaps the single-most important causative factor. Detoxifying the body and reducing inflammation with optimum nutraceutical balance is key to helping you reach the ageless zone. Bioidentical hormone replacement, which is discussed in the next chapter, is the other vital factor to help reduce silent inflammation and optimize cell communication to help you live better longer.

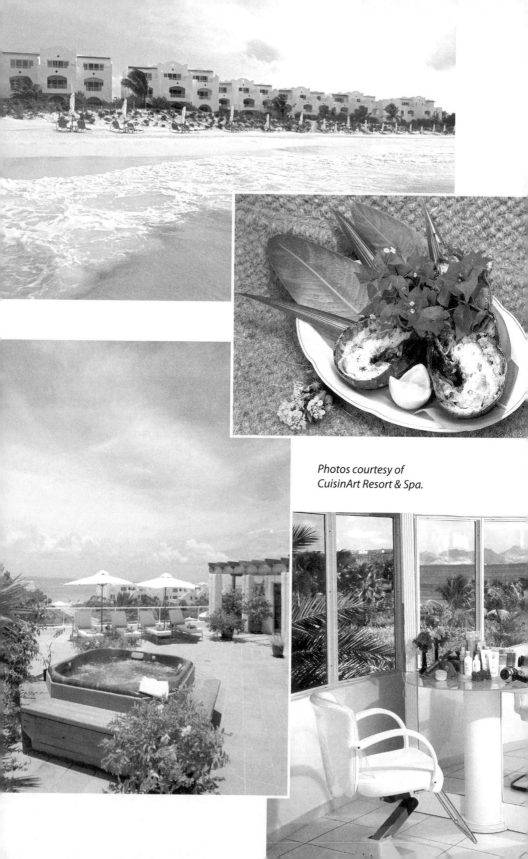

Photos courtesy of CuisinArt Resort & Spa.

Chapter 9

Secret Three —
Hormonal Therapy

There is no need to dread menopause. The work I have done
to understand this time of my life has brought me to a place of
absolute joy. I am balanced and on track, and—no kidding—
this passage has become the most glorious time of my life.

—SUZANNE SOMERS, *THE SEXY YEARS*

There is so much misinformation and ignorance about andropause and menopause. Although these are life-changing events in the lives of men and women, they are the least understood medical mystery. Considering that we are all living longer than our predecessors, and knowing that as baby boomers, we have always demanded a better quality of life, it becomes extremely important to understand and learn how best to deal with both conditions. This is where natural bio-identical hormones come in. They are an important secret for handling this passage of life better, and you can learn more details about them in introductory books on the topic, including *The Superhormone Promise,* by Dr. William Regelson and *The Sexy Years,* by Suzanne Somers.

In this chapter of *Spa Medicine,* we will cover the latest scientific research on all eight of the major hormones vital to our health and well-being. If you have an interest in a particular hormone, feel free to jump ahead and review its role in your health.

THE HYPOTHALAMUS

The hypothalamus located in the brain controls the release of hormones from various glands in the body (*see* Figure 9.1 on page 167). As we age, the hypothalamus loses its ability to regulate hormone production, with the result that hormone secretions decline after age thirty to thirty-five. As well, hormonal receptors lose their sensitivity and thus their ability to function effectively.

In addition to toxins and free radicals, loss of regulation within the hypothalamus may be due to the damage done by cortisol, which is one of the few hormones known to *increase* with age. We know that one of the main reasons for this increase is chronic stress. It raises cortisol levels, which then damages the hypothalamus and other brain structures, thereby impacting greatly on the quality of life, an important example of how a particular worldview—the way a person assigns meaning to stressful events—can either help or hurt that person's health.

We will begin with an overview of the important hormones regulated by the all-important hypothalamus and will discuss the changes taking place in 40 million women (menopause) and 40 million men (andropause) in the United States alone, not to mention the 80 million people who are also going through somatopause (decreased growth hormone). Throughout, we will discuss how restoring hormonal functioning can help combat the negative effects of aging.

Hormones are the real juice of life. In our practice we are always astonished by how men and women are revitalized in as little as six to eight weeks after beginning hormonal replacement. Trust your experience and you will soon be convinced of the benefits of bio-identical hormonal replacement therapy (HRT).

Once we restore a client's hormones to their youthful levels (age thirty to thirty-five), the client feels a greater sense of well-being and vitality because her or his balance is reinstated, and their receptor-site sensitivity is improved. To be done properly, the type of hormonal replacement therapy that we practice must be done under the supervision of a physician who follows a few simple rules. The doctor must:

1. Replace each hormone deficiency present.

2. Individualize all doses.

3. Use only bio-identical hormones.

4. Make polytherapy (multihormones) the treatment of choice.

5. Monitor the client frequently.

These guidelines are intended to ensure a safe and effective slowing, halting, or even reversing of many diseases related to aging.

HORMONES REGULATED BY THE HYPOTHALAMUS

These important hormones can help combat the negative effects of aging.

1. DHEA

Dehydroepiandrosterone, or DHEA, is a steroid hormone produced by the adrenal glands and is the most abundant natural steroid found in the bloodstream. Many research scientists consider high levels of DHEA in the body to be an excel-

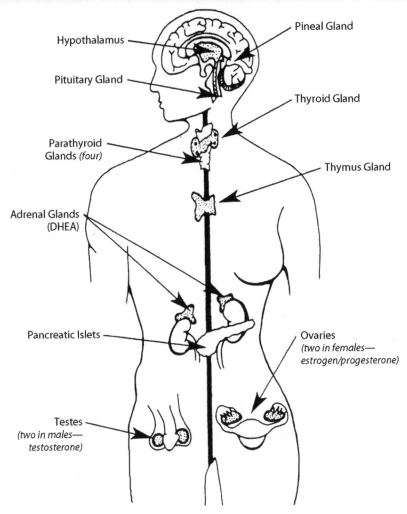

Figure 9.1. Major Endocrine (Hormone) Glands of the Body

lent marker of health. Studies indicate that DHEA has significant antiaging, anticancer, and antiobesity effects and that it enhances mental abilities. As we get older, DHEA levels decline—by age seventy-five, DHEA levels are only 10 to 20 percent of what they were at age twenty (*see* Figure 9.2 on page 168). Here is strong reason to think that DHEA supplements may make us feel more youthful.

DHEA—Protection from Dementias

Brain tissues contain, on average, six and a half times more DHEA than any other body tissue, and it is known to protect brain cells from Alzheimer's disease and

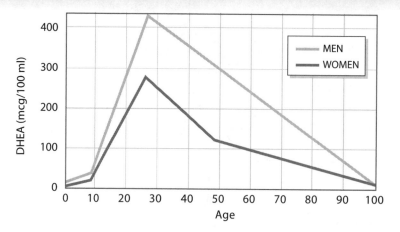

Figure 9.2. Average Age-Related Decline of DHEA Blood Levels

other degenerative conditions. Nerve degenerations are found to occur more rapidly when DHEA conditions in the body are low.

When researcher Dr. Eugene Roberts added low concentrations of DHEA to nerve-cell cultures, he found that it augmented both the number of neurons (nerve cells) and their ability to establish contacts. In other studies, DHEA has boosted long-term memory in mice, and similar effects have been shown in humans. Dr. Samuel Yen, from the University of California at San Diego, feels that DHEA is "a drug that may help people age more gracefully."

Alzheimer's Disease and DHEA

In controlled scientific studies, DHEA is now being administered to people with Alzheimer's disease who are found to have 48 percent less DHEA than similar people of the same age without the disease. Unfortunately, it is not yet clear what to conclude from these results—whether Alzheimer's disease decreases DHEA supplies, or whether low DHEA concentrations are responsible for Alzheimer's disease. They are still working to find the answer.

DHEA—Protection from AIDS

Recent research has shown that DHEA may be able to prevent HIV-infected people from developing full-blown AIDS. People infected with HIV do not experience immune-system suppression until their adrenal output of DHEA declines.

In an AIDS study performed by the University of California at San Francisco, blood samples were drawn from HIV-infected men and frozen. The samples were then tested for DHEA and the men's rate of progression from HIV to AIDS was monitored. The results showed an association between low DHEA levels in the blood and a steady progression to full-blown AIDS. Those men with low levels of DHEA had twice the risk of developing full-blown AIDS as those with normal DHEA levels.

Because of its immune enhancement and its antiviral properties, DHEA is now being used by a great number of HIV-infected people. Further evidence of its benefits is provided by a report in *AIDS Research and Human Retroviruses,* which points to the fact that maintaining high levels of DHEA can inhibit the progression of HIV-1.

DHEA and Heart Disease

One study conducted over twenty years showed that DHEA levels were far lower in men who died of heart disease. DHEA is known to reduce plaque and decrease sticky platelets. DHEA can also lower cholesterol, especially LDL cholesterol, by an average of 18 percent, without any modification of lifestyle. DHEA levels are, in fact, an accurate indicator of blockage in the arteries, hypertension (high blood pressure), LDL cholesterol (the bad cholesterol), and other risk factors.

DHEA and Cancer

DHEA is known to help prevent breast and ovarian cancer. Scientists now believe that a person's risk of cancer can be correlated with their DHEA levels.

DHEA and Osteoporosis

Menopause is also associated with a low level of DHEA. Research shows that the lower a woman's DHEA level, the lower her bone density, and the higher that her risk for developing osteoporosis (due to her reduced bone mass) will be.

DHEA and Diabetes

A high-carbohydrate diet will increase insulin levels, which will, in turn, drive down DHEA levels. DHEA will increase the sensitivity of anyone with diabetes to insulin (as well as increase the RMR, the resting metabolic rate).

DHEA—The Youth Steroid?

Reports have indicated that DHEA levels normally start to decline after the age of twenty-one, and that, by age forty, DHEA levels are often down to 30 percent of what they are in our twenties. At present it is unclear why the adrenal gland reduces its output of DHEA as we age. But individuals, bodybuilders in particular, are discovering the effects of DHEA supplements and the reason why DHEA has been nicknamed the youth steroid.

The initial excitement was sparked by a medical report from Dr. William Regelson that was conducted under double-blind placebo-controlled conditions (in other words nobody was aware of who was receiving DHEA or a placebo). The scientists tested 1,600 milligrams of DHEA (or a dummy capsule) supplements daily on ten normal, healthy individuals, and everyone was instructed to continue their normal lifestyles. After twenty-eight days, the five receiving the placebo had no noticeable differences; however, the five receiving the 1,600 milligrams of DHEA daily had lost 31 percent of their body fat. Their actual weight hadn't changed; fat had just been replaced by lean muscle, and there were no side effects noted.

Another study published in the *Journal of Clinical Endocrinology and Metabolism* found that, in a group of men between ages sixty and eighty, those with the highest levels of DHEA were younger, leaner, more fit, and had higher levels of testosterone. DHEA appears to be a powerful immune booster and may also be beneficial in lupus and other autoimmune diseases.

Different Forms of DHEA

DHEA was originally synthesized using a sulfate base, which is the most common form of DHEA circulating in blood. It now appears that this process, which is a much cheaper way of producing DHEA, could be less effective, as the body can utilize little of the DHEA itself. DHEA in a pure micronized free-base form without sulfates is more effective.

Whichever form is used, the simplest way to introduce any hormone is to let it dissolve under the tongue or apply it transdermally (through the skin) in creams. Either way, the substance will reach the bloodstream more quickly and effectively and will place far less load upon the liver than swallowing a supplement would. DHEA creams appear to convert readily to a form of DHEA called 7-keto. This process takes place within the skin and 7-keto DHEA is estimated to be two and a half times more potent than the other forms. It also appears that 7-keto DHEA does not convert to testosterone or its precursors, which could be important for anyone who wishes to avoid both testosterone and potential estrogen increases when testosterone is broken down.

DHEA Precautions

Although no serious side effects have been noted in short-term use, the use of DHEA can still be considered somewhat experimental. Some women have reported slight increases in facial hair, and livers in DHEA-treated rats and mice have enlarged slightly, possibly because DHEA can convert to testosterone. There is also a risk that testosterone can convert to estradiol, a potent estrogen. This is why the 7-keto form of DHEA is important. It doesn't convert to testosterone (therefore, not to estradiol), and it also appears to have even more potent immune-enhancing properties than other forms.

DHEA Dosages and Side Effects

DHEA dosage can be as much as 1,200 milligrams a day, with some reported cases even higher at 2,000 milligrams daily. However, such high dosages should be used only when there is a serious immune disorder syndrome, such as HIV, and then only under the guidance of a physician.

For those on long-term antiaging programs, more recent evidence would indicate that the use of a low-dosage long-term approach is preferable. Somewhere in the region of 10–50 milligrams daily (maximum 100 milligrams), which mimics normal DHEA production in the adrenal glands, is generally recommended. The use of more potent forms of DHEA—sublingual (under the tongue) or transdermal (through the skin)—could reduce this dosage significantly.

2. Melatonin

Melatonin is produced in the dark while we sleep, and it wanes at daybreak. Melatonin is made from the amino acid tryptophan, which is converted into serotonin, then converted into melatonin.

Until fairly recently it was believed that the pineal gland was to the brain what the tonsils are to the throat, a superfluous accessory. But the pineal gland excretes the hormone melatonin, and it is now known that melatonin has a number of important functions. It plays an important role in regulating sleep, acts as an antidepressant, is a potent antioxidant, helps jet lag, and may even help improve alertness. It has also been shown to slow the aging process in animals. With no noted side effects in clinical trial dosages, melatonin is likely to become a very widely used nutritional supplement.

Melatonin's Role in Treatment of SAD

The changing flow of melatonin appears to control the daily cycle of wakefulness. The pineal gland takes its cue from the light levels surrounding it. It increases the output of melatonin in the dark and diminishes the melatonin level with the sunlight in the morning. If this cycle gets out of sync for any reason, it can lead to SAD (seasonal affective disorder), which produces a depressed or run-down feeling. Shift work, jet lag, or any other major disturbances in sleep patterns can also cause fluctuations in melatonin levels.

Melatonin and Aging

Dr. Walter Pierpaoli, from Italy, has shown that the life span of mice can be extended as much as 25 percent when treated with melatonin. His groundbreaking research demonstrates that old mice may be rejuvenated by replacing their pineal glands with the pineal glands of young mice.

Seasonal Affective Disorder (SAD)

Psychiatrists have been baffled by the increases in suicides, depression, and anti-depressant drug prescriptions in September and continuing until March. Research by the British psychiatrist Dr. Ronald Kay of the West Bank Clinic in Falkirk, Scotland, suggests that the explanation may lie in magnetic storms. He and other scientists investigating changes in the environment and their effects on human behavior are concentrating their studies on the pineal gland. Each year, the earth is wracked by dozens of geomagnetic storms (sudden changes in the earth's magnetic field caused by explosions of particles from the sun). Since these storms are most common around the end of September and the end of March, Dr. Kay was prompted to investigate and see if the correlation was coincidence or not. He gathered the medical records of patients admitted for depression to the Lothian Hospital, Scotland, between 1976 and 1986, and compared the number of admissions to records of geomagnetic storms. What he found was a striking correlation between individuals admitted for psychotic depression and increases in geomagnetic storm activity. In some years, the admissions during peak times of geomagnetic storms were up more than a third over average admissions.

Given this correlation, Dr. Kay is also concerned that electrical appliances could affect some individuals with depression, as 50 hertz electrical appliances have an effect similar to geomagnetic storms, by causing small electromagnetic fields (EMF) to occur within the home or office. Since any EMF can reduce melatonin levels in the body, we recommend removing as many electrical appliances from the bedroom as possible.

The pineal gland somehow senses that we are too old to reproduce around forty-five years of age, and it begins to produce far lower levels of melatonin. This signals all other systems that the aging process has begun. (Some scientists believe that a woman's larger pineal gland is the reason why women age more slowly than men and why they live longer.)

Dr. Pierpaoli has found that by taking melatonin we can mimic a more youthful state. One of the key glands stimulated by melatonin is the thymus, which is vital for our immune system. One of the reasons we lose our ability to fight disease as we age is that, by the time we reach age sixty-five, the thymus has degenerated by 90 percent. Melatonin helps reverse this trend.

Restoring melatonin levels also helps counter the immune-suppressing effect of the stress hormone cortisol and restores our youthful ability to handle challenges with grace and resilience. Melatonin also keeps the sex hormones at a youthful level and is a potent antioxidant.

Melatonin and Cancer

According to Dr. Steve Hill at Tulane University, more than half of all women with breast cancer have lower levels of melatonin. Several recent studies have indicated that increasing levels of melatonin might help prevent or treat breast cancer. Breast cancer in women has been linked to a cumulative exposure to estrogen. Because a woman stops ovulating every time she becomes pregnant, she gets a break from estrogen production, and this is one reason why it is believed that women who have few or no children are at greater risk for breast cancer. Another cause, mentioned earlier, is industrial pollutants. They have potent estrogenic effects called xenoestrogens that contribute to breast cancer.

Melatonin seems to combat the negative effects of estrogen in the body, stopping the tumors from growing and ultimately shrinking them. Melatonin also increases the survival rate for people with lung cancer, prostate cancer, and other solid tumors.

Conclusions about Melatonin

It appears that disturbances in the sleep pattern or the effects of electromagnetic fields can influence the ebb and flow of melatonin release by the pineal gland, with tiredness and depression resulting from irregular levels of this important hormone. Anecdotally, melatonin has received a great deal of praise. Regular supplements appear to help prevent jet lag, improve alertness in the day by providing a good night's rest, and alleviate depression caused by seasonal affective disorder (SAD).

People who do shift work or go on long-distance flights, as well as those who may feel depressed without any particular reason, may well benefit from melatonin supplements.

Melatonin Dosages and Side Effects

Melatonin supplements have not shown any side effects, and anecdotal evidence supports this safety record. Beneficial results appear to differ greatly from person to person. We have heard of those who need only 1–3 milligrams daily, while others feel they need 12–18 milligrams daily to achieve satisfactory results. Some experimentation may be necessary, starting out with low dosages and gradually increasing them over a period of time. Some people have become drowsy an hour or so after taking melatonin. Because of this potential for becoming drowsy, it is recommended that melatonin only be taken before bedtime.

3. Pregnenolone

The use of pregnenolone may be one of the most effective broad range, and yet safe, antiaging therapies at our disposal today. In its decades of safe, effective clinical use, the scope of treatments have included its acting as an antidepressant, alleviating stress, enhancing memory, improving and extending energy levels, and reducing arthritis.

Figure 9.3 below shows the production of pregnenolone from cholesterol and then the pathways for androgen and estrogen biosynthesis (the formation of chemical compounds from more simple chemicals).

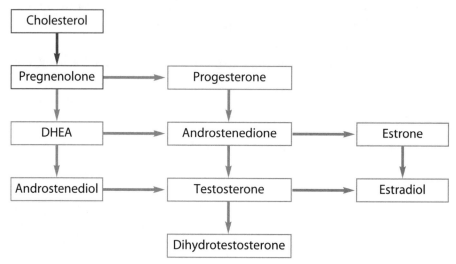

Figure 9.3. Pregnenolone Production from Cholesterol

Pregnenolone—The Grandmother of Hormones

The reason that pregnenolone can have such different uses is because it is the first steroid hormone derived from cholesterol. In fact, as a precursor, it is the grandmother of all the steroids and neurosteroids and it forms their basic material. Without a plentiful availability of pregnenolone, there is likely to be an imbalance of other steroids. For example, DHEA, estrogen, progesterone, and testosterone all originate from pregnenolone—less pregnenolone, less of these substances.

As we age, the secretion and availability of pregnenolone are diminished. Levels of pregnenolone are estimated to be 60 percent less at age seventy-five than at age thirty-five, and this age-related lack of pregnenolone may well lead to a failure to convert other necessary hormones, such as estrogen and progesterone.

Osteo- and Rheumatoid Arthritis and Pregnenolone

Back in the 1940s and 1950s, pregnenolone was a frontline treatment for arthritis, particularly rheumatoid arthritis. At the higher doses employed (200–300 milligrams daily), pregnenolone exhibited anti-inflammatory properties when taken for several weeks. In the 1940s and 1950s, some people took a gram-plus daily dose for years, with no serious side effects, making it generally the safest steroid yet discovered. However, with the introduction of the manufactured steroid cortisone in the early 1950s, the anti-inflammatory use of pregnenolone was diminished.

Although cortisone gives a rapid short-term improvement to the condition, it is marred by considerable side effects, including a decline of the immune system and osteoporosis. Of course, there is money to be made with cortisone and its cortico-derivatives because they are patentable drugs, whereas pregnenolone is an unpatentable natural steroid and therefore not profitable to the drug companies.

Pregnenolone for Depression, Memory, Stress, and the Brain

Perhaps one of the most remarkable aspects of pregnenolone is its effect on brain function. Some animal experiments have shown a direct correlation between the level of pregnenolone and cognitive ability. More pregnenolone, more ability—less pregnenolone, less ability. While the presence of DHEA was discovered to be a major factor in the ability of brain neurons to connect, it was shown that pregnenolone plays an even more important role than DHEA, which it helps to create.

As the precursor for DHEA, pregnenolone may be up to ten times more potent than its offspring for brain function abilities. The most frequently reported cognitive benefits of pregnenolone are:

- Enhanced alertness and greater vigilance;

- Improved mood, more well-being;

- Lowered depression;

- Lowered stress and relaxing effects.

As we said, pregnenolone's actions are very wide ranging. The basis of pregnenolone's benefits for the brain derives mainly from its ability to serve as the precursor for the formation of an extensive range of neurosteroids and its interaction with many receptors in the brain. The animal studies by Drs. Flood, Morley, and Roberts concluded that "Pregnenolone is the most potent memory-enhancer yet reported."

Pregnenolone's Side Effects, Dosages, and Contraindications

The paucity of pregnenolone's side effects at normal therapeutic doses is impressive. Some side effects that have been noted (normally when taking more than 50 milligrams daily) are:

- Headaches and nausea;

- Hives and mild rashes;

- Insomnia;

- Overstimulation;

- Tension and irritability.

We are not aware of any serious contraindications for pregnenolone. Due to their potential to increase testosterone, however, neither it nor DHEA are advisable for men with existing prostate conditions.

As a general guide, antiaging protective doses are 5–10 milligrams daily, cognitive enhancement and general well-being doses are around 25–50 milligrams daily, and higher doses of 100–300 milligrams daily may be more effective in treating such disorders as arthritis. Senile dementia patients could require as much as 500 milligrams daily. Doses should be divided between breakfast and lunch. To avoid insomnia, do not take pregnenolone in the evening.

Conclusions about Pregnenolone

To our way of thinking, pregnenolone exhibits such a wide range of positive benefits, with so few side effects, that it rates in the top ten of antiaging medicines. Normal, otherwise healthy, individuals can supplement with low doses of pregnenolone and know they are helping to improve their memory, lower depression, and reduce stress, as well as experience greater perception, more energy, and greater vigilance, all the while slowing the aging process.

4. Thyroid Hormone

One of the most common (but often undiagnosed) causes of a variety of seemingly unrelated symptoms is an underactive thyroid condition known as *hypothyroidism*. Dr. Broda Barnes, a brilliant, intuitive physician and scientist, estimated that 40 percent of the adult population had this condition.

Hypothyroidism—The Clinical Picture

Some common symptoms of hypothyroidism include cold hands and feet, difficulty in losing weight, dry skin, low energy levels, memory disturbances, menstrual problems, mental confusion, overweight, poor concentration, and thin hair. Other symptoms include arteriosclerosis, depression, diabetes, hypertension, hypoglycemia, infertility, migraine headaches, and even acne. In his book *Hypothyroidism: The Unsuspected Illness,* Dr. Barnes described over forty-seven symptoms that may be related to poor thyroid function. Correcting hypothyroidism can restore your body heat, emotional resilience, endurance, energy, mental vigor, and sexuality. It can protect you from cancer and heart disease, and make your hair and skin healthy and strong.

Hypothyroidism—The Diagnostic Failures

Although many people exhibit symptoms of hypothyroidism, they usually don't receive treatment for this condition if their blood tests are normal. Their physicians often tell them their symptoms are due to other causes or that their problem is all in their head. Many are even referred to psychiatrists to treat their so-called *psychosomatic* problems. However, when they are later given thyroid replacement therapy, they improve dramatically. We refer the interested reader to Dr. Stephen Langer's book *Solved: The Riddle of Illness*.

Hypothyroidism—A Better Way

Dr. Barnes realized that the usual blood tests (T_3, T_4, TSH) performed by doctors are generally inaccurate. Consequently, he developed a simple test to confirm suspected low-thyroid function using an ordinary thermometer.

He found that normal underarm or oral temperatures immediately upon awakening in the morning (while still in bed) are in the range of 97.6 to 98.6 degrees Fahrenheit. He believed that a temperature below 97.6 indicated hypothyroidism, and that one above 98.6 suggested hyperthyroidism, an overactive thyroid. Dr. Barnes recommended using the underarm temperature taken immediately upon awakening to diagnose hypothyroidism. For best results, repeat this test daily for three to four days.

Occasionally, it is necessary to take as much as 5 grains of thyroid daily (full replacement therapy) to obtain complete relief of symptoms. It is not really necessary to receive periodic blood tests, as it is more important to treat the patient than to treat the blood test, but the blood tests are wise from a medical/legal perspective. Using natural thyroid hormone is very safe. There is little risk of excessive thyroid dosage as long as:

- You feel well;
- Your temperature remains below 98.6°F;
- Your pulse is less than 75 beats a minute;
- Your thyroid function tests remain normal (don't be fooled because most hypothyroid people feel best with TSH levels that are below normal).

Hypothyroidism—Why Natural Thyroid?

Synthroid is the most commonly prescribed hormone for hypothyroidism, but it contains only a fraction of the thyroid hormone T_4 (the less active form), which is normally converted by the body into T_3 (the active form). Many doctors believe that most hypothyroid people are not able to efficiently perform this conversion, so Synthroid is not the best choice. (We have found it is very difficult to provide adequate thyroid supplementation with Synthroid without causing our patients to develop a toxicity to thyroid.) Natural thyroid, on the other hand, is a desiccated preparation of porcine thyroid, containing all thyroid hormone factors of T_2, T_3, and T_4. Most of our patients who switch from Synthroid to natural Armour thyroid report that they feel much better with the natural product. The dramatic improvements that many of them have achieved on natural thyroid therapy often appear miraculous. For the physician, it is very gratifying to hear people who have experienced the debilitating symptoms of hypothyroidism for decades express how their life has been totally turned around by a few cents worth of thyroid. Often, they are able to lose weight for the first time in many years.

The downside is that most physicians have been bamboozled by the manufacturers of synthetic thyroid hormones, such as Synthroid, into thinking that the natural thyroid products are an inferior, nonstandardized drug. Nothing could be further from the truth. As we said, most of our patients who switch from Synthroid to natural thyroid find that they feel much better when taking the natural product.

5. Thymic Hormones

The thymus gland has a very important regulatory function in the immune system. This was first recognized in the early 1960s, when its experimental removal in animals resulted in a distinct and progressive depression of the immune system and, more often than not, ended with the death of the animal from an uncontrollable infection. When thymus tissue was reimplanted into such animals, partial or complete recovery took place.

A shrinking of the thymus coincides with a rise in the diseases associated with aging, including autoimmune diseases, cancer, and infectious diseases. More recent research has demonstrated that the hormones of the thymus gland have a marked effect on the maturation and differentiation of T cells, those immune-system cells that are on patrol for disease-causing bacteria and viruses. Dr. Hirokawa from Tokyo attributes the age-related change in T cell-dependent immune functions to the decline of the thymus. While increasing age is associated with a generalized weakening of all the immune defenses, the decreased functioning of the T cell system appears to play the greatest role in the overall decrease in immune function.

Thymic Hormones

It has been shown that a single thymic hormone cannot be isolated. Several thymic hormones, such as thymosin, thymopoietin, and serum thymic factor are all released from the thymus at the same time. For this reason, it is appropriate to produce and administer a natural, complex mixture of extracted thymic hormones.

Thymus Hormone Thym-Uvocal

It has been shown that the German product Thym-Uvocal is an effective thymus hormone. It is very well tolerated and has an impressive action in diseases associated with impaired immune defenses, including old age.

THYM-UVOCAL—IMMUNE SYSTEM AND CANCER

Thym-Uvocal works to strengthen the immune defenses of people with malignant diseases, such as cancer. The immune system is partially or completely impaired in those with malignant tumors, particularly if they are also being treated with drugs or radiation. When Thym-Uvocal has been administered along with the orthodox medical treatment, it has reduced many undesirable side effects. A good number of physicians have also reported an improvement in the underlying disease itself. The positive effects with Thym-Uvocal include:

• Regression of an existing tumor;

• Delayed metastasis (spreading of the cancer);

• Prolonged remission time;

• Improvement in the quality of life.

THYM-UVOCAL AND RHEUMATOID ARTHRITIS

Thym-Uvocal can bring about a lessening of pain in this autoimmune disease, in which the body attacks itself, due to its positive effect on the autoimmune processes. The possible improvements in rheumatoid arthritis are:

• Reduction in joint pain;

• Reduction in morning stiffness;

• Increased ability to move around;

• Positive changes in laboratory findings.

Many practitioners, specialists included, have reported less disability, better mobility, and reduced swelling in the joints when their patients with rheumatoid arthritis have taken this form of the thymus hormone. And there have been frequent reports that Thym-Uvocal has led to lower doses of nonsteroidal anti-inflammatories (NSAIDs), and that long-term use of the product has allowed doctors to wean their patients with rheumatoid arthritis off steroids. There is a dramatic improvement in six weeks and a continued benefit up to seventy-four weeks later.

THYM-UVOCAL AND CHRONIC DISEASES

As mentioned in the introduction, there is a close correlation between the decreasing activity of the thymus, the decreasing competence of the immune system, and an increasing susceptibility to disease as we grow older. Since blood thymus levels decline after the age of twenty-five, this is a good reason why older people, more than any other age group, need to supplement with thymus factors, such as Thym-Uvocal.

Because of the way that Thym-Uvocal stimulates the immune system, it has been used in a number of other conditions involving compromised immune systems, including AIDS, aging skin, allergies, fatigue or exhaustion, infections (bacterial and viral), and lack of vitality.

THYM-UVOCAL—SIDE EFFECTS

Thym-Uvocal, a German thymus product made from cows, is manufactured to such high standards that, in over twenty-five years of use, there have been no known contraindications. Side effects are very rare, and those that have occurred have generally been associated with the injectable form of thymus and have been limited to itching, prickliness, and rashes, usually at the site of the injection.

6. The Hormones Estrogen and Progesterone— Menopause and HRT

There is a growing population of some 40 million women in mid-life today, and it would be presumptuous of us to pretend that we fully understand the menopausal process women go through at this time. We are much more comfortable dealing with the 40 million men who are going through the same mid-life changes as ourselves. We would, however, strongly encourage women who would like more information on this subject to read the excellent books *The Wisdom of Menopause,* by Christiane Northup, M.D., and *Heart Sense for Women,* by Dr. Stephen Sinatra.

Menopausal symptoms usually occur between forty and fifty-five years of age as a direct result of the falling levels of the female sex hormones estrogen (*see* Figure 9.4 on page 181) and progesterone, plus testosterone. And they are reflected by the increased levels of FSH and LH—two hormones that attempt to correct this deficiency. Even though the symptoms of menopause (listed in Table 9.1 on page 181) can be helped with several nonhormonal remedies, such as

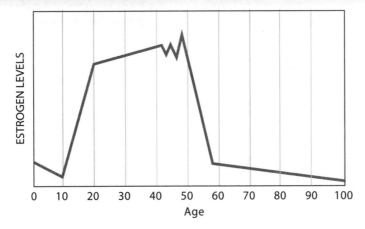

Figure 9.4. Age-Related Estrogen Decline in Women

black cohosh, dong-quai, ginseng, licorice root, omega-3 fatty acids, red clover, and so on, we believe that to eliminate such menopausal signs of aging as degenerative diseases, immune disorders, memory impairment, or osteoporosis, it is essential to have bio-identical hormone replacement therapy (HRT).

TABLE 9.1. Symptoms of Menopause		
Estrogen Deficiency	**Progesterone Deficiency**	**Testosterone Deficiency**
Hot flashes/night sweats	Premenstrual migraine	Decreased libido
Vaginal dryness/thinning	PMS-like symptoms	Decreased energy
Mood swings	Irregular/excessive periods	Impaired sexual function
Headaches/mental fuzziness	Anxiety and nervousness	Thinning pubic hair
Incontinence/urinary infections		Decreased well-being
Decrease sexual response		

Menopause and Osteoporosis

One of the very important problems that shows up in women after the onset of menopause is osteoporosis, thinning porous bones that put a person at risk for fractures. Bone building is the result of a dynamic balance between osteoblasts (cells that increase bone density) and osteoclasts (cells that decrease bone density) as can be seen in Table 9.2 on page 182.

Commonly, less than 20 percent of women in the United States get adequate amounts of calcium every day, not to mention all the other nutrients that are needed to build healthy bone. Even with a good diet, your daily core supplement

TABLE 9.2. Building Bone/Breaking Down Bone

OSTEOBLASTS Stimulated by:	OSTEOCLASTS Stimulated by:
Estrogen	Depleted hormones
Exercise	Depression
Isoflavones	Immune system disorders
Progesterone	Inactivity
Selective estrogen receptor modulators (SERMs)	Nicotine
Testosterone	Nutrient-poor diet
Vitamin D	Steroid drugs

program should include boron, calcium, copper, manganese, magnesium, vitamins C, D, and K, and zinc. Also, bear in mind that there are many good sources of calcium besides dairy products.

Bio-Identical Hormone Replacement

Although the choice of taking hormones is a personal one, we encourage men and women to engage in a hormonal replacement program since, in our experience, it helps clients do better, physically, emotionally, and mentally. And we strongly agree with Dr. Christiane Northup's belief that bio-identical hormones are superior to synthetic hormones. As Dr. Northup writes, "In contrast to Premarin and Provera, the hormones that I recommend are exactly the same as those found in the female body. Though they are synthesized in the lab from hormone precursors found in soybeans or yams, their molecular structure is designed to be an exact match of the hormones found in the human body. Hence, we call them bio-identical, a term that is far more precise than natural, which can be used in confusing and ambiguous ways, as for example, Premarin is said by some people to be a natural product because it is made from horse urine." As Dr. Joel Hargrove, a pioneer in the use of bio-identical hormones, and the medical director of the Menopause Center at Vanderbilt University Medical Center in Tennessee, says, "Premarin is a natural hormone if your native food is hay."

The four main questions that must be answered before beginning HRT are:

1. How will HRT help me?

2. How will HRT hurt me?

3. Is it right for me?

4. How do I take it?

Bio-identical hormones have a long list of benefits that are supported by strong scientific research, primarily including relief from menopausal symptoms, such as hot flashes; prevention of osteoporosis; and decreased urinary incontinence. Other benefits to be derived from the use of bio-identical hormones include more emotional stability, less depression; a decreased risk of Alzheimer's disease or senile dementia; an improved sense of well-being; an increase in the thickness of skin; improved verbal and memory skills; and a decreased risk of colon cancer.

There have been reports of an increased risk in breast and endometrial cancer in some women, although we feel this might well be related to the type of hormone replacement therapy received. To date, there is no evidence as to whether bio-identical estrogens cause breast cancer or not, because no controlled studies have yet been done on them.

After many years of prescribing unopposed estrogen (estrogen with no accompanying hormones), physicians finally discovered that they could decrease the risk of developing endometrial cancer due to estrogen replacement by also replacing the missing progesterone. Progesterone can block or oppose estrogen-causing problems.

Premarin Is Horse Estrogen from Horse Urine

For the last several million years, the female reproductive system has been running quite well on three separate estrogens: estriol (90 percent), estrone (3 percent), and estradiol (7 percent) as seen in Figure 9.5 on page 184. Compare that with Premarin, which consists of estrone at 75 to 80 percent, equilin at 6 to 15 percent, and estradiol and two other equine estrogens at 5 to 19 percent. Notice that, in addition to having disproportionate amounts of estrone and estradiol, Premarin also contains equilin and two other forms of estrogen found exclusively in horses.

A woman's body contains all the enzymes and cofactors it needs to process estriol, estrone, and estradiol when they occur in their natural human proportions. On the other hand, it has *none* of the enzymes and cofactors (factors necessary for the enzymes to function) required to metabolize equilin and the other horse estrogens, nor does it have enough of these important substances (enzymes and related cofactors) to deal with the excessively large amounts of estrone and estradiol found in Premarin (or in the 100 percent estradiol patch). A horse, of course, does have them and is therefore well equipped to handle these. The difference in reproductive hormones is just one of many differences between horses and humans.

It should come as no surprise, then, to learn that the presence of Premarin in a woman's body leads to a hormonal imbalance that can have important adverse consequences. For too many physicians who prescribe Premarin, however, this hormonal imbalance doesn't seem to carry much weight. After all, they reason, the drug works. But, as two leading reproductive physiologists point out, when women take Premarin, "Levels of equilin can remain elevated for thirteen weeks or more posttreatment, due to storage and slow release from adipose (fat) tissue." As a result, Premarin produces estrogenic effects that are *much more potent* and longer lasting than those produced by natural, weaker human estrogens.

This explains why so many women feel unnatural on Premarin, why Premarin can cause the extensive side effects and discomforts that are listed on the manufacturer's box as follows: Breast tenderness, headaches, leg cramps, gallstones, worsened uterine fibroids and endometriosis, vaginal bleeding, high blood pressure, blood clots, nausea and vomiting, fluid retention, impaired glucose tolerance, increased risk of endometrial cancer, and increased risk of breast cancer.

It even explains why Premarin has been associated with a significant risk of breast and endometrial cancer, because one of the primary effects of equilin, estradiol, and estrone is to promote the growth of tissue in the endometrial (uterine) lining and the breast. This growth is important to prepare the premenopausal body for pregnancy and lactation, but the danger comes if some of that tissue becomes cancerous or precancerous in menopause. According to Premarin's official labeling, taking it for a year (without also taking progesterone), increases a women's risk of endometrial cancer by as much as 14 percent.

Most conventional physicians, not to mention the self-serving pharmaceutical industry, are quick to rationalize cancer and other risks of horse estrogens.

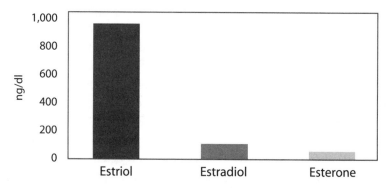

Figure 9.5. Normal Concentrations of Three Major Estrogens

Hormones and the Business of Menopause

If bio-identical triple estrogen is so much better than Premarin, why have so few people heard about it? The answer to this question can be summed up in one word: patentability. Premarin is patentable, which means it can be sold exclusively by its manufacturer and licencees, whereas the less pricey, bio-identical triple estrogen is a natural product, like vitamin C, and can be sold by anyone.

Patentability has made Premarin a huge moneymaker for its manufacturer, Wyeth-Ayerst Pharmaceuticals. For over thirty years, it has been at, or near, the top of the drug bestseller list. In just the first half of 1997, pharmacists filled 22.1 million prescriptions for Premarin, amounting to revenues of $388.2 million in the United States alone. Add in the rest of the world's women, and you get a sense of the high stakes involved in the business of menopause. These enormous financial resources have provided Wyeth-Ayerst the muscle to practically corner the estrogen market. Through advertising, sponsorship of clinical trials and conferences, free samples, and other common marketing techniques, they have created an atmosphere in which physicians virtually equate estrogen replacement with Premarin.

Estriol—The Missing-in-Action Hormone

You may have noticed that one estrogen, estriol, is completely absent from Premarin and other forms of conventional estrogen replacement regimens, although it comprises as much as 80 to 90 percent of the bio-identical triple estrogen. This is not an insignificant omission. Most conventional physicians and pharmaceutical researchers have long dismissed estriol as a weak and unimportant estrogen. They have considered it to be primarily processed from estradiol and estrone, which are far more potent in producing estrogenic effects, such as inducing endometrial tissue growth. "Why go through all the trouble of putting estriol into a pill if you don't really need it?" seems to be their reasoning. Well potency isn't everything. In fact, estriol is vitally important precisely because it *is* a weak estrogen. A number of studies, published over four decades, have demonstrated that estriol's unique, and perhaps most important role, may be to *oppose* the growth of cancer, including cancer promoted by its more potent cousins, estrone and estradiol.

Estriol plays more than just a defensive role though. European physicians have been more open to the potential benefits of estriol in menopausal women than those in the United States. As a result, most of the clinical research evaluating estriol has been conducted in Europe. In general, these studies show that menopausal women who use natural estriol to replace their estrogen experience a reduction in such typical menopausal symptoms as hot flashes and thinning of the vaginal tissue (vaginal atrophy).

In one of the major trials, twenty-two practicing gynecologists from eleven large hospitals in Germany treated 911 premenopausal women with estriol and evaluated them regularly for five years. They found estriol to be "very effective" against common menopausal symptoms and "well-tolerated with no significant side effect."

A Swedish study evaluated forty postmenopausal women with urinary incontinence (leaky bladders) for up to ten years. The researchers found that estriol treatment resulted in significant improvement in 75 percent of the women, including eight whose ability to regulate urination completely returned to normal. The study also found that symptoms of vaginal atrophy disappeared in 79 percent of the women after just four months of estriol treatment. After twelve months, all but one woman were symptom-free.

Built-in Cancer Protection with Estriol

There is no doubt that doses of horse estrogens and 100 percent estradiol patches and creams stimulate excessive proliferation of endometrial cells, a precursor to endometrial cancer. It is to reduce this risk that any woman with a uterus taking these drugs must also take natural progesterone substitute. This is in stark contrast to estriol, which appears to actually antagonize the proliferative effects of estrone and estradiol, while having far less tendency to stimulate endometrial proliferation itself.

Estriol apparently accomplishes its protective role by binding to estrogen receptors in the uterine lining and possibly the breast. Unlike the more potent estrogens though, it does not stimulate growth nearly as much. When the estrogen receptors are covered by estriol, they are shielded from the more carcinogenic estrogens, estrone and estradiol. This is thought to be the same way that other weak estrogens, such as those found in soy products, protect against cancer. In laboratory animal studies totaling more than 500 rat years, estriol has been shown to be the most protective estrogen ever tested against cancers of the breast induced by several potent carcinogenic agents, including radiation.

There is important evidence dating back to the 1960s which suggests that estriol may protect against breast cancer as well. At that time, Henry Lemon, M.D., head of the division of gynecologic oncology at the University of Nebraska College of Medicine, was the first to hypothesize that some women who develop breast cancer have too little estriol relative to the estradiol and estrone circulating in their bodies.

To test this hypothesis, Dr. Lemon ran a preliminary study in which he employed a urinary estrogen quotient (EQ), which was simply a measure of the ratio of estriol to the total of estradiol and estrone in the urine over a twenty-four-hour period. The higher the quotient, the more estriol there is relative to estradiol and estrone.

In a small study of thirty-four women with no signs of breast cancer, Dr. Lemon found the EQ to be a median of 1.3 before menopause and 1.2 after menopause. Only 21 percent of the women had an EQ less than 1.0 (that is, estriol was less than estradiol and estrone combined). For twenty-six women with breast cancer, however, the picture was quite different. Their median EQ was 0.5 before menopause and 0.8 after menopause; 62 percent of these women had an EQ less than 1.0.

The conclusion reached was that the women with breast cancer seemed to be making substantially less estriol than the other group with no breast cancer.

Following this discovery, the bio-identical triple estrogen was first formulated by pharmacist Ed Thorp at the Kripps Pharmacy, in Vancouver, British Columbia, and the rest is history. In the twenty years since triple estrogen was first prescribed, thanks to thousands of other progressive physicians, many grateful women have found that it works as well as, or better than, conventional ERT (estrogen replacement therapy) regimens, while producing far fewer unwanted side effects.

Clearly, much more research, including large-scale, long-term studies are needed for the many unanswered questions regarding estriol's role in cancer. In the meantime, there can be little doubt that an estrogen replacement regimen that includes the three human estrogens in triple estrogen (estriol, estrone, and estradiol) in bio-identical proportions is a superior choice for premenopausal and postmenopausal women, especially when compared with the horse estrogens and the 100 percent estradiol patches and creams the pharmaceutical industry promotes.

This belief was echoed by Alvin H. Follingstad, M.D., in a 1978 editorial, "Estriol, the Forgotten Estrogen?" in the *Journal of the American Medical Association*. He bemoaned the lack of large clinical trials on estriol that would earn it an FDA stamp of approval. "Do we as clinicians have to wait the years necessary for the completion of these trials before estriol becomes available to us?" he asked. "I think not; enough presumptive and scientific evidence has been accumulated that we may say that orally administered estriol is safer than estrone and estradiol." Two and a half decades later, we are still waiting for those clinical trials, and what Dr. Follingstad said then is even truer today. There is nothing to be gained by waiting. If a woman is concerned about her risk of cancer from estrogen replacement (and who wouldn't be?), then the logical choice is an estrogen formula containing a majority of estriol, in other words, the bio-identical triple estrogen. And both current scientific research and the hundreds of thousands of years during which humans have produced and metabolized estrogens makes this an especially suitable choice.

Bio-identical natural hormone formulations like triple estrogen are normally available in the United States only from compounding pharmacies (those that make up preparations containing several ingredients) with a physician's prescription; they cannot be found at standard pharmacies.

Natural Progesterone Protects against Cancer, Heart Disease, and Osteoporosis

Women who replace estrogen also need to replace progesterone, especially if they have a uterus, because estrogen and progesterone are closely linked in the normal menstrual cycle. Each month, as estrogen levels rise, progesterone levels fall, and vice versa.

Unfortunately, this was not always obvious to physicians and pharmaceutical companies. In the early days of ERT, tens of thousands of women developed endometrial cancer as a result of taking Premarin without progesterone. In the absence of progesterone, the estrogen in Premarin can cause excessive proliferation of endometrial tissue, which, in an alarming number of instances, can turn malignant.

Natural bio-identical progesterone largely prevents this excessive growth. But conventional medicine being as obdurate as it is, most physicians do not prescribe natural progesterone for their menopausal patients. Instead, they prescribe a synthetic progesteronelike drug, or progestin, called Provera (medroxyprogesterone), or one of its clones. Synthetic progestins are not the same thing as progesterone. But, thanks to the drug industry's promotional abilities and physicians' willingness to take their words at face value, few physicians ever take the time to investigate and discover that distinction.

Women who take Provera pay a high price for the so-called protection it affords against Premarin-induced endometrial cancer. That price includes an increased risk of cardiovascular disease (CVD), because progestins strip away most of the protection against CVD that they gain from estrogen replacement. In our clinical experience, we have found that many cases of unexplained chest pain, shortness of breath, and high blood pressure have resolved after Provera was discontinued. Since this protection is one of the main reasons women take Premarin in the first place, and since Provera causes a long list of unpleasant side effects—breakthrough bleeding, breast tenderness, depression, and weight gain, to name just a few—you have to wonder whether they wouldn't be better off not taking anything!

On the other hand, natural progesterone, which comes from the same source as the natural bio-identical estrogens in triple estrogen, is a completely different story. As with the bio-identical triple estrogens, it too is structurally and functionally identical to the progesterone the body produces, and replacing missing progesterone with natural progesterone puts the same hormone back into the body that it is accustomed to having. When used properly, natural bio-identical progesterone affords the same protection against cardiovascular disease as the natural progesterone produced by our bodies.

This was most clearly demonstrated in a large-scale, federally sponsored clinical trial, known as PEPI (postmenopausal estrogen progestin interventions). In this PEPI study, 875 postmenopausal women were randomly placed in one of four treatment groups: placebo; estrogen (Premarin) only; Premarin and Provera; or Premarin and natural progesterone (oral). The relevant measure was the subject's level of HDL cholesterol, known as the good cholesterol, since it protects against cardiovascular disease. The results clearly demonstrated that when Provera was added to Premarin, HDL levels dropped to nearly baseline. (With HDL, *higher* levels are better.) By contrast, when natural progesterone was added to Premarin, there was no significant loss of HDL-based protection against cardiovascular disease.

If this weren't enough to recommend natural progesterone, there's also the protection it provides against osteoporosis. This ability has been clearly shown by the work of John R. Lee, M.D.

Osteoporosis is the bone-thinning disease that commonly occurs following menopause. It appears to be due to a loss of both estrogen and progesterone. Replacing estrogen will usually help slow or even halt bone that has already been lost.

Dr. Lee took regular bone-mineral density measurements of sixty-two postmenopausal women who were taking Premarin plus progesterone (in a cream base) or progesterone alone for a period of at least three months. The women also took calcium supplements and maintained a diet and lifestyle designed to minimize bone loss. He found that natural progesterone replacement resulted in a remarkable increase in bone-mineral density. Some of Dr. Lee's patients increased the density of their lumbar vertebrae by 20 to 25 percent in the first year. Over the three years of the study, the mean increase in bone mineral density was 15.4 percent (*see* Figure 9.6 on page 190).

Other studies (similar to the PEPI study) show that a 4 to 5 percent decrease in bone density would have been expected in women not using natural progesterone. Not surprisingly, Provera appears to provide no protection against osteoporosis and definitely does not enhance bone growth. As Jonathan Wright, M.D., stated at the 2000 Monte Carlo Anti-Aging Conference, "We physicians don't have to be rocket scientists. All the work has already been done for us. We just have to copy nature."

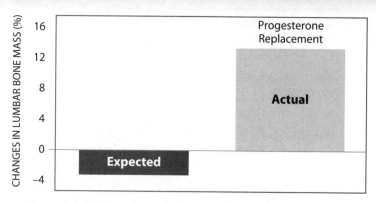

Figure 9.6. Progesterone Restores Bone Loss in Osteoporosis

7. Andropause and Testosterone

Andropause is the technical term for the changes that men go through as they age. Between the ages of forty and seventy, a typical American male loses about twenty pounds of muscle, 15 percent of his bone mass, and nearly two inches in height. After age forty, the testicles begin to shrink so that many men become impotent in their later years.

In 1889, Dr. Charles Brown Sequard, a famous neurologist, gave himself crushed animal testicles and claimed that he became stronger, developed more stamina, and had a better memory. This is one of the earliest cell-therapy treatments (*see* Appendix G). Although widely accepted as a theory, we do not believe that andropause is related only to a decline in testosterone levels because higher testosterone levels by themselves do not always mean there is increased sexual prowess. Other hormones, such as DHEA, growth hormone, and thyroid hormone are also very important in andropause. Sexual decline may also be related to a decrease in neurotransmitters in the brain. Certain medications can also aggravate the brain neurotransmission and interfere with a man's potency.

It is estimated that testosterone levels will drop to abnormally low levels in more than 20 percent of men after age fifty. Testosterone can not only be affected by medications but also by illness, obesity, stress, and lifestyle factors, such as excessive alcohol intake and smoking.

Technically, the term *andropause* (known in England as *viropause*) involves the progressive decline of testosterone levels with age, coupled with an increased production of sex-hormone–binding globulin (SHBG). Testosterone binds to this protein, reducing its availability to tissues, and thus reducing its effect.

The following is part one of a simple questionnaire for men to determine if their testerone levels are adequate. How do you score?

PART ONE—IS YOUR TESTOSTERONE LEVEL ADEQUATE?		
Do you have:	Yes	No
1. A decrease in your sex drive?		
2. A less strong erection?		
3. A lack of energy?		
4. A decrease in strength and/or endurance?		
5. Lost height?		
6. Decreased enjoyment of life?		
7. Sadness and/or grumpiness?		
8. A deterioration in your sports ability?		
9. A tendency to fall asleep after dinner?		
10. Decreased work performance?		

Men who have answered YES to numbers 1 and 2, or to any four questions, are candidates for possible hormone replacement therapy.

There are more than 40 million men in the United States experiencing andropause, but the vast majority of them don't even realize it. As the tremendous popularity of Viagra suggests, many of these men have symptoms of male sexual dysfunction, while others find themselves fighting more subtle battles against depression, diabetes, fatigue, insomnia, and obesity—all common symptoms of low testosterone that most doctors overlook and attribute to the natural process of aging or stress.

Standard Laboratory Tests for Low Testosterone Have Failed

This is the reason why contemporary medicine is missing the low-testosterone mark. Medical science has determined that while a man's total (protein-bound) testosterone levels remain relatively stable over time, his bioavailable (free) levels gradually decline at an alarming rate of 2 percent each year, beginning at age thirty. This means that a man in his sixties is functioning with only about 40 percent of the testosterone he had in his twenties.

However, when standard laboratory tests are performed, most men typically have only their *total* levels of testosterone evaluated. Their more important bioavailable levels go unchecked. To make matters worse, most practitioners require a diagnosis of hypogonadism (a medical term used to classify total testosterone levels that fall below a specified laboratory limit) prior to prescribing any testosterone-replacement medication. As a result, millions of American men who have symptoms of low testosterone are walking around undiagnosed and untreated.

Detection of Low Testosterone—A Necessary First Step

When it comes to treating and eliminating the symptoms of low testosterone, detecting the problem is a fundamental first step.

Are your testosterone levels low? The following is part two of the questionnaire, which can alert you to andropause.

PART TWO—IS YOUR TESTOSTERONE LEVEL ADEQUATE?	Yes	No
1. Are you over the age of thirty-five?		
2. Do you have poor muscle tone?		
3. Are you prone to weight gain, particularly around the midsection?		
4. Do you frequently feel weak and tired for no apparent reason?		
5. Is your recovery from exercise slow?		
6. Do you have a low sex drive or symptoms of sexual dysfunction?		
7. Do you feel depressed, irritable, or unmotivated?		
8. Do you have difficulty coping with stress?		
9. Do you smoke cigarettes, drink alcohol regularly, or take prescription medicines?		
10. Have you recently been diagnosed with diabetes?		

If you answered YES to any of these ten questions, chances are your testosterone levels are less than optimal.

But how can you know for sure if your testosterone levels are low? In addition to being more convenient and less costly than standard laboratory tests, recent medical research has proven that hormone testing of the saliva is far more accurate when it comes to measuring bioavailable testosterone and a number of other key male hormones.

Benefits of Testosterone

- Enhances muscle mass and strength;

- Enhances sex drive and function;

- Improves cardiac health and blood pressure;

- Improves memory, concentration, and visual acuity;

- Improves mood and overall sense of well-being;

- Improves overall energy;

- Increases bone strength;

- Increases tolerance for stress;

- Promotes protein-building;

- Reduces cholesterol and blood sugar.

Produced in the testes, testosterone is the end result of a series of biochemical steps that all start with, and fundamentally depend on, cholesterol. Testosterone also regulates prostaglandin, which seems to keep the growth of the prostate under control. Testosterone also nourishes all the tissues in the male urinary and reproductive systems.

Rising Estrogen in Men

Men are usually surprised to learn that estrogen is present in their bodies (just as women are surprised to learn their bodies have testosterone). It is produced in very small amounts as a byproduct of the testosterone conversion process. In fact, balanced levels of estrogen in men are essential to encourage a healthy libido, improved brain function, cardiac protection, and strengthening of the bones. But due to aging, body fat, excessive alcohol intake, hormonal replacement, nutritional deficiencies, pesticides, and prescription medicines, many men experience too-high levels of estrogen, which are detrimental to their health. In fact, studies have shown that, because of all the above, the estrogen levels of the average fifty-four-year-old man are higher than those of the average fifty-nine-year-old woman. These high levels of estrogen can cause reduced levels of testosterone, with the resulting symptoms of an enlarged prostate, fatigue, increased body fat, loss of libido and sexual function, and loss of muscle tone.

Testosterone and Estrogen Balance in Men

When there is less testosterone present, estrogen moves in and attaches to testosterone cell-receptor sites throughout the body. As these estrogen levels increase with age, testosterone is not able to stimulate the cells, which causes reduced sexual arousal and sensation, as well as loss of libido. Excess estrogen can also do the following.

- It can shut down normal testosterone production. Excess estrogen saturates testosterone receptors in the hypothalamus in the brain, thereby reducing the testosterone signal sent to the pituitary gland, which, in turn, reduces the secretion of luteinizing hormone, the necessary trigger the gonads need to produce testosterone.

- It can increase the body's production of sex hormone–binding globulin (SHBG). SHBG binds testosterone in the blood, which reduces the amount of free bio-available testosterone in the blood.

- It can reduce the effectiveness of the testosterone replacement therapy by converting testosterone medications to estrogen. This conversion is known in medical circles as aromatization.

- It can increase the long-term risk of diabetes, heart disease, and some cancers (possibly prostate).

Obviously, men who are concerned about healthy aging, or are experiencing the unpleasant symptoms of low testosterone, or are undergoing testosterone replacement therapy, need to test their estrogen levels. If these are too high, they need to reduce the excess estrogen to a safe range as they increase their testosterone levels.

Testosterone Replacement Therapy

Although there is no perfect method for supplementing testosterone in a way that mimics normal secretion, the five principle methods that are available follow:

1. Intramuscular injection;

2. Lozenges to take by mouth;

3. Patches;

4. Gels;

5. Implantation of pellets under the skin.

The method of choice often depends on preference for one reason or another. The pros and cons of each technique are summarized below.

1. Injection

Pros: Once-a-week administration.

Cons: Short-term, high-peak concentrations of testosterone, therefore, more conversion to estradiol, which causes an imbalance between testosterone and estradiol; requires an intramuscular injection.

2. Lozenges

Pros: A good method of supplementing testosterone blood levels; easiest and most convenient method.

Cons: Short duration of action (five to six hours); must be taken three times a day.

3. Patches

Pros: Provide a slow, steady release; can be almost anywhere on the body; free of side effects.

Cons: Rash from the adhesive in the patch leaves embarrassing red circles on the skin; must be changed daily; difficult to get testosterone levels above 600 nanograms/deciliter—some men need levels in the 800–900 range.

4. Transdermal gels or creams

Pros: Convenient and very effective; rapidly absorbed through the skin; no residual left on the skin.

Cons: Discipline and accuracy are required in measuring the amount applied each day.

5. Pellets

Pros: Offer long-term treatment with minimal inconvenience; pellets are implanted once every four to six months; provide slow, steady constant infusion of testosterone; probably the most effective delivery system; estrogen conversion is minimal.

Cons: Implantation in the buttocks with local anesthesia is required; once implanted, the pellets cannot be removed if you wish to stop therapy.

We recommend gel or cream preparations to begin testosterone supplementation. They are painless and easiest to use overall. Gels can be custom compounded to a dose that is specific for your hormone supplementation program, and they can be used by both women and men.

The Pluses of Testosterone Replacement Therapy

Testosterone replacement should approximate the natural youthful production of the hormone. The average man produces 4–7 milligrams of testosterone per day, with maximum levels attained in early morning and minimal levels in the evening. Normally, testosterone is 30 percent higher in the morning than in the evening, which may explain why men are more interested in sex in the morning and partially explain why they have spontaneous morning erections. In fact, the loss of morning erections is a sure sign that testosterone is declining. By using testosterone gel, you are infusing testosterone into your system in a natural manner. By administering a dose at night, your plasma levels are maximized for best results. A dose in the morning maintains a lower, but still elevated, level during the day. Both forms of testosterone treatment, low-dose high-frequency injections and transdermal applications, are effective treatments for low testosterone levels. Again, we recommend applying gel for its ease and convenience.

If you are undergoing testosterone replacement therapy, it is prudent to measure your PSA (prostate specific antigen) levels to see how your prostate is doing. An HDL and hematocrit blood test should also be taken, which is why HRT is best done under the care of a knowledgeable, healthcare professional.

8. Growth Hormone

Growth hormone therapy was, until recently, considered a useful therapy only in children suffering from growth hormone deficiency. The importance of growth hormone becomes clear when we look at the dwarfs of the Spanish royal courts in the paintings of Velázquez. Or, on the other side, we look at the world's tallest man in *Guinness World Records,* which shows what happens when there is an excess of growth hormone. Not only is growth hormone necessary to make children grow into adults, but growth hormone must be maintained at good levels to provide adequate functioning of adult tissues and organs.

It was Dr. Daniel Rudman's article in the *New England Journal of Medicine* on July 5, 1990, that really aroused the medical communities' interest in growth hormone. He studied twenty-one healthy men who had low IgF-1 levels (insulin growth factors—good measures of growth hormone deficiency). Twelve of these men received growth hormone injections over a six-month period, which produced remarkable results. Dr. Rudman showed that the signs of aging and those of growth hormone deficiency were nearly identical, and that by providing growth hormone to these men it was possible to achieve improvement in these functions (*see* Table 9.3 on page 197). Growth hormone has a wide range of potent effects on adipose tissue, bones, liver, muscle, nervous system, and more. This broad spectrum of favorable effects helps us understand how different symptoms of growth hormone deficiency appear in adults.

More than 20,000 clinical studies from around the world document the benefits of HGH therapy. In August 1996, the FDA approved HGH for use in adult patients. HGH declines with age in every animal species that has been evaluated. Dr. Rudman considered an IgF-1 level under 350 evidence of a deficiency of growth hormone.

Growth Hormone Deficiency and Aging
Lead to a Similar Decline in Function

The intriguing similarity between growth hormone deficiency and aging outlined by the late Dr. Rudman became even more interesting when Rudman and others showed how growth hormone can improve those declining structures and physiological functions of aging.

TABLE 9.3. Growth Hormone Changes in Aging

Function	Change with Age	Growth Hormone Deficiency	Growth Hormone Treatment
Adipose mass	Increases	Increases	Decreases
Bone density	Decreases	Decreases	Increases
Bone mass	Decreases	Decreases	Increases
Cardiac index	Decreases	Decreases	Increases
Glomerular filtration rate	Decreases	Decreases	Increases
Kidney size	Decreases	Decreases	Not known
Liver size	Decreases	Decreases	Not known
Mandible size	Decreases	Decreases	Increases
Maximal breathing capacity	Decreases	Not known	Increases
Muscle mass	Decreases	Decreases	Increases
Muscle strength	Decreases	Decreases	Increases
Renal blood flow	Decreases	Decreases	Increases
Spleen size	Decreases	Decreases	Not known

Growth hormone is a protein hormone of about 190 amino acids that is synthesized and secreted by cells in the anterior pituitary gland, which lies at the base of the brain and is controlled by a brain area just above it called the hypothalamus. The hypothalamus sends messages to the pituitary to increase or decrease the formation and release of HGH into the bloodstream. Growth hormone is a major participant in the control of several complex physiological processes, including growth and metabolism.

Physiological Effects of Growth Hormone

A critical concept in understanding growth hormone activity is that it has two distinct types of effects in the body, direct and indirect:

1. Direct effects are the result of growth hormone's actions on the receptors of tar-

get cells. Fat cells (adipocytes), for example, have growth-hormone receptors, and growth hormone stimulates them to break down triglycerides, while it suppresses their ability to take up and accumulate circulating fats.

2. Indirect effects come primarily from an insulinlike growth factor (IGF-1), a hormone that is secreted from the liver and other tissues in response to growth hormone. IGF-1 is also known as somatomedin C. A majority of the growth-promoting effects of growth hormone are actually due to IGF-1 acting on its target cells.

Effects on Growth

Growth is a very complex process and requires the coordinated action of several hormones. The major role of growth hormone in stimulating body growth is to stimulate the liver and other tissues to secrete IGF-1, which then stimulates the proliferation of cartilage cells, resulting in bone growth. Growth hormone appears to have a direct effect on bone growth. IGF-1 also appears to be the key player in muscle growth. It stimulates the absorption and utilization of protein, which helps to build stronger muscle.

Metabolic Effects of Growth Hormone

Growth hormone has important effects on protein, fat, and carbohydrate metabolism. In some cases, a direct effect of growth hormone has been clearly demonstrated; in others, IGF-1 is thought to be the critical factor, and in some cases, it appears that both direct and indirect effects are at play.

Protein metabolism: In general, growth hormone stimulates the building of protein in many tissues. This effect increases the body's ability to absorb protein more efficiently without causing it to make free radicals.

Fat metabolism: Growth hormone helps to break down fat more efficiently and keeps it from generating free radicals.

Carbohydrate metabolism: Growth hormone is one of a battery of hormones that serves to maintain blood glucose within a normal range.

Integration of all the factors that affect growth hormone's action in the body results in a time-release pattern. Basal concentrations of growth hormone in blood are very low. In children and young adults, the most intense period of growth hormone release is shortly after the onset of deep sleep. This is why many physicians prefer to administer it at night.

Benefits of HGH Replacement

- Sustained improvement in body composition, specifically:
  - Decreased percent body fat;

- ▪ Increased lean body and muscle mass;
- ▪ Increased total body water and fat-free body mass.

- Decreased need for assistance with daily activities in more mature people;

- Decreased use of healthcare resources;

- Improved cholesterol profile;

- Improved measures of balance and physical performance in older men;

- Improved psychological well-being;

- Increased muscle IGF-1 gene expression;

- Reduced bone loss;

- Reduced carotid-artery thickness;

- Rejuvenated immune system—leading to regrowth of the thymus gland.

More important, these changes can occur without side effects if normal blood levels of IGF-1 are maintained. Side effects, if any, are few and include mild fluid retention and joint discomfort, which disappear in four to six weeks. There is no reported occurrence of cancer with HGH administration. HGH should not be given to people with diabetes or to anyone who has a history of cancer.

Let us look at what happens to growth hormone levels as we age.

Daily Production of Growth Hormone Declines with Age

The maximum daily production of growth hormone peaks in late puberty and begins to decline at about twenty. Each decade after this time shows a clear decline in GH. As can be seen in Figure 9.7 on page 200, total HGH secretion declines with advancing age. Obese men seem to produce less than lean men. A great part of the effects of GH depend on insulinlike growth factor 1 (IgF-1) as an intermediary. This hormone declines with age (as do most of the other major hormones in the body).

Optimum levels of blood IgF-1 seem to occur in adults between twenty and thirty years old. Replacing GH to those levels in people with physical signs and complaints of aging appears to act as a potent rejuvenation therapy.

Growth Hormone Therapy

A Belgian study of forty-eight adults conducted by Dr. Thierry Hertoghe found that the following physical signs (in order of frequency) were improved after just two months of GH therapy. Average dosage was 0.75 IU per day.

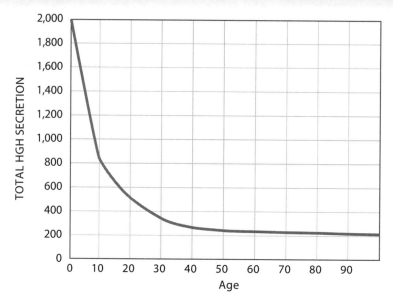

Figure 9.7. Growth Hormone Decline with Age

1. Sagging cheeks (get tenser) (75.5 percent)

2. Wrinkled face (less wrinkled) (71 percent)

3. Pouches under the eyes (less visible) (65.8 percent)

4. Loose folds of skin under the chin (tighten) (62.5 percent)

5. Sagging body silhouette (straightens up) (62.5 percent)

6. Dropping triceps (tighten) (60.7 percent)

7. Bagging inner side of the triceps (tightens) (60.7 percent)

8. Floppy stomach (flattens) (48 percent)

9. Less muscled shoulders (muscles return) (44 percent)

10. Less muscled buttocks (muscles return) (42.3 percent)

11. Meager, wrinkled buttocks (muscles return) (41.6 percent)

12. Fatty cushions above the knees (decrease) (41.2 percent)

13. Thinned skin (thickens) (34.5 percent)

14. Obesity (decreases) (33.3 percent)

15. Thin hair (thickens) (28.1 percent)

16. Thin lips (thicken) (25 percent)

17. Gum retraction (less important) (20 percent)

18. Thinned jawbones (thickens) (9.5 percent)

The same study also shows the frequency of improved psychological symptoms in the same forty-eight people mentioned above.

1. Permanent fatigue (decreases or disappears) (86.8 percent)

2. Easy exhaustion when physically busy (recovery better) (86.04 percent)

3. Poor resistance to stress (improves) (83.7 percent)

4. Depression (fades away) (82.7 percent)

5. Low resistance when staying up after midnight (improves) (82.5 percent)

6. Low self-esteem (improves) (79.2 percent)

7. Sense of powerlessness (subject gets sense of empowerment) (77.8 percent)

8. Poor sociability (person opens up to others) (77.8 percent)

9. Anxiety (decreases greatly) (73.5 percent)

10. Insufficient aggressiveness (subjects get firmer) (73.1 percent)

11. Inappropriate hyperemotionality (person calms down) (71.4 percent)

12. Sharp verbal retorts (speech softens) (71 percent)

The results of this study show that GH not only improves physical signs of aging, but also improves psychological well-being. Anxiety, depression, fatigue, and insomnia all improve. Indirect evidence suggests that growth hormone therapy, started at the right time, when we are aging, can also prolong our lives. For example, adults deficient in GH double their mortality from cardiovascular disease compared with normal people. We have found that, by age fifty, most adults become sensitive to the benefits of GH. The more an adult advances in age, the more this person benefits from GH supplementation.

HGH also does something that no weight-loss regimen does—it recontours the body, melting away fat and building muscle. In every study, HGH reduces body fat and increases lean body mass. What is even better, the greatest fat loss is in the deep belly fat, which is a marker of risk for heart disease.

High blood sugar and increased risk of cancer should not occur with use of mild to moderate doses of GH. In fact, studies show that the immune system is greatly improved with GH.

Just as menopause and andropause are now considered syndromes, which result from the lack of sexual hormones in women and men respectively, GH deficiency is being accepted more and more as a distinct medical condition (somatopause).

More astute physicians are now recognizing the intermediate degrees of GH deficiency, which result as we slowly age (before extreme deficiency is reached in the very aged). GH therapy is providing these people with a new sense of well-being and youth. HGH appears to be the silver bullet of life extension.

What Dose of GH Should a Person Take?

1. **Monotherapy.** Here treatment consists only of GH. In this case, the dose of GH varies between 0.5 and 2 IU per day.

2. **Polytherapy.** In this case, GH is combined with other hormone replacement therapy, including melatonin, sex hormones, thyroid hormones, and so on. In this mixed form of therapy (our preference), we can provide a lower dose of GH (0.5–1 IU per day). Not only do we see a synergistic effect of hormones with this combination, but also there is more rejuvenation and greater safety. Treatment is best provided daily just before bedtime, which helps mimic the time surge of GH.

Good nutrition (especially protein); decreasing coffee, nicotine, and alcohol; regular exercise; and sleep will also improve GH levels.

How Is HGH Administered?

Because HGH is a protein, it cannot withstand the trip through the digestive system where stomach acids and enzymes will break it down. Also, there is no evidence to support the theory that it can be absorbed through the skin or the mucous membranes of the mouth. In the freeze-dried form, it can be kept at room temperature, but once dissolved, it must be refrigerated and has a shelf life of two weeks. So, as with insulin, HGH must be injected. It is usually administered at night, or at least two hours before or after a meal, for six days out of seven.

Risks of GH Therapy

The most frequent problems are retention of fluid, such as swelling feet, carpal-tunnel syndrome, and (rarely) joint pains. If any of these symptoms appear, the daily dose should be decreased.

TABLE 9.4. Our Recommended Basic HRT Program

WOMEN		MEN	
Melatonin	40–50 years: 1 mg at bedtime 50–70 years: 2 mg at bedtime 70+ years: 3 mg at bedtime	Melatonin	40–50 years: 1 mg at bedtime 50–70 years: 2 mg at bedtime 70+ years: 3 mg at bedtime
Thyroid*	$1/2$–1 g Armour thyroid (if temperature less 97.6)	Thyroid*	$1/2$–1 g Armour thyroid (if temperature less 97.6)
DHEA	10 mg in A.M.	DHEA	25 mg in A.M.
Pregnenolone	100 mg (micronized) in A.M.	Pregnenolone	100 mg (micronized) in A.M.
Thymus extract	(Individual measure needed)	Thymus extract	(Individual measure needed)
Estrogen/ progesterone*	(Individual measure needed)		
Testosterone*	(Individual measure needed)	Testosterone*	(Individual measure needed)
Growth hormone*	(Individual measure needed)	Growth hormone*	(Individual measure needed)

* Denotes hormones that should be measured. HRT with these hormones needs to be individualized under the supervision of a practitioner skilled in hormone replacement therapy. All hormones mentioned can be ordered from Medaus Pharmacy or Eternity Medicine (*see* Resources and Medi-Spa Directory).

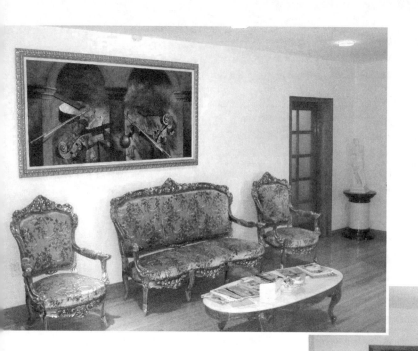

*Photos courtesy of MeSuá
Dermocosmetic Spa.*

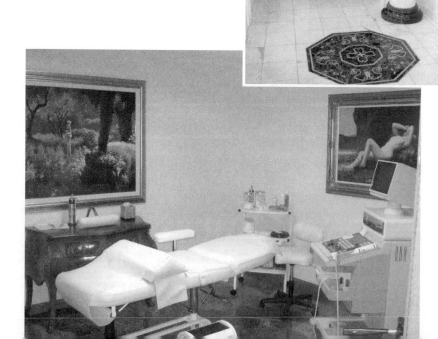

Chapter 10

Secret Four —
Beauty Inside Out

The most effective way to reduce wrinkles
is to reduce inflammation in the skin.

—Dr. Barry Sears

In this last chapter, we want to share our spa-medicine beauty program with you. Our clients, including those at Miami's MeSuá Dermocosmetic Spa directed by Dr. Suárez-Menéndez, most often not only want to feel better, but also want to look better. First, we introduce you to the skin and let you know the main reasons why the skin ages and wrinkles, and then we show you what you can do to manage this.

The skin is the largest organ of the human body. It is 15 percent of the total body weight. On average, one square inch of the skin is made up of the following:

- 65 hairs;
- 100 sebaceous glands;
- 78 yards of nerves;
- 1,300 nerve endings;

- 20,000 sensory cells;
- 650 sweat glands;
- 19 yards of blood vessels;
- 9,500,000 cells.

ANATOMY OF THE SKIN

The skin consists of three layers: (1) the epidermis; (2) the dermis; (3) the subcutaneous (fat) layer. (*See* Figure 10.1 on page 206.)

1. The Epidermis

The epidermis is the outermost layer of skin. It is one-tenth of one millimeter thick (half the thickness of a regular sheet of paper). The major purpose of the epidermis is to form the stratum cornium, a layer of dead cells that acts as a barrier between the body and the environment. Essentially, it acts as a barrier to water loss and is resistant to chemical, physical, and bacterial insults.

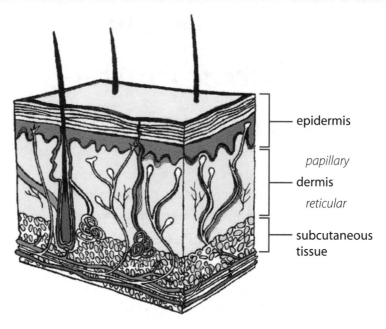

epidermis

papillary
dermis
reticular

subcutaneous
tissue

Figure 10.1. Anatomy of the Skin

Eighty to 90 percent of the epidermis is made up of cells called *keratinocytes*, which are formed in the basal (bottom) layer, one of four layers in the epidermis. Approximately half of these cells migrate up to the top layer, the stratum corneum, where they are known as *corneocyte cells*. The keratinocyte cells develop in a process called *mitosis* (cell reproduction), which occurs at the same rate that the corneocyte cells are lost. The usual time for this migration from the basal layer to exfoliation at the skin's surface is six weeks. If the skin is injured (peels, dermabrasion, etc.), the production of keratinocyte cells at the base level increases dramatically.

Melanocytes (melanin pigment cells) are also found in the basal layer of the epidermis and are connected to approximately thirty or forty keratinocyte cells by fingerlike projections. When the melanin pigment cells move through these projections into the keratinocyte cells, they form a protective cap over the nucleus (DNA) of the cells and protect them from UV light.

Two other cell types are found in the epidermis. Langerhans cells (3 to 5 percent of the cells) originate in the bone marrow and are important for immune regulation. They play a role in delayed skin hypersensitivity, as do Merkel's tactile cells, which are felt to play a role in skin sensation generally.

Types of Epidermis and Exposure to the Sun

There are six common ways that different types of epidermal layers react to sun exposure.

Type 1. Always burns—doesn't tan;

Type 2. Easily burns—doesn't tan;

Type 3. Can burn, but tans gradually;

Type 4. Burns minimally and tans easily;

Type 5. Rarely burns and tans quickly;

Type 6. Never burns.

UV Index Scale for Exposure to the Sun

- 0–2 Minimal UV: One hour of repeated sun exposure will produce sunburn on the average person's skin.

- 3–4 Low UV: 45 minutes of repeated sun exposure will produce sunburn on the average person's skin.

- 5–6 Moderate UV: 30 minutes of repeated sun exposure will produce sunburn on the average person's skin.

- 7–8 High UV: 15 minutes of repeated sun exposure will produce sunburn on the average person's skin.

- 10+ Very High UV: 10 minutes of repeated sun exposure will produce sunburn on the average person's skin.

The Three Types of UV Rays

There are three types of UV rays—UVA, UVB, and UVC.

UVA rays. These are the *second* strongest burning rays of the sun (320–400 nm long wavelength—an nm is a nanometer, which is one-billionth of a meter) and they penetrate through the skin's epidermis into the dermis (*see* Figure 10.2 on page 208). Through free-radical action, they primarily damage the dermis. They also break down collagen and elastin, which are the connective tissues that keep skin firm and young. UVA rays, which penetrate deeper into the skin's layer than UVB rays, are associated with premature aging, skin cancer, and wrinkling of the skin. UVA rays maintain their intensity and wrinkle-causing effects throughout daylight hours all year long.

UVB rays. These rays damage the epidermis (*see* Figure 10.2 on page 208). It is the UVB wavelength (290–320 nm medium wavelength) that causes the tanning

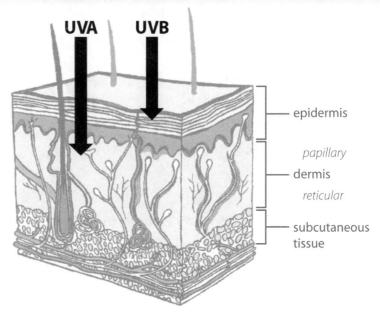

Figure 10.2. Skin Penetration of UVA and UVB Rays

response, and is responsible for sunburn and skin cancer. The UVB medium wavelength rays, the *third* strongest type of rays, are most pronounced between 10 A.M. and 3 P.M. They can cause premature cataracts and disrupt circulation and blood flow, which eventually leads to the clumps of darkened cells that cause age spots on the skin. UVB rays also increase the potential risk for multiple types of skin cancer. They are more intense during summer months, at higher altitudes, and in locations closer to the equator.

UVC rays. These are the worst, most dangerous types of rays (200–270 nm short wavelength). We are protected from their damage by the ozone layer, without which we would not be able to exist on earth. However, 2 to 3 percent of the ozone layer has already been depleted as a result of pollution. With time, it is hoped that this depletion can be reversed and that the layer can be regenerated to its full protective strength.

2. The Dermis

The dermis consists of two layers—the upper papillary dermis (blood supply) and the lower reticular dermis (strength and elasticity). Unlike the epidermis, the dermis has few cells—its master cells are called fibroblasts—and is composed mainly of connective tissue, collagen fibers, and elastin fibers. In addition to producing collagen, elastin, and connective tissue, the fibroblasts also control the turnover of connective tissue by producing enzymes that degrade collagen (collagenases), elastin (elastases), and glycosaminoglycans (GAGs—glyosomal hydrolases) to make room for new versions of these substances, important because their presence is paramount in maintaining youthful skin.

3. The Subcutaneous (Fat) Layer

The innermost layer of the skin contains a single layer of fat that helps protect the internal organs. Blood vessels, nerves, and lymph vessels can be found here.

WHY SKIN AGES

As we age, a number of changes take place in the skin. Beginning at birth with the transition from a water to an air environment, and going on to changes in hormonal levels, diet, and antioxidant levels, environmental toxins, illness, photo-aging (sun damage), trauma, and other lifestyle factors—all these play a role in aging the skin. And all this aging (blemishes, pigmentation, sagging skin, wrinkles, etc.) can be slowed, and often reversed, by using our spa-medicine beauty program.

When we look at children, we notice that their skin is firm, smooth, and supple. This is because the skin is well-hydrated, well-oxygenated, and well-nourished. All the skin cells function properly and epidermal turnover occurs every two to four weeks (as compared to nine to twelve weeks in adults). This is partly due to blood flow and partly due to the higher concentrations of glycosaminoglycans (GAGs) in the basement membranes of the epidermis and dermis. These

Types of Skin Cancers

Basal cell carcinoma. This is the most common type, affecting close to 95 percent of all those with skin cancer. As the prevalent type, it affects more than 1 million people per year.

Squamous cell carcinoma. This is the second most common type of skin cancer and is more serious than basal cell carcinoma. Squamous cell carcinoma can be responsible for facial deformity and also has the ability to spread to the rest of the body.

Melanoma. This is the third, and most serious, type of skin cancer, causing over 10,000 deaths a year in the United States. It manifests as a regular mole or nevi (birthmark) with tan or brownish spots and irregular borders. It has a hard texture and may cause itching and slight bleeding. More than accidents or cancer, this is the number-one killer of females between the ages of twenty-five and thirty.

complex sugar-protein molecules can bind up to 1,000 times their weight in water and thereby keep the skin well-hydrated. In addition to their water-binding characteristics, they also provide a pathway for the diffusion of nutrients throughout the body.

As noted, skin aging is mostly the result of inflammation and decreasing blood flow as, in fact, are most chronic diseases of aging in general. Inflammation and decreased blood flow are primarily the result of poor diet and hormonal imbalance. So, in addition to good skin care, a comprehensive skin program must focus on improving these essential elements.

Inflammation

The major cause of skin aging is inflammation. As a medical student, dermatologist Nicholas Perricone was intrigued when he saw biopsies of skin that showed signs of aging. In every such case, inflammation was present, and skin that showed no signs of aging also showed no inflammation.

To understand this, we have to take a look at how and why we age. The most widely accepted theory of aging is the free-radical theory. Its originator, Denham Harman (*see* Chapter 6), first postulated that, at a cellular level, free radicals (unpaired molecules, missing one of their two electrons, that roam the body to try and take another electron from any nearby molecule, leaving damage in their wake) were responsible for severe damage. Most scientists believed then that the cystosol (inner core of the cell) was the site of this free-radical damage. Dr. Imre Zs-Nagy, a Hungarian scientist (*see* Chapter 6) came along and disagreed. He felt that free radicals were doing the most damage on the *outside* of the cell—on the cell's membrane. He knew that the cell membrane must remain fluid to function properly, but that, as we age, these membranes stiffen and lose their fluidity so that receptors for hormones and neurotransmitters cannot function—nutrients cannot get in and waste products cannot get out. This is how the cell ages.

When Nicholas Perricone studied the situation, he recognized that, although the cell membrane is a free-radical shield, it is also a source of inflammatory chemicals that are very destructive if they get inside the cell. When the phospholipids (fats containing phosphorous in the cell membrane) break down, they produce a fatty acid called *arachidonic acid* that oxidizes the fats. Some of these fats convert to aldehydes (chemical compounds obtained by oxidation) and other toxic chemicals that trigger an inflammatory cascade.

In summary, a threefold cyclic process occurs:

1. A burst of free radicals attacks the cell membrane;

2. The cell membrane produces proinflammatory chemicals;

3. These proinflammatory chemicals produce more free radicals.

A Note of Caution

The cosmetic industry's solution to aging skin is a mass-marketing campaign that encourages women to apply moisturizers, which are in reality very damaging to the skin. These cosmetic products lack the ability to penetrate cells, a result of poor delivery systems. Because of these faulty delivery systems, moisturizers clog the pores and sebaceous glands, which causes acne, prevents exfoliation of the skin, and leads to a dramatic slowdown in cell turnover, which causes the skin to thin out. Inferior moisturizers also hinder the skin's ability to breathe, and dramatically decrease the number of GAGs. The final result is that the deeper layers of the skin dehydrate, and the transfer of nutrients is hindered by the degeneration of GAGs. It is, instead, recommended that results-oriented skin products be used, such as the MeSuá Dermasystem, which contains two patent-pending elements—one for its formulation, and the other for its delivery system. For more information, visit www.mesua.com.

When free radicals penetrate the cell membrane in the skin and overwhelm the cell's defenses (oxidative stress), certain factors are activated that produce toxic chemicals. These include collagenases, which will digest collagen and result in microscars in the skin that lead to skin aging. By protecting the cell membrane and the cell itself from oxidative stress, inflammation can be minimized and we can prevent the skin from aging. Proper nutrition, supplements, and hormonal balance are essential for this protection.

Decreased Blood Flow

Arteries, veins, and millions of capillaries in your body total over 60,000 miles in length and equal the area of a football field. This blood-vessel system has the task of providing oxygen and nutrients to literally every cell of the body. If blood flow to the skin is impaired, millions of its cells cease to function properly.

Heart disease is the number-one killer of American men and women, and the real underlying cause of heart disease is not cholesterol but, like aging skin, a decrease in blood flow and inflammation. Fifty percent of the people hospitalized for heart attacks have completely normal cholesterol levels, and 25 percent have no traditional risk factors at all.

Both inflammation and blood flow result from an increased production of bad eicosanoid hormones, as mentioned previously, and you can decrease them by eating a moderate-carbohydrate diet (such as the Zone) and supplementing with high-grade fish oils. (The idea that fish oils decrease inflammation was first proposed by studies on Eskimos in Greenland who had virtually no heart disease, even though they consumed a very high-fat diet.) Outside of high-quality fish oils, no other nutrients can promote regeneration of the skin and improve blood flow to it as quickly or as profoundly as hydrophobic GLA. This is a key ingredient in all Zone skincare products, and it can dramatically stave off the biomarkers of aging.

Certain other nutrients, such as vitamins C and E, beta-carotene, coenzyme Q_{10}, grapeseed extract, and Pycnogenol, all help decrease inflammation through their antioxidant function. (Aspirin and statin drugs reduce the risk of heart disease primarily by decreasing the inflammation at a cellular level; aspirin also increases certain good eicosanoids).

YOUR SPA-MEDICINE BEAUTY PROGRAM

This program has benefits for your inner and your outer beauty.

I. Inner Beauty

The eight categories outlined below are designed to help you bring out your inner beauty.

1. Detoxify

As part of the comprehensive spa-medicine beauty program (*see* Figure 10.3 on page 213), it is essential to detoxify the body on a regular basis. Many of these principles have been outlined in Chapter 2. You should review those detox therapies, especially those dealing with the skin.

2. Zone Diet

Once you accept that your everyday lifestyle choices affect the way you age, you are on your way to restoring your beauty and vitality. Food is your single most powerful antiaging tool. Sugar and high-glycemic, refined carbohydrates create inflammation on a cellular basis throughout your body. Whenever sugar increases, you get insulin release, storage of body fat, and an excess of bad eicosanoids (free radicals). As certain foods rapidly convert to sugar in the bloodstream, they cause browning, or glycating, of proteins. When glycation occurs in your skin, sugar molecules attach themselves to the collagen fibers and cause cross-linking, which also causes a major loss of skin elasticity. Healthy collagen strands normally slide over each other, which keeps the skin elastic.

Sugar can also attach to components in the cell membrane, forming chemicals called *advanced glycosalation end products,* producing free radicals, therefore

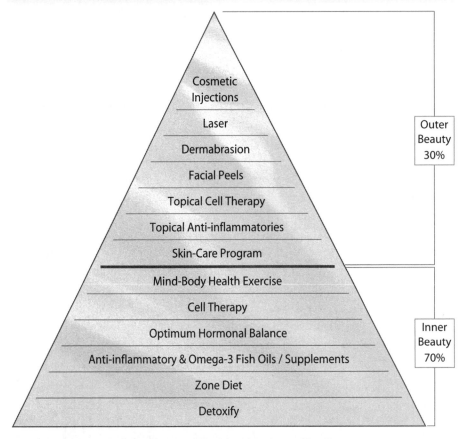

Figure 10.3. Spa-Medicine Beauty Program

inflammation and premature aging. A Zone diet will control excess insulin and the inflammation associated with it. To stay young and beautiful, we need to have a slow, steady release of insulin in our bodies. Tobacco and alcohol are proinflammatory—alcohol should be kept to a minimum and tobacco should be eliminated. Finally, most of us are constantly dehydrated. If we are even mildly dehydrated, our metabolism drops, which will result in a pound weight gain every six months. It is therefore vital to drink at least six to eight glasses of water a day.

Healthy skin, like a healthy heart, starts with a good diet. There is a mountain of evidence to show that certain foods can indeed help delay skin aging. In one particularly intriguing study, investigators compared the skin evaluations of Greek subjects living in Melbourne, Australia; Greeks living in rural Greece; Anglo-Celtic Australians living in Melbourne; and Swedes living in Goteborg,

Sweden. The data in these evaluations was collected through interviews, viewer-administrative questionnaires, clinical histories, and physical examinations. Participants were asked how frequently they ate specified foods over the previous year. When all the data were in, there were some interesting correlations. For example, the top three foods for skin health, according to studies, were prunes, apples, and black tea. The top three for your heart, according to other research, were onions, apples, and tea. This is really no coincidence. Prunes and dates contain some of the highest antioxidant levels of any foods. Meanwhile, apples and tea are abundant in quercetin, a vital phytonutrient (plant nutrient) that interrupts the oxidation of LDL cholesterol. An analysis of the pooled data from this skin study indicated that a high intake of olive oil, legumes, fish, vegetables, and dried fruits that some participants ate appeared to be protective against the accelerated aging of the skin that occurs from long-term sun damage.

By contrast, a high intake of processed meats, dairy products, and sugar that others ate appear to be the most detrimental to the skin. It was also interesting to note that the older Swedish people, who consumed more vegetable dishes and eggs, and drank mostly water, while eating very little bread, had the least amount of skin damage. Based on this data, researchers speculate that olive oil, beans, and vegetables protect skin from excessive oxidation.

To summarize, foods associated with the least amount of photo-aging are apples, asparagus, celery, cherries, dried fruits, eggplant, eggs, fish, garlic, grapes, leeks, legumes, lima beans, melon, nuts, olives, onions, pears, prunes, spinach, tea, and water. The worst offenders, in terms of premature aging, or the food associated with the greatest amount of photo-aging, are cakes and pastries, cordials, full-fat milk, potatoes, processed meats, and soft drinks. So if you believe in clinical research, avoid the cakes, pastries, sugars, and soft drinks and you'll enhance the health not only of your skin, but also of your heart.

3. Anti-Inflammatory Supplements (Nutraceuticals)

Certain nutrients and antioxidants can penetrate into the cell where they can combat free radicals and decrease inflammation. The right supplements are an essential part of your skin and longevity program. Core Zone nutraceutical supplements contain (in addition to many multivitamins and minerals) some ingredients that are especially beneficial to the skin. They include the fourteen supplements listed below.

1. Acetyl L-carnitine

2. Alpha-lipoic acid

3. Coenzyme Q_{10}

4. Gamma linolenic acid

5. Glucosamine

6. Glutamine

7. Grapeseed extract

8. L-carnitine

9. Mucopolysaccharides

10. Oral collagen

11. Pycnogenol

12. Turmeric

13. Vitamin C

14. Vitamin E

4. Omega Oils

The omega-6 oils found in borage oil and evening primrose oil are also good for the skin. Their active ingredients are derived from linoleic acid, and one component, gamma linolenic acid (GLA), has been shown to lower triglycerides and raise the good HDL cholesterol. Both omega-6 and omega-3 oils, in the ideal one to one ratio, help control hormones, such as the bad eicosanoids, cortisol, and norepinephrine, which, like cortisol, is elevated by stress, again demonstrating that food acts as a powerful drug, affecting all aspects of our cells. GLA is rapidly converted to prostaglandin E_1, a potent anti-inflammatory agent.

5. Optimum Hormonal Balance

Many of the hormones discussed in Chapter 9 play an important role in slowing the skin's aging rate. They include DHEA, estrogen, progesterone, melatonin, testosterone, thymus, and thyroid hormones. Growth hormone has been shown to increase both skin texture and thickness, and improve skin elasticity. In some cases, even gray hair has regained a more youthful, black appearance.

6. Cell Therapy

Biological therapy for the skin is available by injection or by mouth. There is also evidence from clinical studies to show that topical cell therapy (Cellusana—*see ahead* in chapter) can have a beneficial effect on the skin. (*See also* Appendix G.)

7. Exercise and Electrical Stimulation

Studies have shown that exercise will help the skin in much the same way that it benefits muscle and bone health. The skin of athletes is thicker and has more collagen. All aspects of exercise—aerobic conditioning, flexibility, and muscle strength training—can promote skin health as well as an overall sense of well-being. Growth hormone is also released by exercise and it improves skin health. A healthy heart and lungs increase oxygen and other vital nutrients to the skin. A regular, moderate workout is ideal to reduce the level of cortisol and free radicals that can age the skin.

Light electrical stimulation of the muscles of the face also seems to help create beautiful skin. For optimum results, Dr. Suárez-Menéndez particularly recommends a DMAE cream applied with ultrasound at 3 megahertz for five minutes.

8. Mind-Body Health

Someone once said that, after the age of forty, we are all responsible for our face. For example, if you look in the mirror, you could very well have furrows across your brow (worry lines) or between your eyebrows (anger lines). Dealing with stress and maintaining a sense of equanimity is important for skin health.

II. Outer Beauty—Antiaging Remedies

These eight categories of maintenance can give your skin glowing good health and beauty.

1. Skin-Care Program

A good home program pays attention to cleansing, exfoliating, hydrating, repairing, and toning. In addition, you should always protect yourself from sun damage.

Protecting Yourself from the Sun

After years of research, it has been found that the best strategies for sun protection are the following:

1. Avoid sun exposure during the most intense part of the day, from 10 A.M. to 4 P.M.

2. Try to cover up. An act as simple as wearing a broad-brimmed hat can significantly reduce the sun's shining on parts of the body where skin cancer is most common (ears, lips, and nose). Wear long sleeves as well.

3. When the above is inadequate (especially at a pool or the beach), apply a broad-spectrum high or maximum sunblock to your face, each arm, and exposed areas of the shoulders and neck (when wearing an open-necked T-shirt). Apply the equivalent of 1 to 2 teaspoons to each leg, and 2 teaspoons to the upper body when you expose more skin.

4. Be aware of your skin. If you notice signs of short-term reddening or longer-term photo-aging (wrinkling or dryness), it is best to avoid further exposure to sunlight (even in the absence of such signs, it is a good idea to minimize your exposure).

5. Visit a dermatologist or a plastic surgeon on a regular basis.

2. Topical Anti-inflammatories

Alpha-lipoic acid (ALA): This universal antioxidant is both water and fat soluble. This means that ALA is easily absorbed through the skin and works well as a free-radical fighter, both in the cell plasma membranes and in the water interior of the cell.

Vitamin C ester: This consists of basic vitamin C joined with palmitic acid, a fatty acid derived from palm oil. The antioxidant power of vitamin C ester at the cell membrane provides key protection. Research by Proctor & Gamble shows that vitamin C ester is absorbed more quickly, and achieves seven times higher levels of C in the skin, than the basic vitamin C.

DMAE: Loss of skin tone and sagging is due in part to the decline of neurotransmitters, such as acetylcholine, that stimulate muscle contraction. As we age, we lose this tone, which results in sagging skin. Studies have shown that DMAE lotion will tone your skin for eighteen to twenty-four hours, and will cause an immediate reduction in lines and wrinkles.

Olive oil: We have already mentioned the important role of extra-virgin olive oil in your diet. However, since ancient times, olive oil has been used as an emollient that is massaged on the skin. All historical records on the subject indicate that the Romans had beautiful skin, thanks to olive oil's powerful antioxidant and anti-inflammatory properties. Antioxidants known as polyphenols are contained in olive oil. They are stable and protective, and give skin a smoother, more radiant appearance.

Polyenylphosphatidyl choline (PPC): PPC offers protection to the cell membrane. It can rapidly penetrate the skin and soften it while acting as a powerful anti-inflammatory. PPC is a natural moisturizer, which can reduce flaking and cracking in a matter of days.

Sunblock: Since everyone is now aware of how damaging the sun's rays can be, it is vital to use a high-protection sunblock beginning at an early age. This is the key to preventing wrinkling, premature cataracts, and multiple skin cancers (which can cause death). The main ingredients to look for in such formulations are aloe vera, zinc oxide (micronized), phospholipids, titanium dioxide (micronized), grapeseed extract, wine leaf extract, green tea extract, sodium ascorbyl phosphate, vitamin E tocopherol, vitamin A palmitate, and mushroom extract. These ingredients will soften your skin and shelter it from critical moisture loss, while at the same time protecting you from aging and the damaging rays that can cause skin cancer.

Tocotrienols—super vitamin E: This fat-soluble nutrient is a powerful antioxidant and moisturizer. Vitamin E is made up of two separate categories: tocopherols and tocotrienols. This new super vitamin E is proving significantly stronger as an antioxidant than tocopherols. It is able to make hair shinier, reduce redness and flaking in dry skin, and prevent nails from cracking.

Topical vitamins (antioxidants): MeSuá Dermasystem Vita-ACE Reparative

Youth Serum contains, in order of amounts, vitamins A, C, and E; DMAE; zinc; coenzymeQ_{10}; lipoic acid; and retinoic acid. These powerful components increase and stimulate the activity of ATP (adenosine triphosphate), which in turn increases the energy of the tissues in the skin.

3. Topical Treatment—Cell Therapy (Cellusana)

Cosmetic treatment, using Cellusana fresh cell-extract cosmetics, is a scientifically tested biological treatment that uses juvenile components of animals to repair and rejuvenate damaged cells and cell structures. One application a day helps promote the beauty, longevity, and toning of your skin, and reduces the negative effects of aging, pollution, stress, and sun. See www.eternitymedicine.com for information on Cellusana.

4. Facials

It is recommended that extractions, masks, massages, and steam, in addition to the usual cleaning, exfoliation, hydrating, toning, and repair be done by a trained professional aesthetician. A nurturing environment at a medical spa directed by a doctor is ideal.

5. Chemical Peels

There are various facial peels to choose from, such as alpha-hydroxy acids (AHA), beta-hydroxy acids (BHA), Jessner, or Obaji peels. Medical-strength chemical peels, such as the alpha and beta hydroxy, vary in intensity, depending on the different percentages and different pHs used. For example, you are able to achieve a medium peel of the skin after doing a recommended average series of six peels (one per week). This will improve your skin's appearance and texture by removing superficial and medium wrinkles, diminishing acne marks, scars, and stretch marks, and improving depressed pits. This type of peel can also be done on the

A Note on MeSuá Dermasystem and Zone Cosmeceuticals

Spa Medicine recommends these antiaging skin products because they contain many of the nutrients that combat free radicals, and they reduce the inflammation responsible for skin's aging. The latest medical science, and over twelve years of research and testing has produced the line of MeSuá Dermasystem and Zone Cosmeceuticals. They can be reviewed by going to www.mesua.com or www.zonecafe.com.

neck and chest area, and on the hands. With a deeper peel, such as the modified phenol, which uses a lower percentage of phenol, you will be able to remove the deeper facial lines that come with aging. As always, after undergoing any of the above-mentioned procedures, it is highly advisable to use a high-protection facial sunblock.

The MeSuá Peel: This is a combination of dermabrasion, chemical peel, and the infusion of a serum composed of topical antioxidants and applied with ultrasound.

For best results, a series of six treatments is recommended. The benefits of the MeSuá peel include the following:

1. Reduction of acne scars and surgical scars;

2. Reduction of age spots;

3. Reduction of minor-to-moderate early-aging fine lines;

4. Stimulation to promote collagen reproduction;

5. Overall rejuvenation of the skin.

6. Microdermabrasion

Microdermabrasion is a technique that exfoliates the uppermost layers of the skin with precise control. The goal is to progressively treat and promote the cell renewal process, thereby stimulating the production of new cells. This will improve the skin's elasticity and texture, and result in fresher, healthier skin that looks better.

7. Laser Treatments

Laser treatments should be performed by a trained plastic or dermatology surgeon who adheres to the standards set by the American National Standards Institute, the benchmark standards for safe laser use in the United States. The ANSI standards are written up in a sixty-two-page document that covers nine control measures, and is an excellent guide for anyone setting up a laser safety program.

The scientific basis for laser safety is based on the measurement of potential exposure risks identified with each laser's wavelength. Each wavelength interacts differently with different biological tissue, meaning each laser has different risk factors for different tissues. Risk assessment is assigned by how the laser's wavelength interacts with tissue, how it interacts when it strikes a reflective surface, whether it has the potential for flammability, and whether there is potential damage to eye or skin. Each wavelength also has a maximum permissible exposure, which is the amount of light the eye can accept, without eyewear, before injury.

Control measures are required for medical lasers. Standard measures include the appointment of a safety officer, controlled access to the entryway where the laser is used, and wearing protective eyewear.

Depending on the wavelength and pulse duration, there are different lasers for different conditions and treatments, such as for removing acne, birthmarks, lesions, tattoos, or wrinkles, removing bulging leg veins or sun damage, and resurfacing the face.

8. Cosmetic Injections

Plastic surgery remains the cornerstone of facial rejuvenation. However, these are exciting times, and we can now bring in other options, such as the use of dermal fillers between surgical procedures, that can delay surgery and enhance existing surgical procedures with such nonsurgical procedures as collagen injections, fat injections, and Perlane and Restylane, which are fillers for the face, lasting about three months.

Lastly, there are Botox injections. Botox is nothing short of a major breakthrough in fighting the aging process. It is safe, effective, noninvasive, yet long-lasting. In the 1970s, Dr. Alan Scott, a pediatric ophthalmologist, pioneered the use of the drug to treat problems relating to vision. In 1992, a husband and wife ophthalmologist/dermatologist team first published their use of Botox for cosmetic purposes. From here, the field of Botox advanced rapidly. In 2002, there were over 2.4 million Botox injections in the United States alone. On April 15, 2002, Botox received FDA approval. Once clients have followed our antiaging program for a few months, we select them for either a deep chemical peel or Botox to smooth wrinkles from the skin. Botox is one of the few rejuvenating treatments that can benefit patients of almost any age. It is also a preventive procedure against aging because it will prevent the wrinkles that result from constantly frowning or raising the eyebrows.

Afterword

Eternity Medicine

Eternity Medicine is about our awareness of the non-local nature
of our mind; that it is infinite, indestructible, and immortal.

A number of years ago, Dr. Simpson sent his friend, Dr. Larry Dossey, a manuscript he wrote, dividing medicine into three historical eras. He had adapted his idea from John Wheeler, a physicist who once described the development of physics through three major eras. Dr. Dossey reciprocated Dr. Simpson's gesture by sending him a chapter from a book *he* had just finished. Coincidentally, also following Wheeler's conceptual structure, Dr. Dossey had, himself, drawn up three eras of medicine (*see* the table on page 222).

You will see that, unlike ERA I and ERA II medicine, which are grounded in constructs of time, ERA III medicine resides in eternity: a space-free and time-free continuum. We like to call this third era of medicine *Eternity Medicine* because it denotes the infinite nature of consciousness and regards immortality as a given.

Consciousness itself has developed from a simple phase (in animals) to a self-reflective ego consciousness (in humans). At present, it is evolving toward a new integral consciousness, the chief manifestations of which are wisdom, wonder, and joy—very different from the loneliness and alienation felt by most contemporary people in today's world.

Looking at the table, you can see that spa medicine readily embraces ERA I medicine. The wellness pillars of detoxification, exercise, and Zone nutrition all currently exist in the better medi-spas. And the four secrets of longevity (inflammation reduction, nutraceutical supplementation, hormone replacement therapy, and cosmeceutical application) are also found in many medi-spa treatment programs.

Spa medicine embraces ERA II medicine as well. Many spas incorporate various mind-body therapies, such as biofeedback, imagery, meditation, and psychoneuroimmunology, as part of the total spa program.

Few spas, however, utilize ERA III medicine. As individual awareness of this emerging integral consciousness grows, humanity will eventually recognize that the mind is unified and infinite in space and time—thus consciousness is omnipresent, eternal, and, ultimately, one.

MEDICAL ERAS		
ERA I Local	**ERA II Local**	**ERA III Nonlocal**
Mechanical, material, or physical medicine	Mind-body medicine	Nonlocal or transpersonal medicine
Casual, deterministic, describable by classical concepts of space, time, and matter energy. Mind not a factor; mind is a result of brain mechanisms.	Mind is a major factor in *healing within the single person*. Mind has causal power, is thus not fully explainable by classical concepts in physics. Includes, but goes beyond, Era I.	Mind is a factor in healing both *within and between people*. Mind not completely localized to points in space (brain or bodies) or time (present moment or single lifetimes). Mind is unbounded and infinite in space and time, thus omnipresent, eternal, and ultimately one. Healing at a distance is possible. Not describable by classical concepts of space, time, or matter energy.
Any form of therapy focusing solely on the effects of things on the body are Era I approaches—including techniques such as acupuncture and homeopathy. The uses of modern medicine—drugs, surgery, irradiation, CPR, etc. are included.	Any therapy emphasizing the effects of consciousness solely within the individual body is an ERA II approach. Psychoneuroimmunology, counseling, hypnosis, and most type of imagery-based alternative therapies are included.	Any therapy in which the effects of consciousness bridge between different persons is an Era III approach. All forms of distal healing, intercessory prayer, some types of shamanic healing, diagnosis at a distance, telesomatic events, and probably noncontact therapeutic touch are included.

Larry Dossey, M.D. For a detailed description of the three medical ERAS, refer to *Recovering the Soul.*

As physicians, we have come to recognize that this ordering of consciousness, or worldview, may be more important than all the wellness and longevity lifestyle choices a person makes. Worldview, in fact, may be the single most important ingredient for well-being.

Essentially, integral health (*see* Appendix A) is the process through which we humans achieve well-being by the ordering of consciousness. Remembering is central to this process and includes the integration of our species and our own psychohistorical development. (Ontogeny recapitulates phylogeny.)

Just over 500 years ago, during the Renaissance, an unmistakable reorganization in our consciousness occurred. It was the discovery of perspective, which opened up 3-D space. Besides illuminating space, perspective brings to man's (in this context, *man* encompasses both genders) awareness the envisioning of himself. Perspective provides a distance between man and objects. Man's conception of himself as a subject is based on his objectification of the world around him.

Man's previous lack of spatial awareness accompanies his lack of ego consciousness. In order to objectify and qualify space, a self-conscious *I* that is able to stand opposite or confront space is required. From about A.D. 1250 onward, therefore, man has grown: he perceives the world with self-consciousness rather than from a primitive, simple consciousness.

At medi-spas, we often illustrate this abstract process of the ordering of consciousness with art history. Simply pick up any art-history book and leaf through it—perceiving the progression of artistic expression throughout history, note how man's depictions of himself in relation to his surroundings evolve.

Jean Gebser describes this evolution of consciousness in his book *The Ever Present Origin*. Gebser notes that the unperspectival era (the one *without* perspective) is roughly from 5,000,000 to 2,000 B.C., and the perspectival era (the one *with* perspective) runs from 2,000 B.C. to the present. We are just now experiencing a new aperspectival era, he says, writing that, "With each mutation of consciousness, origin acquires an intensified conscious character of presentness; origin, which bears the imprint of the whole and of the spiritual, and is before time and space, becomes time-free *present*. It is the aperspectival world that acquires this ever-present origin and thereby supersedes the perspectival world."

Just as a novel understanding of space gave birth to self-consciousness, a new understanding of time is now giving birth to the integral structure of consciousness. Only where time emerges as pure present and is no longer divided into its three phases of past, present, and future is it concrete. Artists like Picasso and scientists like Einstein recognized this new manifestation of time and space.

For those interested in a more complete understanding of the different structures of consciousness, you can refer to www.eternitymedicine.com. It is a vital part of the goal of every integral physician, who, as an "eternist," seeks to help the client toward a reordering of his worldview. As Larry Dossey has written, we must help clients realize that they exist within a *process* of space-time, they are not isolated entities adrift in linear time, moving slowly to extermination. We wish to impart this knowledge of the interconnectedness in life, and to the extent that we accomplish this task, we are truly healers.

Eternity Medicine can now be recognized and experienced by understanding and integrating the various structures of consciousness. This remembering (anamnesis) results in a space-free/time-free (nonlocal) worldview where the spiritual flowing present is deeply felt and experienced.

With a single, subtle voice, science, art, and the great spiritual traditions all communicate this notion today—that each of us is infinite, immortal, and indestructible. Eternity Medicine is the ageless zone.

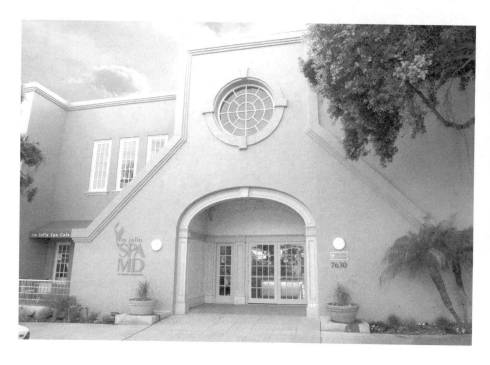

Photos courtesy of La Jolla Spa MD.

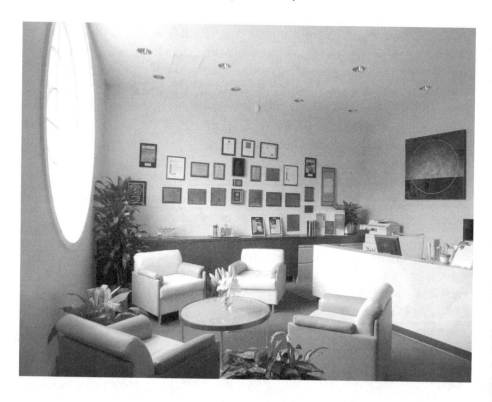

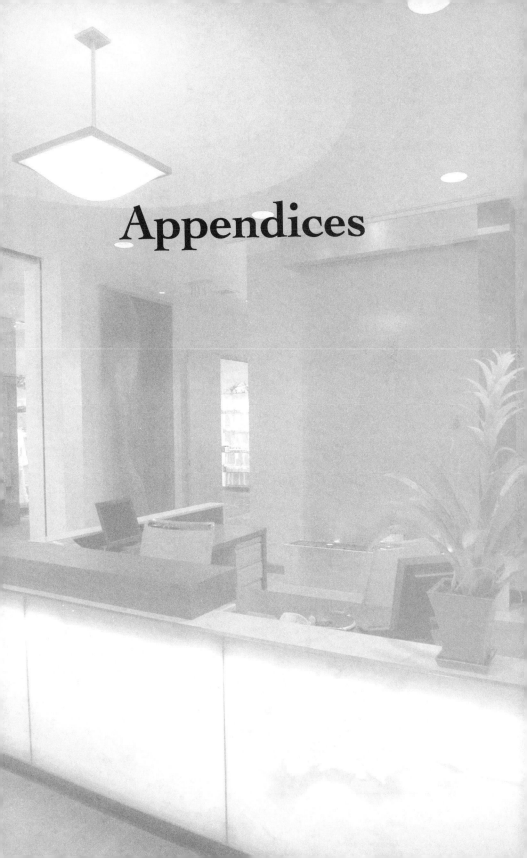

Appendices

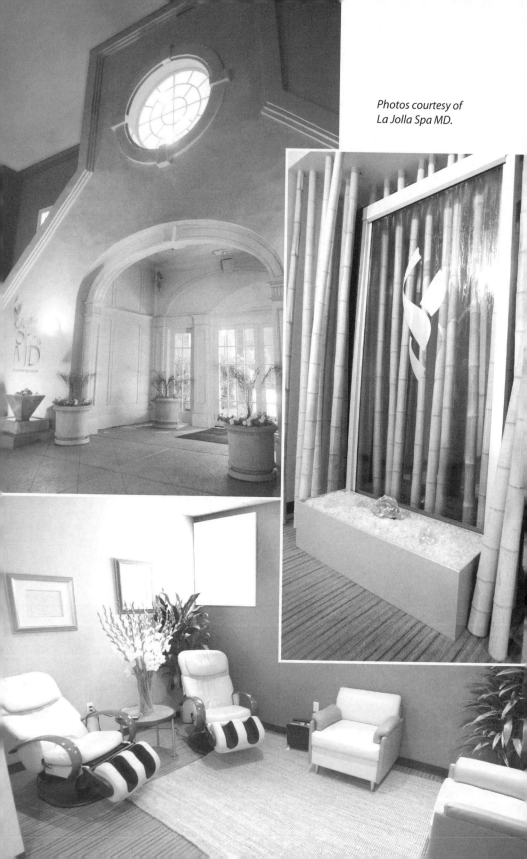

Photos courtesy of La Jolla Spa MD.

Appendix A

The Integral Health Model

Integral Health is the process through which we humans achieve well-being by the ordering of consciousness. This includes the expansion of consciousness (knowledge) and the intensification of consiousness (wisdom).

—GRAHAM SIMPSON, M.D.

For the past decade or so, it has become obvious to many of us health professionals that a new model of medicine is needed. An understanding of integral health will not only assist us in dealing with the ever-increasing incidence of chronic disease, but it will teach us to acknowledge the multidimensional nature of the human being and embrace alternative systems of health delivery that are less invasive and more effective.

In 1977, George Engel wrote in the journal *Science* that psychiatry and biomedicine were in a crisis because they both adhered to a view of disease that was no longer adequate for the scientific tasks and social responsibilities of either medicine or psychiatry. Engel proposed a new *biopsychosocial* method that treats a person, and not just the illness.

The integral health model we wish to present here extends Engel's idea and is patterned after works of Ken Wilber, Jean Gebser, and others.

Humanity has evolved from a simple consciousness to self-consciousness and is now ready for its next major transition, from self-consciousness to integral consciousness. Integral consciousness is an emergent psychohistorical development. With this awareness, the interaction between the physician and his or her patient changes. We can no longer adhere to the mechanistic, fix-it disease mentality that conventional medicine has upheld throughout much of the last century, treating symptoms of illness instead of getting to the root of a person's problem.

Integral health, here, means integrative, inclusive, comprehensive, and balanced. As Wilber writes, "To understand the whole, it is necessary to understand the parts. To understand the parts, it is necessary to understand the whole. Such is the circle of understanding."

The value of any method lies in how useful it is. We have been applying this integral health method with increasing success and would appreciate feedback from other health practitioners engaged in similar practices, as well as clients who share a similar experience in their lives. As Wilber points out, any phenomenon can be approached in an interior and exterior fashion, and also as an individual and a member of a collective. In Figure A.1 on page 229, we have included a key theorist in each of the four quadrants that makes up our integral health model.

Before discussing these in detail, it is important to recognize the power of the Internet in the future of medicine. In conventional medicine, hospitals and doctors are responsible for the medical environment. Now, the consumer is in the driver's seat. Much of what people want—and can have because of the Internet—is self-service. We would like to provide a new context for individuals to serve themselves, for example, with coaching from www.eternitymedicine.com. By integrating the best of conventional and alternative medicine, we can delay, prevent, and in some cases, actually reverse the diseases associated with aging—you can now *live better longer.*

We believe the physicians, chiropractors, and other health professionals who are oriented to preventive medicine can best deliver this method. Certain medi-spas, especially day spas and destination resort-spas, are ideal locations for people interested in incorporating this method into their lives. Moreover, through the Internet, useful products and lifelong learning related to this method can be provided.

Until recently, most of what we know as medicine was largely confined to the upper right quadrant of Figure A.1. In fact, most medicine practiced today is still predominantly from this quadrant. About twenty-five years ago, people began to appreciate wellness medicine and mind-body practices (upper left quadrant); though these practices, too, are incomplete. As Aaron Antonovsky wrote, "And yet, the voluminous writing of—shall we call it the holistic approach to health?—as far as I can tell, shows a near-total absence of reference to, or awareness of, the larger social system in which the mind-body relationship operates."

History, culture, worldview, and social structure are all indispensable (lower quadrants) to understanding the roots of health and well-being. Systems theory (lower right quadrant) provides us with a framework for alternative medicine. As Ranjan pointed out in *Advances in Mind-Body Medicine*, "The notion of relativity, that the same element can assume a different identity according to the context in which it operates, points to one of the most salient differences between bio-medicine and other medical systems. In biomedicine, pharmacology, for exam-

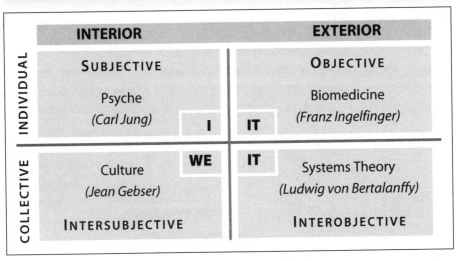

Figure A.1. Integral Health Model

ple, emphasizes an *active ingredient* regardless of context. Herbalism, on the other hand, emphasizes context, with the impact of the whole not only being greater, but even being different from the sum of the individual parts."

Von Bertalanffy writes, "The existence of laws of similar structures in different fields enables the use of systems which are simpler or better known as models for more complicated and less manageable systems."

Ranjan concludes that it is precisely within this kind of conceptual scheme that Ayurveda, traditional Chinese medicine, and other alternative medical systems have been developed. In Ayurveda, the simpler and better known method is called *doshas*. In Chinese medicine, there are the five elements and yin and yang; in homeopathy, there is the law of similars.

If we look at Figure A.1 again, we can see how a particular medical system will have a strong influence on the cultural worldview, which will set limits to individual thoughts that register in the brain. And, as Wilber points out, we can go around that circle in any direction. They are all interwoven. They are all mutually determining. They all cause, and are caused by, the others, in concentric spheres of contexts within contexts indefinitely.

The integral health method we have introduced attempts to deliver a new model for health that honors all four quadrants.

EXTERIOR OBJECTIVE

The first step after a client has decided to enroll in an integral medi-spa program is to complete a meta-analysis. This includes a comprehensive physical exam, fitness test, organ analysis, and biomarker analysis, together with select laboratory and other testing that may be necessary.

The client's completed meta-analysis then becomes part of what we call a Lifetime Health Assessment and Monitoring Program (LAMP). And, for each client, a personal wellness and longevity program is designed to complement the LAMP, including detoxification, fitness, lifestyle, and nutrition recommendations.

INTERIOR SUBJECTIVE

Self-assessment information, which includes several hundred studies over the past three decades, indicates that peoples' reports of their own health are a global measure of the quality of their lives. They predict survival more powerfully than any clinical assessments based on examinations by physicians and laboratory tests (exterior objective). Thus, a person's perspective about her or his life influences the health and longevity of that person.

Well-being is emerging as the best measure of individual health based on the 1991 U.S. Surgeon General and the Public Health Services' *Healthy People 2000*. Since well-being is a subjective quality, health under this quadrant also becomes a subjective state.

Ellen Idler and Stanislav Kasl conclude from the Yale Health and Aging Project that self-evaluations of health predict mortality above and beyond the presence of health problems, physical disability, and biological or lifestyle risk factors. What a person believes about him- or herself is by far the greatest measure of health. Physical ailments are generally symptoms of greater issues within the whole person and her or his relation to the surrounding world.

Our interest is in discovering what allows individuals to go beyond the physical for their sense of well-being. Our belief is that a sense of the spiritual and an integral worldview are the common sources of inner health and wholeness. Well-being is clearly an interior subjective and intersubjective state.

The fundamental meaning of spiritual, as taken from the Greek word *pneuma* and the Latin *spiritus* is breath. Spiritual is thus anything that gives us a second breath, a feeling of wholeness and being fully alive. This is consistent with the original meaning of health, which comes from the old English and early German terms for a state of being whole. Guided imagery, lifelong learning, meditation, prayer, psychology, relaxation, and yoga can be used to assist each client in the *individuation* process. Individuation, a term coined by Carl Jung, and not to be confused with the selfish individualism of the past decade, is a lifelong process through which a person becomes increasingly whole. Individuation entails the gradual expansion and intensification of consciousness. The individual recognizes that the ego is not the center of one's being, or as Jung writes, "One could say, with a little exaggeration, that the persona is that which in reality one is not, but which oneself as well as others think one is."

The recognition of the higher self, or the spiritual self, is a valuable aspect of the integral health model. Various assessments on the interior subjective state and lifestyle patterns of the individual are also done and are included as part of the LAMP. Finally, several mind-body health tools are given to each client as part of their wellness program.

INTERIOR INTERSUBJECTIVE

It is not enough for information to flow through the senses. To make sense of sensory data, using a context that organizes the information conveyed is essential. Cognitive development is cumulative; cultivating meaning in life is a reflective process.

The work of Jean Gebser best articulates this necessary context. In 1943, Gebser, political historian Eric Voegelin, and psychoanalyst Carl Jung each independently recognized that the mounting crisis for Western civilization was in fact a fundamental restructuring of consciousness (part of the new integral health model). Prior to the initial recognition of perspective in Europe around A.D. 1250, the human lacked spatial awareness and thus lacked an ego-consciousness or a definite sense of self. Giotto was one of the first painters in Western civilization to show us this objectified world in his work.

We live today in this world, or what Gebser terms the perspectival era. (*See* Table A.1 below.) Prior to this, there was the unperspectival era, consisting of the archaic, magical, and mythical periods. Gebser was very aware of the new era dawning for humanity beyond these—the aperspectival era.

TABLE A.1. The Basic Schema*

Time	Space	Sense Organ	Structure	Spirit	Era
5 Million–200,000 B.C.	0	Body-kinesthetic Smell	Archaic	Mystique	Unperspectival Era
200,000–10,000 B.C.	1 D	Ear	Magical	Ritual	Unperspectival Era
10,000–2,000 B.C.	2 D	Mouth	Mythical	Gods/symbols	Unperspectival Era
2,000 B.C.–Present	3 D	Eye	Mental	God/dogma	Perspectival Era
Future	4 D	Meta-sense	Integral	Overself/transcendent	Aperspectival Era

*Modified after Jean Gebser

Within each structure of consciousness, there is a distinct understanding of space and time coupled with a predominate sense organ. The integration of these five structures in each of us prepares the ground for the much-needed transformation that humanity (and medicine) must undergo at this moment. We need to assimilate the entirety of our human existence into our awareness. With this integration, people will develop an integral worldview and a greater sense of well-being. They will exhibit what Aaron Antonovsky called a "sense of coherence," and will see the world as comprehensible, meaningful, and manageable. Culture (worldview) is nothing more than collective shared meaning.

Again, assessments are made to determine the primary structure (worldview) of the client and these become part of the LAMP.

EXTERIOR INTEROBJECTIVE

This quadrant is about functional fit. It is clear that a systems approach is needed to integrate alternative systems of medical practices with conventional medicine. We use:

- Anthroposophic medicine;

- Ayurvedic medicine;

- Chiropractic medicine;

- Environmental medicine;

- Homeopathic medicine;

- Naturopathic medicine;

- Traditional Chinese medicine (TCM).

Each method is unique, and we vary their use, depending on the needs of the client.

THE VALUE OF INTEGRAL HEALTH

We believe that as much as 90 percent of all illness can be addressed and taken care of by individuals who understand this new context for health. The transition from our current mental structure to the emerging integral structure of consciousness (*see* Table A.2 on page 233) will allow for this revolutionary means of healing.

The single most important lesson in life is that we are here to learn and grow into whole healthy human beings who are not merely clever or successful, but are

TABLE A.2. Example of Two Structures of Consciousness

Mental Structure (Current)	Integral Structure (Emerging)	Mental Structure (Current)	Integral Structure (Emerging)
Domination of nature	Ego transcendence	Boredom	Dialogue
Ego fulfillment	Reverence for life	Discussion	Meaning
Knowledge	Space freedom	Dis-ease	Sufficiency
Obsession with time	Time freedom	Lack of meaning	Well-being
Parts	Whole	Scarcity	Wonder
Space fixity	Wisdom		

also in touch with our deepest roots. These roots are anchored in the ultimate reality itself. The institution that is most suited to bringing about this transformation, believe it or not, is the healthcare industry.

The details of the evolution of human consciousness, through the five distinct periods mentioned above, are well described by Gebser in his 1943 book *The Ever Present Origin.* A summary of some of Gebser's work can be found in the monograph, *Remembering the Future,* by Dr. Graham Simpson, available at www.eternitymedicine.com.

These same stages must be integrated as phases of our own psychological growth. Of central importance for this ordering of consciousness and emergent sense of well-being is *anamnesis,* or the remembering of both our own personal and collective (as a species) psychohistorical development. (Ontogeny recapitulates phylogeny.)

The same context that defines the integral health model also delineates the transformation presently occurring in all our institutions, and underlies the deep ecological movement now underway, since we recognize that well people cannot exist on a sick planet.

We are now ready to expand this integral health model and invite both healthcare professionals and those interested in learning more about integral health to join us.

Appendix B

Detoxification

DETOXIFICATION BATHS

These are soaking baths intended to draw toxins out of the body.

For the first two weeks of detox bathing, put $\frac{1}{2}$ cup baking soda in the tub filled with a water temperature that is pleasant.

Soak in this for ten to twenty minutes twice a week, keeping at least a couple of days between each bath. In addition to these detox baths, continue bathing or showering as usual.

After two weeks, depending on how you feel, choose from one of the following.

1. When feeling strong: Put $\frac{1}{4}$ cup of Epsom salts into a tub of water and soak for ten to twenty minutes.

2. When feeling OK (average): Combine $\frac{1}{4}$ cup of Epsom salts and $\frac{1}{4}$ cup of baking soda in a tub of water and soak for ten to twenty minutes.

3. When feeling tired and fragile: Put $\frac{1}{2}$ cup of baking soda into a tub of water and soak for ten to twenty minutes.

4. Basin bathing: Put $\frac{1}{4}$ cup of baking soda or Epsom salts in a sink of warm water and wipe this detox water on body with a washcloth. Pat dry.

After your detoxification bathing, shower off, using a washcloth and soap to remove any toxins that may be on the surface of the skin. After your shower, put on clean clothing so you are not exposed to toxins in your clothing.

STEP-BY-STEP METHODS FOR CLEANING FOODS

This method has been reprinted with permission from *Live Better Longer: The Parcell's Center 7-Step Plan for Health and Longevity*, by Joseph Dispenza.

Procedure to Eliminate Bacteria, Fungus, Metallics, and Sprays

Formula: Use $\frac{1}{2}$ teaspoon of Clorox to 1 gallon of water obtained from the usual supply. (Use regular Clorox only. Do not try to use any other product, as it will not work!)

Into this bath, place the fruits and vegetables to be treated. The thin-skinned fruits and leafy vegetables will require ten minutes. The root vegetables and heavy-skinned fruits will require fifteen to thirty minutes. Apples and potatoes will take thirty minutes. Timing is very important. (Refer to time schedule below.) Make a fresh bath for each group.

Remove from the Clorox bath and place into a freshwater (only) bath for five to ten minutes. Now the food is ready to finish cleaning and prepare for storage. Let the food drain very well before placing it into the refrigerator.

A Caution

Do not use more Clorox than instructed, and do not leave the fruits or vegetables in it longer than the given time, especially the green leafy vegetables, as they will turn brown due to oxidation. There is no known harm, but the eye appeal is spoiled.

Follow the timing instructions for both the Clorox bath and the rinse bath. Some people are afraid that soaking the vegetables will make them lose their mineral content, but this cannot happen in fifteen to thirty minutes. As you will find, the mineral activity is only increased. You will destroy many parasites, as well as many forms of fungus found in the soil for which our bodies may become the host. It is better to be safe than sorry.

Timing Instructions for Treating Foods with Clorox Bath

Separate the foods into groups.

Vegetables

Leafy vegetables	5–10 minutes
Root vegetables, heavy-skinned, or fiber vegetables	10–15 minutes

Fruits

Thin-skinned berries	5 minutes
Medium-skinned fruits	10 minutes
Thick-skinned fruits	10–15 minutes
Citrus fruits and bananas	15 minutes

Eggs

Eggs are at the top of our list of allergy-causing foods. This may be due to the pesticide sprays used around the pens and nests. The eggshell is porous and can absorb these poisons very quickly. Salmonella bacteria may also be present in the egg, as it is often found in the fowl. By putting the eggs (with shells intact) through the Clorox bath for twenty to thirty minutes, you will find the egg has a better flavor and it will lose its tendency to create allergies.

Meats

Meats are heavy carriers of many toxic materials, from shots to poisons ingested in the food consumed by the animal. You will find that by placing meats in the Clorox bath, all of this will be eliminated, the flavor will be improved, and the tissue tenderized. This applies to all flesh foods, including fish, which carry a heavy mercury content. Today, there are many other toxic materials that will respond to this type of treatment, making your food more enjoyable. If your meat is frozen, you will find it will not lose its juices if placed in the Clorox bath, using the same formula. The timing for this would be fifteen to thirty minutes for a two to five pound weight. Frozen turkey or chicken should remain in the Clorox bath until thawed. With the exception of ground meats, all meats should be treated.

Benefits of This Treatment for Foods

There are several advantages to this treatment. Fruits and vegetables will all keep much longer. The wilted ones will return to a fresh crispness. The faded color will vanish and the faded flavor will be gone. For your efforts, you will be rewarded with fresh, crisp vegetables that will keep twice as long. The flavors of both fruits and vegetables will be greatly enhanced, tasting like they have just been taken from the garden—plus all the harmful possibilities have been removed. The dangers from these sprays and other materials used is, in so many ways, greater than you know.

Note: This section on clorox baths for food was modified from *Whole Body Dentistry*, by Mark Breiner, D.D.C. (*See* References—Chapter 2.)

Appendix C

Glycemic Index

RAPID INDUCERS OF INSULIN

Glycemic Index Greater than 100 Percent

Grain-based foods

Corn flakes

French bread

Instant potato

Instant rice

Microwaved potato

Millet

Puffed rice

Puffed wheat

Simple sugars

Glucose

Maltose

Snacks

Puffed rice cakes

Tofu ice cream

Glycemic Index of 80 to 100 Percent

Grain-based foods

Brown rice

Grapenuts

Instant mashed potatoes

Muesli

Oat bran

Rolled oats

Shredded wheat

White rice

Whole-wheat bread

Vegetables

Carrots

Corn

Parsnips

Fruits

Apricots

Banana

Mango

Papaya

Raisins

Snacks

Corn chips

Ice cream (low fat)

Rye crisps

MODERATE INDUCERS OF INSULIN

Glycemic Index Between 50 and 80 Percent

Grain-based foods

All-bran cereal	All pastas, including white and whole-wheat spaghetti	Pumpernickel bread

Fruits

Orange	Orange juice

Vegetables

Baked beans	Navy beans	Pinto beans
Garbanzo beans (canned)	Peas	

Simple sugars

Lactose	Sucrose

Snacks

Candy bar*	Potato chips (with fat)*

LOW INDUCERS OF INSULIN

Glycemic Index Between 30 and 50 Percent

Grain-based foods

Barley	Oatmeal (slow cooking)	Whole-grain rye bread

Fruits

Apple	Applesauce	Peaches
Apple juice	Grapes	Pears

Vegetables

Black-eyed peas	Kidney beans (dried)	Tomato soup
Chickpeas	Lentils	
Kidney beans	Peas	

Dairy products

Ice cream (high fat)*	Milk (whole)*	Yogurt
Milk (skim)		

Glycemic Index of 30 Percent or Less

Fruits

| Cherries | Grapefruit | Plums |

Simple sugars

Fructose

Vegetables

Soy beans*

Snacks

Peanuts*

*High-fat content will slow the rate of absorption of carbohydrates into the body.
A little olive oil at the beginning of a meal will help you feel full.

Hydroponic Farm • *Photo courtesy of CuisinArt Resort & Spa.*

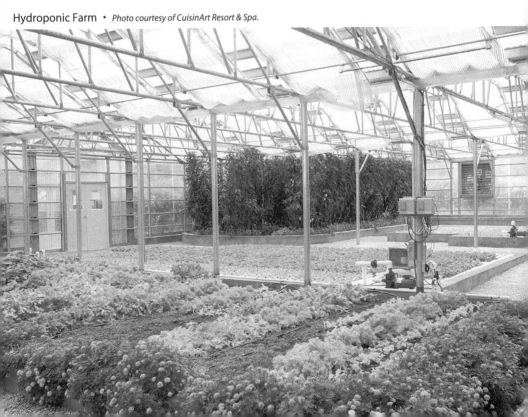

Appendix D

Hydroponic Farming

CUISINART'S HYDROPONIC FARM

Dr. Howard Resh is one of the world's leading experts in hydroponic farming. It is interesting to note how similar the requirements are for the proper growth of both people and plants—it is essential to supply each with the most optimum nutrients possible. As Dr. Resh writes, concerning the objectives of his hydroponic farm:

> The first objective of the CuisinArt hydroponic farm is to grow garden-fresh produce for its restaurants. This produce is to be of the highest nutritional value. It is to be clean and free of synthetic pesticides, and be picked at its optimum ripened state in order to be both flavorful and highly nutritious. These nutritional objectives can also apply to any hydroponic farm.

Productivity in the Hydroponic Farm

The average hydroponic greenhouse occupies 18,000 square feet. Different growing techniques are used, depending on the various crops. With the exception of lettuce, the hydroponic systems are designed to utilize the maximum available space by growing most of the plants vertically. For example, by growing bok choy and herbs in vertical plant towers, our farm increases its productivity by a factor of eight over normal horizontal bed cultivation.

We use greenhouse varieties of cucumbers, lettuce, peppers, and tomatoes that have a good yield under controlled environmental conditions. Through ongoing trials for this tropical climate, we select the vegetable plants that produce the best flavor and texture. This is evident by the tenderness of the Bibb (buttercrunch) lettuce and the very flavorful cherry tomatoes that have become so popular in the marketplace for their distinct flavor.

Plant Nutrition

In order to produce a fresh fruit or vegetable (cucumbers, peppers, tomatoes) of the highest nutritional value for people, we must start with the most optimum diet for the plants. All plants require thirteen essential plant minerals—most important are calcium, magnesium, nitrogen, phosphorus, potassium, and sulfur, all in relatively large amounts. In addition, the principal trace elements required include boron, chlorine, copper, iron, manganese, molybdenum, and zinc. Without any one of these essential elements, the plant is unable to grow in a healthy manner. If any of these substances are lacking, or not in the correct ratios, the plants will undergo stress that will make them unable to synthesize the vitamins and minerals they are genetically capable of doing.

Unless you are very experienced and analyze your soil on a regular basis, this imbalance, or deficiency, of certain plant nutrients is the usual situation in soil growing. You must add the correct amendments at the correct rates, or your plants will suffer from nutritional, and possibly water, stresses that lead to less-than-optimum production of the nutrients vital to our wellness. In our hydroponic systems, we add all these essential elements to the irrigation water in the correct concentrations and ratios for the specific crops. Every time we make up a stock of nutrients, we send a sample to a laboratory for atomic-absorption analysis, to determine the level and ratios of each essential element. In this way, we can adjust the formulation to its optimum every two weeks.

The vine crops, such as cucumbers, tomatoes, and peppers, are grown in buckets of perlite, which is fired volcanic pumice. Each plant is fed by its individual drip emitter from the irrigation system. Irrigation cycles are operated from a central controller that determines the time and duration of each cycle. To conserve water, drainage is piped to a central gray-water system for its use on the outside landscape. Water conservation is important, as all our fresh water must be generated from a reverse osmosis (RO) system of purification. The lettuce growing in the hydroponic ponds has its own system, and formulation for it is different from that of the vine crops. Known as raft culture, the name comes from the lettuce floating on Styrofoam boards on top of the nutrient solution. The herbs and bok choy grow in a layer of perlite in Styrofoam pots stacked ten feet high to form a plant tower. These foods are fed with several irrigation drip lines at the top and one in the middle of the tower.

Organic versus Inorganic Growing

Organic growing is a misnomer, as all plants are organic. The real issue here is pesticide-free. The hydroponic greenhouse industry has the safest product on the market as it uses integrated pest management (IPM), which is the introduction of beneficial predators or parasites that eat or parasitize the pests. Specific *beneficials* are introduced at the early stage of the crop, and they multiply to levels that will keep the pest populations in check. This use of beneficials is supplemented with the use of natural bioagents. For example, we use Dipel or XenTari, trade names for *Bacillus thuringiensis,* a bacterium that controls various larvae (worms) on the crops. This safe biological control is also used in organic farming.

In terms of plant nutrition in soil growing, the soil compost (organic matter) and its inorganic components (sand, rock, etc.) release the basic elements in their ionic (charged) atomic state to the soil water that contacts the plant roots, at which point an electrochemical exchange takes place to actively allow the plant to take in the nutrients. Large organic compounds cannot enter the plant roots, only elements in their ionic state can do so. In hydroponics, we add the plant nutrients from highly purified greenhouse-grade salts to the water to form the nutrient solution. This nutrient solution, like the soil solution, contacts the roots of the plants where the uptake occurs.

The difference with hydroponics is that we know exactly what is in the solution and we can balance all the elements in their optimum concentrations and ratios to give the plants the most nutrient-dense diet. This in turn enables the plants to produce the most nutritious fruits and vegetables they are capable of producing in the processes of photosynthesis and respiration.

Nutrition of the Vegetables

As explained earlier, by harvesting the vegetables at their prime ripe stage, the highest nutritional value of the product will be attained. It is generally true that if fruits or vegetables reach their fully mature state, they will have absorbed and synthesized the maximum amount of vitamins and minerals they are capable of producing. Studies with tomatoes have shown that vine-ripened fruits have from two to five times as much vitamin A and in excess of five times as much vitamin B_6 in comparison to immature green ones. You may purchase red tomatoes in a supermarket, but they may in fact have been picked green and gassed with ethylene to turn them red. And, even if it is red, the gassed fruit does not have the same nutrition or flavor as that of vine-ripened. Similarly, with sweet bell peppers, the final stage of the ripened fruit is their red, yellow, or orange color, depending on the variety.

Here at the hydroponic farm, we allow all of our vegetables to reach their optimum ripeness before picking. In this way, they are most nutritious and have that backyard-garden flavor. This is how the hydroponic farm fits into the overall CuisinArt wellness program.

Appendix E

Calorie Value for Ten Minutes of Activity

Activity	125 pounds	175 pounds	250 pounds
PERSONAL NECESSITIES			
Sleeping	10	14	20
Sitting (watching TV)	10	14	18
Sitting (talking)	15	21	30
Dressing or washing	26	37	53
Standing	12	16	24
LOCOMOTION			
Walking downstairs	56	78	111
Walking upstairs	146	202	288
Walking at 2 mph	29	40	58
Walking at 4 mph	52	72	102
Running at 5.5 mph	90	125	178
Running at 7 mph	118	164	232
Running at 12 mph	164	228	326
Cycling at 5.5 mph	42	58	83
Cycling at 13 mph	89	124	178
HOUSEWORK			
Making beds	32	46	65
Washing floors	38	53	75
Washing windows	35	48	69
Dusting	22	31	44
Preparing a meal	32	46	65
Shoveling snow	65	89	130

Activity	125 pounds	175 pounds	250 pounds
HOUSEWORK (cont.)			
Light gardening	30	42	59
Weeding garden	49	68	98
Mowing grass (power)	34	47	67
Mowing grass (manual)	38	52	74
SEDENTARY OCCUPATION			
Sitting	15	21	30
Light office work	25	34	50
Standing, light activity	20	28	40
Typing (electric)	19	27	39
LIGHT WORK			
Assembly line	20	28	40
Auto repair	35	48	69
Carpentry	32	44	64
Bricklaying	28	40	57
Farming chores	32	44	64
House painting	29	40	58
HEAVY WORK			
Pick and shovel work	56	78	110
Chopping wood	60	84	121
Dragging logs	158	220	315
Drilling coal	79	111	159
RECREATION			
Badminton	43	65	94
Baseball	39	54	78
Basketball	58	82	117
Bowling (nonstop)	56	78	111
Canoeing (4 mph)	90	128	182
Dancing (moderate)	35	48	69
Dancing (vigorous)	48	66	94
Football	69	96	137
Golfing	33	48	68

Activity	125 pounds	175 pounds	250 pounds
RECREATION (cont.)			
Horseback riding	56	78	112
Ping-pong	32	45	64
Racquetball	75	104	144
Skiing (Alpine)	80	112	160
Skiing (cross-country)	98	138	194
Skiing (water)	60	88	130
Squash	75	104	144
Swimming (backstroke)	32	45	64
Swimming (crawl)	40	56	80
Tennis	56	80	115
Volleyball	43	65	94

Calorie values are approximate.

Appendix F

Zone Café

THE CONSCIOUS CHOICE

It is no secret that a worldwide obesity epidemic threatens to handicap our healthcare system, as well as contribute to numerous health complications, including cancer, diabetes, and heart disease. Notably, about half the money used to buy food in the United States is spent at restaurants, predominantly fast-food establishments—in 2001, Americans spent over $110 billion on fast food.

MISSION

Zone Café is positioned to become the number-one quick and casual healthy restaurant chain in America. With a unique menu based on the Zone diet, we serve delicious, high-quality, affordable cuisine, providing a nutritious alternative to traditional fast food.

PHILOSOPHY

Hippocrates said, "Let food be your medicine." Centuries later, his timeless wisdom is not only simple to implement, but may also be integral in combating obesity while reversing the aging process. The key to applying this strategy for health management is to consciously choose the most ideal foods to enhance optimal health and well-being.

Perceiving food as preventive medicine is the first step in taking responsibility and caring for the body. With this in mind, we have designed Zone Café cuisine to be not only your healthiest food option, but also the tastiest. In developing these meals, we offer you a trustworthy option crafted by leading scientists and doctors.

MENU

Based on the Zone diet, as created by Dr. Barry Sears, Zone Café meals consist of specific combinations of quality macronutrients (proteins, carbohydrates, and fats). Our chefs prepare creative medleys of lean protein and monounsaturated fats to accompany generous portions of low-glycemic carbohydrates (ones that do not provoke an excess-insulin response). With unique spice combinations to delight even the most discriminating palate, Zone Café meals provide the variety and quality necessary for sustaining a healthy dietary regimen.

The intention behind our light, yet hearty, meals is to create hormonal equilibrium in the person who eats them. Hormonal imbalance, usually the result of chronically elevated insulin levels (characteristic of a diet filled with breads, pastas, and processed foods), is the culprit behind obesity and many related degenerative diseases.

The Zone Café menu highlights a vast selection of gourmet foods that you may combine as you like, according to the 30/40/30 principle: 30 percent lean protein (fish, chicken, tofu, turkey, steak), 40 percent low-glycemic carbohydrates (vegetables and most fruits), and 30 percent healthy fat (avocados, nuts, and olive oil dressings). Our menu items are made with the freshest ingredients to ensure maximum delectability as well as superior nutritional content.

In addition, we have developed a selection of low-carbohydrate Zone-compliant breads from which you may make sandwiches, and we offer Zone ice cream for your sweet tooth. Zone smoothies, as a snack or meal replacement, are also available, complete with essential omega-3 infusions to guide you on the road to greater health.

SERVICE

Zone Café employees not only cater to your food preferences, but are equipped to educate you further about the science behind the food and help you choose which Zone nutraceuticals and other Zone products may best support your individual health needs. Our quality staff guarantees that your dining experience at the Zone Café will be pleasant and satisfying, and they are readily available to address any questions or needs you may have.

LOCATIONS

Zone Cafés will be conveniently situated in superstores throughout the nation. And freestanding cafés will be centrally located within communities, in close proximity to business hubs, shopping areas, universities, and Zone Wellness Centers to give you the greatest access to our Zone cuisine and products.

PRODUCTS

Besides offering the most delicious food medicine you will ever take, Zone Cafés also serve as your one-stop shopping source for nutraceuticals, beauty products, and related literature. Zone nutraceuticals and cosmeceuticals have been specially designed by board-certified medical doctors to suit your health needs and provide the additional preventive measures against age-related degenerative disease. Zone and other health-specific books will be available for your in-store perusal or to purchase for your home library.

If you have any interest in partnering with Zone Café, LLC, to open your own Zone Café, please contact us at:

Zone Café, LLC
1495 Ridgeview Drive, Suite 230
Reno, NV 89509
Ph: 775-673-ZONE (9663)
Fax: 775-825-6447
website: www.zonecafe.com
e-mail: info@zonecafe.com

Appendix G

Cell Therapy

What do Pope Pius XII, Pablo Picasso, Winston Churchill, Frank Sinatra, and Sophia Loren have in common? All have lived, or are still enjoying, long, productive lives. Part of their legendary longevity might be attributed to the fact that they all availed themselves of cell therapy. In fact, for more than seventy years, cell therapy has been used by millions of people with allergies, arteriosclerosis, dementia, diabetes, eye problems, hormone and immune dysfunction, hypertension, impotence, obesity, Parkinson's disease, premature aging, prostatic hypertrophy, wrinkles, and varicose veins.

WHAT IS CELL THERAPY?

Cell therapy is an implantation of the fetal or juvenile cells or tissues of animals in a solution that is administered orally or by injection. The principle of healing through the injection of animal organs and tissues has been known in medicine for a long time. This therapeutic principle is mentioned in some of the oldest medical documents, such as the Ebers Papyrus from Egypt. *Glandular therapy* is based on the ancient principle of *like cures like,* which first found expression in the teachings of Hippocrates, the father of Western medicine. Aristotle, and later Paracelsus, also taught that *like cures like,* as in heart heals heart, kidney heals kidney, and so on. More recently, a branch of homeopathy called *organotherapy* uses minute concentrations of glandular or organ tissue to achieve a similar therapeutic effect.

The cell therapy of today (the same principle that is used in bone marrow transplants) can be traced back to 1931, when the Swiss surgeon Professor Paul Niehans injected his first cells into a woman with acute hypoparathyroidism. Then, after successfully treating the gravely ill Pope Pius XII in 1953, Niehans became known worldwide, and the grateful Pope appointed him to the Papal Academy of Sciences, where he succeeded Sir Alexander Fleming, the discoverer of penicillin.

THE EVIDENCE FOR CELL THERAPY

Cell therapy is based on solid biological principles. This field of biological medicine is well known in Europe, and there is now a growing awareness of this important rejuvenation therapy in the United States and South America.

When Dr. Paul Niehans, considered the father of cell therapy, treated the above-mentioned dying woman, whose parathyroid glands had failed after an unsuccessful operation, he injected her with the tissue from a calf's parathyroid gland. Thanks to his cell therapy, the woman recovered and remained free of symptoms for many years. As he treated others, Niehans eventually came to realize he didn't need a whole organ because all it took to elicit a healing response was small amounts of the cell tissue. In the forty years following his first cell-therapy injection, Niehans applied his method more than 50,000 times without any major side effects. His patients included kings, presidents, artists, actors, and many other prominent people.

In 1949, Niehans developed the process of injecting lyophilized (freeze-dried) cells because he recognized that to obtain cells of constant quality and quantity, 70 to 80 percent of the water content must be removed. Niehans developed this method with scientists from Nestlé, and these preparations are still used by many physicians throughout the world today.

Another giant in the field of cell therapy was Dr. Franz Schmid. While teaching at Heidelberg University in 1951, he was doing research to find out how the cells know where to go once they were injected. The way he determined this was by staining the donor spleen cells of animals, injecting them into animals, and then examining the organs of the injected animals. The only place these injected stained cells were found was in the spleen of those animals. Schmid went on to show that liver cells migrate to the liver, brain cells migrate to the brain, and so on. This research is documented in his 1984 textbook, *Cell Therapy*, in which he states, "The material is incorporated specifically where the structures are of use and where they are needed." Similar experiments were done with bone marrow transplants in the United States over thirty years ago. In another book, "*Das Down Syndrome*" (1987), he documents his experience in treating over 3,000 children with Down syndrome.

Oral cells and ultrafiltrate extracts (very small molecules), based on the work of Dr. Niehans and Dr. Schmid, are currently produced in Germany and are useful adjuncts to injected freeze-dried cells. For better absorption, these are best taken under the tongue (sublingually).

A. Kment and his coworkers in Heidelberg, Germany, have conducted extensive experiments with animals to prove the effectiveness of cell therapy. Having performed tests on over 94,324 animals, they published over 472,000 results, though most are available only in German.

THE BASIS FOR CELL THERAPY

In classic cell therapy, the cells (tissue) are deep-frozen and vacuum-dried without any additives. In the journal *Nature* in 1961, Medawar (who received a Nobel Prize in 1960) established that during the process of freeze-drying (lyophilization), the cells lose their ability to produce antibodies and therefore pose no danger of provoking an immunological (allergic) reaction. This method does the least damage to the fine structure of these freeze-dried cells. They also found that fetal tissues were preferable because they are more easily tolerated and have a stronger therapeutic effect than older cells. The use of human tissue in cell therapy can be dangerous because of the possibility of transferring disease, and its use is considered ethically unacceptable in any case. German research has shown that cells from any mammalian source, besides human, can be used, since the therapeutic value is the same.

ULTRAFILTRATES

Organ ultrafiltrates are obtained from the fetal or juvenile organs of sheep by a special manufacturing process that involves extraction with organic acids. The separation level is determined by the size of the filters. The finished product, considered a nutritional supplement, is cell-free and is mixed with 5 milliliters of sterile solution. Except for the topical agent, Cellusana, these supplements are all taken orally. The commonly held opinion in many textbooks is that, taken orally, fats, carbohydrates, and proteins are completely broken down by acids and enzymes, but this notion must be revised as a result of overwhelming medical research. For example, it is well known that during the normal digestion process, solid particles (the proportion may exceed 20 percent) from the intestine can be introduced into the bloodstream, without being broken down, via the thoracic duct in the chest. This has important physiological and immunological consequences. For example, 150 years ago, researchers observed that American Indians ate toxic ivy leaves in order to protect themselves from the skin rash caused by these leaves.

In 1990, Howard Weiner from the Harvard Medical School fed people with multiple sclerosis 300 milligrams of myelin from bovine brain and there was significant improvement, especially in the men (estrogen was felt to inhibit some of the effect in the women).

In 1994, other scientists showed that, by simply feeding myelin-based proteins to animals with experimental allergic encephalitis (EAE), you can prevent or reverse paralysis. These results indicate that the organ capsules produced by Cytobiopharm may also be quite useful.

APPLICATION OF CELL THERAPY

Until recently, taking advantage of this medicine of the past and future meant traveling to Switzerland, to a clinic such as La Prairie where the cost would range from $10,000 to $15,000. Now, however, cell therapy is available in the United States, but the downside is the same old story: Since the use of natural glandular tissue negates any chance for a patent, the American drug companies have little economic incentive to develop and market these products.

Dr. Michael Murray, an authority on biological medicine writes, "The biologically active material, such as enzymes, soluble proteins, natural lipid factors, vitamins, minerals, and hormone precursors are destroyed or eliminated if the glandular products are not prepared properly. Thus, making sure the product is freeze-dried (lyophilized) greatly preserves their active ingredients." It is important to emphasize the key concept that glandular tissues are organ specific, not species specific. These animal cells from other mammals have enough genetic similarity to be able to assist similar weakened cells in the human body. Liver cells go to liver, sex cells go to sexual organs, heart cells to the heart, and so on. Radioactive isotope tracings have recently confirmed Dr. Schmid's findings from the 1950s, that when these cells enter the bloodstream they are deposited in the corresponding organs and tissues.

USES OF CELL THERAPY

Cell therapy is one of the most exciting rejuvenating therapies now available. Its effectiveness is recognized in at least four major subdivisions.

1. Adjuvant tumor therapy, where there is powerful immune stimulation with medulla, Resistocell, spleen, thymus, etc. cells.

2. Congenital disorders, such as Down syndrome or Noonan's syndrome.

3. Dysfunction due to disease, such as Crohn's and other autoimmune diseases.

4. Revitalization for premature aging, with loss of vitality from hormonal and diminished organ functions.

METHODS OF TREATMENT

In the past, when fresh cells were used, scientists recognized it was not the freshness that determined its effectiveness, but rather the composition and quantity of the cells' biochemical contents (the substrates, the material on which enzymes act, and the enzymes themselves, which amount to more than thirty different compounds). The faster this tissue is preserved, the more the active ingredients remain intact. Lyophilization (freeze-drying) is the safest method of guaranteeing this in the fetal tissues, and also the most effective. This freeze-dried cell preparation is given in doses of 100–150 milligrams.

The German Federal Health Gazette, an official publication, contains the rules for the production of all these therapeutic cell preparations. Cattle, pigs, and sheep must be proven safe for humans through careful inspection, in order to ensure that there is no transmission of animal diseases to humans. With such dangerous diseases as mad cow around, it is obvious why this is important.

The normal way to administer these preparations is by deep subcutaneous or intramuscular injections. Up to five or six preparations (500–800 milligrams of the freeze-dried cells) may be injected at a single session. Hard physical work should be restricted for seven to fourteen days after an injection, and its positive effects usually appear between the third and fourth week. The best time to start cell therapy is when a person is in his or her fifties because that is when the body is in its catabolic (breakdown) phase. The injection site should be covered for several days to prevent infection, and for the same reason, it is also best to avoid sitting in a hot tub for those first days.

SIDE EFFECTS OF CELL THERAPY

Freeze-dried tissues are usually well tolerated.

1. Local reactions include some redness and swelling, with discomfort seen 5 to 10 percent of the time.

2. Nonallergic erythema (redness) is more common after injections with placenta cells.

3. One in 5,000 implantations will results in an abscess, so cleanliness at the injection site is important.

4. Hypersensitivity is very rare, but immediate reactions can occur, especially if there is already an infection or if there have been frequent implantations.

5. Infections from animals have, so far, never been reported, either from the original fresh cell or the freeze-dried preparations.

6. Nonspecific symptoms can occur. A small percentage of people experience flu-like symptoms, accompanied by a slight rise in temperature, which last a few days.

As for taking the oral ultrafiltrates, in our experience over the past decade, we have not seen any side effects. As with enzymes, the ultrafiltrates need to be taken in large enough doses, and for several months, to produce the best effects. (Only about 40 percent of these oral therapies are thought to be absorbed.)

CONTRAINDICATIONS FOR CELL THERAPY

It is best not to undergo cell therapy if any of the following conditions apply:

1. Acute and chronic bacterial infections;

2. Acute viral infections;

3. A history of acute allergic hypersensitivity;

4. An acute stress condition (a recent heart attack, for example);

5. Following a vaccination (four-week waiting period needed).

Today, there are over 2,500 scientific publications and more than 50,000 medical reports that record and document the effectiveness and success of cell therapy. Cell therapy can be part of an integral medi-spa program focused on the whole person to provide the most optimum results for clients wishing to *live better longer.*

Appendix H

Losing Weight Is Easy in the Zone

Losing weight is easy, but keeping weight off is tough. There are hundreds of diet plans. Many are helpful in shedding pounds, but within a year most people have regained the weight they lost. Some people spend untold hours searching for the ideal diet, one that will work for a lifetime. However, it is not the particulars of a diet that determine whether a person is successful in sustaining long-term weight loss, it is learning to change your eating behaviors and manage your lifestyle. And this is what the OmegaZone Dietary Program is all about. These lifestyle and behavior changes not only help keep your weight off long-term but can also move you toward greater wellness. The following is a discussion of various weight-loss strategies to be implemented in the OmegaZone Dietary Program. Their use does not guarantee success, but it does increase the likelihood that the difficult problem of losing and maintaining weight has a better chance of succeeding.

One of the most important things to understand from the start is that weight loss does not involve willpower. Too often, people beat themselves up and use guilt as the only impetus for change, blaming a lack of will for failure. Ask yourself, what is willpower as it applies to behavior change, and how do you come by enough determination to take on the difficult task of long-term weight loss? Do you need to lock yourself in a room and simply make up your mind to be serious once and for all? Or does successful behavior change involve something very different and possibly more straightforward?

The problem with blaming everything on willpower is that when failure occurs, as it often does, you end up blaming yourself for being weak or inadequate. Willpower is not sprinkled on like fairy dust or granted to the few lucky souls born with the right stuff. Instead, willpower comes from the ways people structure things to stimulate the will—*where there is a way, there is a will.* This twist of a common expression carries important implications for any effort to change behavior because it means in essence that you can create the way by using strong incentives, changing beliefs and behaviors, and adopting skills to secure the foundation for behavior change. Success comes from stirring the will rather than assuming that willpower will sit in reserve ready to rescue you simply because you desire behavior change. Bob, for example, wanted to lose weight rapidly. He wore a full sweatsuit in the heat of summer and ran around the inner-city lake several times daily. His plan, however, was doomed to failure from the start, for several reasons. Wearing a sweatsuit is not only dangerous, but so uncomfortable in the heat that Bob looked for any and every excuse to avoid running again. He needed to create a better way that was more fun and rewarding. Using a Discman or an iPod, wearing more comfortable clothing, and exercising at a time that was convenient for him would have increased his chances for success. He also could have created a better way by starting his exercise program gradually, and stretching beforehand to reduce tightness in his muscles. These efforts would have helped more than anything to stimulate willpower, and definitely more than simply relying on his free will to rescue him in his hour of need.

The bottom line is that successful behavior change requires setting the stage with environmental, mental, and social changes to support behavior change. Essentially, the goal is to minimize the behavioral cost associated with behavior change and maximize the gains. Make the task of changing much pleasanter and more rewarding, rather than believing that a simple commitment will succeed.

Another way to overcome the challenge of behavior change is to recognize that whatever people do, however good or bad, represents what is most reinforcing for them—things that will move them toward rewarding consequences and away from punishment. Why does Mary have problems staying away from rich foods high in sugar? Simple: she likes cakes, candies, and cookies, and her efforts to change will be met with resistance because there is always the inherent pull to return to what is most reinforcing. The essence of human nature is to return to ingrained habits until their consequences make it less and less comfortable to do so. People use a variety of sometimes very creative excuses and a fair dose of denial in order to maintain the status quo, and this allows them to continue practicing their usual habits, however unhealthy. A case in point are those people who continue to smoke despite full knowledge of how cigarettes threaten them. Only when the costs outweigh the gains for continuing the habits are people sufficiently motivated to seek change. Unfortunately, it is usually through an accident or an accumulation of uncomfortable consequences, such as getting sick or gaining too much weight, that people become motivated to change. However, people who create the way, making it more reinforcing to want to quit, are the people whose stronger willpower will be supporting the gains they seek to make.

With these background issues in mind, below are some practical steps for achieving long-term weight loss using the OmegaZone Dietary Program and changing old habits that work against successful behavior change.

Effective weight loss should never involve absolutes. No one is perfect and everyone fails. It is important for you to be flexible and work toward realistic goals because, when your goals are unrealistic, your efforts at behavior change will collapse. If you shun certain foods completely, can you extend this commitment, not just for a few weeks but for a lifetime? Absolute goals are meaningful, but they rarely work except to sabotage an otherwise workable diet.

It is important that you shape your behavior gradually. Expectations usually exceed what is realistic, but gradually molding your behavior is more successful. For example, if you eat bread every day and the goal is to reduce your intake of bread and starches, you might start by cutting them out one or two days a week at the beginning, and progress gradually from there to your ultimate goal.

Success is more likely to be achieved if you are aware of what psychologists call *competing reinforcers*. Specifically, if you are surrounded by enticements at every turn, reaching even your modest goals could be difficult, if not impossible. Opening the refrigerator door and finding a chocolate cake is asking for trouble. Since there is no reason to tempt willpower, it is important to keep foods you want to stay away from out of reach and make their preparation difficult and troublesome, thereby reducing your likelihood of experiencing a setback. In the same vein, it is important to avoid hunger pangs. This is why the OmegaZone Dietary Program, which encourages three meals a day with two healthy snacks, is ideal. With it, you never become overwhelmed by urges or susceptibility to foods you want to stay away from, but it will require a bit of planning and foresight on your part, since busy schedules make eating three meals difficult. Carrying healthy snacks, for example Zone Bars, and scheduling lunches at healthy restaurants, such as the Zone Café, will increase your likelihood of success.

Like many habits, managing urges is an important skill in long-term weight loss. It is important for you to have a game plan for dealing with urges that sometimes can strike unexpectedly and be triggered by something as simple as a commercial or a magazine ad. Most urges are short-lived and subside quickly, especially with effective distraction, such as quickly consuming foods that are permitted or healthy. For example, if you get an urge to urge to drink soda, try drinking a glass of water instead—it could be a quick way to dissipate your urge. Similarly, a handful of almonds can replace the donut you want. Zone meals are designed to help you out by producing the ideal hormonal response so you do not get hungry between meals.

Successful behavior change requires your getting the right kinds of information about effective weight loss. Knowing it is important to regulate insulin and eat balanced meals with moderate protein, carbohydrates, and fat will increase your commitment and will for change. You need to be aware of what foods are permitted and how much exercise is recommended, but you don't need to overwhelm yourself with information. Just knowing the basics can go a long way toward solidifying your efforts. Uncertainty and ignorance can, on the other hand, breed anxiety and doubt, increasing your vulnerability to excuses and a desire to return to old habits. Information on all of this can be found at Zone Cafés.

Keeping it simple is important for any behavior change. The simpler, the better. Counting calories, following difficult daily schedules, and eating a very restricted range of foods most often fails. Complicated and cumbersome regimens make eating and dieting a chore. They require so much effort that the diet plan is soon dismissed.

Change should be a rewarding experience. Unless you make the effort for behavior change rewarding and minimize the discomfort, success is unlikely. In other words, the idea is to choose the right kinds of foods, avoid hunger, and take guilt out of the equation. If failure occurs, you should see it as an opportunity to return to the drawing board to implement stronger reinforcers, thus shaping your behavior toward more realistic goals. Instead of failure being attributed to a lack of willpower and inner strength, you should question whether or not your plan for creating the way to stimulate the willpower was adequate. Revamping your plan is expected and anticipated.

Long-term weight loss is a commitment for life, not a two-to-four-week, or six-month hiatus from the usual fare. You should not even attempt to lose weight and change habits unless you are willing to make that commitment. The Omega-Zone Dietary Program is not really a diet, it is a lifestyle choice.

You should expect no more than a two-pound weight loss per week. Any more can be celebrated as long as drastic attempts are not being made. The reason for this is that quick weight loss usually means you are not engaging in behaviors you can commit to for a lifetime. Anyone can lose weight; but it is the long-term maintenance of that weight loss that determines your success. Changes that are gradual, more reinforcing, and less punishing are ten times more likely to succeed in the long run.

Guilt is not the answer to successful weight loss. No one achieves long-term weight reduction by using guilt as the prime motivator. In fact, if guilt is the stimulus for your weight loss, your plan is almost guaranteed to fail. The reason is that minor relapses will inevitably occur, and if your guilt is pronounced and your efforts at behavior change are associated with it, you would avoid any future behavior changes because they could they result in low self-esteem. Remember, it is not a fighting inner free spirit that determines your successful behavior change, it is *the way that stimulates the will* for you to continue forging ahead with your plan.

Again, watch for excuses and denials. There is always a tendency to return to your old habits; otherwise, you would never have practiced those habits that made you comfortable in the first place.

Although the ultimate goal is weight loss, try to avoid daily weigh-ins. Weight fluctuates, especially at the beginning, and one or two pounds up or down is expected. If you must know how you're doing, then weekly weigh-ins are recommended. This said, some anecdotal evidence suggests that some people do better weighing themselves more frequently. Remember, your emphasis is on behavior change. If your goals are achieved, then weight loss is inevitable.

No weight program is successful without exercise. Exercise increases the metabolic rate and adds significantly to the success of any long-term weight-loss program. Besides, as this book shows, exercise has many other positive benefits. Eating on a regular basis also increases your metabolic level and hence your energy level, helping you in your desire to exercise. All the points above regarding weight loss should have exercise following them. Don't start too quickly or you will get discouraged and fail. Exercise is rewarding, but initially, until you get acclimated, it can make you feel uncomfortable.

There are no magic pills, but you *can* achieve successful long-term weight loss. People who are successful at it have created the way to support the gains they want to make. They may even have done this accidentally, but their efforts worked because they successfully abolished the excuses and denials that most people use to return to old comfortable habits. Create the way, make it strong and reinforcing, keep it simple and uncomplicated, and you can achieve any long-term behavior change you want.

Glossary

acetylcholine. A neurotransmitter that causes muscles to contract.

adenosine triphosphate (ATP). The primary source of energy found in all cells that fuels essential biochemical reactions in the body.

advanced glycosylation end products (AGEs). Modified proteins created from the cross-linking of sugar and proteins. The more AGEs in the body, the faster you age; excess blood sugar and free radicals exacerbate the production of AGEs.

aerobic exercise. Energy expenditure that facilitates enough oxygen transfer to muscles without a buildup of lactic acid; useful for lowering blood glucose and reducing insulin levels.

aging. The general deterioration of the mind and body with increasing age.

anabolic. Pertaining to the building up or growth phase of metabolism (anabolism) in which the body builds up new tissue for growth and repair.

anthroposophy. A system of medicine developed by the Western mystic Rudolph Steiner, maintaining that by correct training and personal discipline one can attain experience of the spiritual world.

antioxidants. Agents produced naturally within the body, as well as taken in the form of vitamin and mineral supplements, that help counteract the effects of free radicals on cells and help repair cellular damage.

arachidonic acid (AA). An essential fatty acid (EFA) found in fatty red meats, egg yokes, and organ meats that is the immediate precursor of prostaglandins and bad eicosanoids (AA indirectly causes inflammation).

articular. Associated with the joints between bones.

ascites. Accumulated fluid, and subsequent swelling, in the lining of the abdominal cavity.

autogenic training. A technique developed in Germany by Dr. Johannes H. Schultz that is designed to produce a relaxation-type response to counteract the fight-or-flight response.

autonomic nervous system (ANS). The part of the nervous system that is concerned with control of involuntary bodily functions, such as the heartbeat, salivating, and sweating. The sympathetic and parasympathetic systems are subdivisions of the ANS.

biological response modifiers. Natural compounds, such as enzymes, that act to speed up or slow down body processes.

biomarkers. Predictive biological indicators of aging. Each biomarker of aging usually decreases 2 to 6 percent every decade after age thirty-five.

calorie. A unit for measuring energy. The more calories a food has, the more energy-producing value it has. Proteins contain 4 calories per gram. Fats contain 9 calories per gram. Carbohydrates contain 4 calories per gram.

calorie restriction. The reduction of calories that maintains adequate levels of proteins, carbohydrates, and essential fats while supplying adequate amounts of micronutrients (vitamins and minerals).

carbohydrates. Various forms of sugar that, when converted into glucose, are the primary source fuel for the body. Simple carbohydrates are absorbed more quickly into the bloodstream than complex carbohydrates, such as whole grains and fibers.

catabolic. Pertaining to the breakdown phase of metabolism (catabolism) in which the body breaks down complex substances into simpler ones, or in terms of aging, degenerates.

cavitation. A factor of periodontal disease characterized by the formation of cavities, or holes, in the jaw bones where teeth once were, causing unnecessary oxidative stress and toxicity.

cholesterol. A fatty, waxlike substance, necessary in small amounts for cell function, though harmful to the heart if too much is consumed or produced by the body. HDL (high-density lipoprotein) is considered good cholesterol because it lowers your risk of heart disease, while LDL (low-density lipoprotein) is considered bad cholesterol as it places you at risk for heart disease.

cirrhosis. Chronic disease of the liver in which liver cells, which detoxify the body and convert glucose into stored energy, no longer function correctly.

corticosteroids. (1) Hormonal substances the adrenal gland releases as adaptation responses to chronic stress. (2) Pharmaceutical drugs (prednisone) prescribed for various medical conditions.

cortisol. Hormone produced in the adrenal gland to help control stress by inhibiting the formation of both good and bad eicosanoids. Too much or too little cortisol production accelerates the aging process.

cosmeceuticals. Skin-care products that contain vital nutrients to combat the damage of free radicals and reduce inflammation, keeping skin in a youthful condition.

cross-linking. The binding of sugar to protein in the presence of oxygen, caused by free radicals, which can create problems because the protein becomes damaged and thus accelerates aging.

deoxyribonucleic acid (DNA). The unique genetic code each living being is born with.

diabetes. A condition in which blood glucose (sugar) is not well-controlled. People with type-1 diabetes, a condition that often develops in childhood, require insulin, usually via injection. People with type-2 diabetes overproduce insulin and their target cells do not respond to insulin (insulin resistance). By controlling insulin release through dietary measures, people with type-2 diabetes can help bring balance back to their hormonal systems. Most people with type-2 diabetes, which is more common than type-1, are obese.

docosahexaenoic acid (DHA). An omega-3 essential fatty acid found in coldwater fish that helps decrease inflammation.

EDTA. A weak synthetic amino acid that works to detoxify as a chelating agent, pulling unwanted mineral deposits from blood vessels. It is given as Sodium EDTA (Edathamil Calcium-Disodium Acetate) intravenously. It can also be given orally.

eicosanoid. A hormone made by every cell in the body. The type of eicosanoid produced depends on which essential fatty acid it comes from. A good eicosanoid is anti-inflammatory; a bad eicosanoid causes inflammation.

eicosapentaenoic acid (EPA). An omega-3 fatty acid found in coldwater fish and fish oil; a precursor to good eicosanoids.

enzymes. Proteins that serve as powerhouses of cells and are catalysts for every metabolic process in the body.

endermologie. A massaging technique that delivers intermittent suction and rolling to improve the appearance of cellulite. Invented in the 1980s by Louis Guitay, a French engineer.

epidemiology. Study of causes and distribution of diseases.

essential fatty acids (EFAs). Omega-3 and omega-6 EFAs are fats the body cannot make and therefore must be part of the diet.

eternity medicine. A space-free, time-free concept of integrative medicine; it is about our awareness of the nonlocal nature of mind—that is infinite, indestructible, and immortal.

extracellular space. The area outside the cells, as opposed to the matter inside the cells (intracellular space).

fats. Compounds composed of carbon, hydrogen, and oxygen atoms that serve as stored fuel for the body. (*See also* definitions for hydrogenated, monounsaturated, polyunsaturated, and saturated fats.)

free radicals. Highly reactive, imbalanced molecules that are the byproducts of normal metabolism and are associated with the degenerative aging process. Free radicals are also produced by exposure to cigarette smoke, smog, and other environmental pollutants, harmful chemicals, toxins, and even sunlight.

functional medicine. A practice by which doctors examine symptoms in the body to diagnose particular ailments and determine the patient's overall state of health. By detecting symptoms early on, doctors can help the patient heal and avoid severe manifestations of degenerative illness.

gene expression. The dominant manifestation of a particular characteristic in an individual's genetic code; other traits that exist remain recessive.

general adaptation syndrome. The long-term physiological changes the body makes to adapt to chronic conditions, such as stress or environmental toxicity, and their subsequent complications (the release of the harmful hormone cortisol is among them).

glomerular filtration rate. The amount of blood per minute that gets filtered by the kidneys; this determines the amount of urine produced every day.

glucagon. The hormone from the pancreas that causes the release of stored carbohydrates in the liver to restore blood glucose levels.

glucose. The simplest form of sugar that circulates in the bloodstream and is used as fuel by cells. Glucose is the primary fuel used by the brain and is stored in the liver and muscles as glycogen.

glycation. The process of cross-linking in which sugar attaches to protein and causes loss of elasticity and decline in skin tone and other organs.

glycemic index. The measure of the rate at which a carbohydrate will enter the bloodstream as glucose. The faster a carbohydrate enters the bloodstream, the higher its glycemic index. The higher the glycemic index of a carbohydrate, the greater the increase in insulin levels, and thus the more inflammation. Fruits and vegetables tend to have a low-glycemic index, whereas breads, pasta, refined grains, and starches tend to have a high-glycemic index.

glycemic load. The measure of the density and digestion speed of carbohydrates (the glycemic index of a food multiplied by the amount of carbohydrates per serving). A higher glycemic load indicates that a food is more carbohydrate-dense; pasta has a high glycemic load, while carrots do not, though they both respectively have high glycemic indices.

glycogen. The form in which carbohydrates (glucose) are stored in the liver for future energy use.

glycosylation. A damaging process in which the linkage of sugars and proteins in collagen causes skin inflexibility and age spots (similar to glycation). The same process can occur in many organ systems, contributing to degenerative diseases.

heart rate variability (HRV). An assessment of the balance or imbalance of the sympathetic nervous system (SNS) and parasympathetic nervous system (PNS) to determine the health of the cardiovascular system.

helicobactor pylori (H. pylori). The bacteria thought to cause most ulcers.

high glycemic. Foods that are high glycemic are broken down rapidly into glucose and enter the bloodstream more quickly than low-glycemic foods.

hormones. Biological compounds that communicate information throughout the body; A substance, usually a peptide or steroid, produced by one tissue and conveyed by the bloodstream to another to effect physiological activity, such as growth or metabolism.

hydrogenated fats. Considered the unhealthiest fats of all, these have an added hydrogen atom to make them solid at room temperature and increase the shelf life of the processed foods and commercially baked goods containing them.

hydroponics. The cultivation of fresh produce in water, rather than soil, to ensure maximum nutritional value.

hypothalamus. A walnut-sized gland in the brain responsible for regulating body temperature, water balance, sugar and fat metabolism, and the release of hormones for other glands in the body.

insulin. A hormone that drives incoming nutrients into cells for storage; excess insulin is the cause of inflammation, weight gain, and many other degenerative diseases.

insulin resistance. A condition in which cells no longer respond well to insulin. As a result, the body chronically secretes more insulin into the bloodstream in an effort to reduce blood-sugar levels.

integral health. Integration of the best of alternative and conventional medicine to enhance wellness and longevity in the body, emotions, mind, and spirit. Connects mental, physical, and spiritual energies for healing purposes, and the expansion and intensification of consciousness.

integrative physicians. Doctors who practice whole-person medicine, combining alternative and conventional methods to treat the body, emotions, mind, and spirit.

low glycemic. Foods that are broken down into glucose less quickly than high-glycemic foods and enter the bloodstream at a much slower rate.

macronutrients. Foods that contain calories and can therefore generate hormonal responses. Proteins, fats, and carbohydrates are the macronutrients found in food.

macrophages. The scavenger white blood cells of the immune system.

metabolic syndrome. A condition in which the body's rate of metabolism is altered as a result of chronically high insulin levels. Symptoms of metabolic syndrome include decreased HDL cholesterol, elevated triglycerides, high blood pressure, high insulin levels, and weight gain (apple shape).

metaplasia. Process through which cells go from normal to abnormal, often a forerunner of cancer.

micronutrients. Vitamins and minerals that have no caloric value and little direct impact on hormonal response, but are a vital means of achieving optimal health.

mindfulness. A state of awareness practiced during meditation that raises consciousness; experiencing reality for what it is, rather than operating on autopilot.

monounsaturated fats. Produced by plants, these are the healthiest fats. With a lower number of hydrogen atoms, they tend to be liquid at room temperature.

natural killer (NK) cells. Infection-fighting white blood cells.

neuroendocrine. Pertaining to the nervous and endocrine systems' functioning as a unit.

neuropeptides. Transmitters in nerve tissue composed of two or more amino acids.

nutraceuticals. Concentrated natural components of foods or supplements that have medicinal or therapeutic effects.

obesity. A condition characterized by the excessive accumulation and storage of body fat. A weight more than thirty pounds over what is considered normal.

omega-3s. Essential fatty acids (EFAs) found primarily in coldwater fish and purified fish oils; omega-3s are the building blocks for good eicosanoids.

omega-6s. Essential fatty acids (EFAs) found in protein and most seed oils; omega-6s can generate both good and bad eicosanoids.

omega-9s. Essential fatty acids (EFAs) that have neutral effects on hormone production—they do not produce good or bad eicosanoids.

opioids. Naturally occurring substances in the body, such as endorphins, that act on the brain to decrease the sensation of pain.

oxidative stress. A condition in the body in which antioxidant defenses are overwhelmed by free radicals.

parasympathetic nervous system (PNS). A subdivision of the automatic nervous system responsible for calming and relaxing the body (by constricting the bronchioles and pupils, slowing the heart rate, and so forth).

periodontitis. Degeneration or inflammation of dental bones and the surrounding areas as a result of chronic gum disease, poor dental hygiene, or other complications in the mouth.

phytonutrients. Nutrients derived from plants.

pituitary. The gland at the base of the brain that controls and regulates most endocrine (hormonal) functions in the body (the pituitary has strong connections with the hypothalamus).

policosanol. A nutraceutical that helps lower cholesterol.

polyunsaturated fats. From plant sources. These fats have the lowest number of hydrogen atoms and are liquid at room temperature.

psychohistorical. The way the mind has evolved over time. Distinct mental *structures of consciousness* have developed at certain times over the last 5 million years of evolution. Each structure of consciousness has its own understanding of space and time along with a predominate sense organ.

psychoneuroimmunology (PNI). The study of the interrelation between the mind, the nervous and hormonal systems, and the immune system.

receptors. Molecules on the surfaces of cells that bind to specific factors (for example, insulin receptors). Sensitivity of receptors tends to diminish with aging.

resting metabolic rate (RMR). The rate at which the body burns calories each day; the higher the rate, the faster calories are burned. A person's RMR tends to get slower with age.

saturated fats. Found in most animal products and tropical oils. With a high proportion of hydrogen atoms, they are solid at room temperature and are converted to cholesterol in the body.

silent inflammation profile (SIP). A lab test that measures the ratio of arachidonic acid (AA) to eicosapentaenoic acid (EPA) to determine the levels of good and bad eicosanoids, and therefore, the level of silent inflammation in the body; perhaps the single best evidence-based wellness test as of now.

static balance. A measure of the state of equilibrium and balance in the internal environment of the human body that is maintained by various feedback controls.

stealth bacteria. Minute bacteria (microbes) that remain undetected while flourishing and causing chronic health complications (for example, nanobacteria, or the Lyme spirochete).

substrates. Material acted upon by enzymes.

sympathetic nervous system (SNS). A large part of the automatic nervous system consisting of nerves, mostly motor but some sensory, that supply the involuntary muscles. The SNS causes arousal responses with results opposite to the parasympathetic nervous system. Chronic overstimulation can lead to cardiac problems.

syndrome X. (*See* metabolic syndrome.)

T cells. Cells of the immune system that patrol for foreign substances that can cause disease and that help the body fight infection by attacking and destroying diseased cells. T cells orchestrate, regulate, and coordinate the overall immune system response.

telomeres. A sequence of nucleic acids in DNA that extend from the ends of chromosomes; important to the longevity of cells.

toxic blood. A state of the blood characterized by increased coagulation, heavy metals, infections, and other toxins, causing inflammation and sluggish blood flow.

vital capacity. The volume of air expelled by a forced maximal expiration (breathing out) from a position of full inspiration (breathing in).

vitamins. Organic substances essential to the nutrition of most animals and plants. Though we produce some vitamins in our bodies, we need to obtain others via the foods we eat.

Wobenzym. An enzyme preparation from Germany that is available in oral form or by injection.

worldview. How a person perceives her or his role in the world as it relates to life and humanity.

xenobiotics. Synthetic petrochemical substances that can mimic estrogen. They are found everywhere—in dry cleaning, gasoline vapors, hair spray, household cleaners, perfumes, plastic food containers, plastic wraps, soaps, and industrial toxins, such as DDT and insecticides.

xenoestrogens. Synthetic estrogen compounds not produced naturally in the body that can cause health problems, including cancer. Contained in dairy and meat products.

Resources and Medi-Spa Directory

RESOURCES

American Academy of Anti-Aging Medicine (A4M)
1510 West Montana St.
Chicago, IL 60614
Ph: 773-528-1000 or 773-528-4333
Fax: 773-528-5390
website: www.worldhealth.net
e-mail: info@worldhealth.net

American Academy of Biological Dentistry
P.O. Box 856
Carmel Valley, CA 93924
Ph: 408-659-5385
website: www.biologicaldentistry.com
e-mail: info@biologicaldentistry.com

American Holistic Medical Association
12101 Menaul Blvd, Suite C
Albuquerque, NM 87112
Ph: 505-292-7788
Fax: 505-293-7582
website:www.holisticmedicine.org
e-mail: info@holisticmedicine.org

Doctors Data
3755 Illinois Ave
St. Charles, IL 60174-2420
Ph: 800-323-2784
Fax: 630-587-7860
website: www.doctorsdata.com
e-mail: inquiries@doctorsdata.com

Eternity Medicine
13704 Treviso Court
San Diego, CA 92130
Ph: 858-720-0046
website: www.eternitymedicine.com
e-mail: info@eternitymedicine.com

Far Infrared Sauna
High Tech Health, Inc.
1919 Seventh Street, Suite 100
Boulder, CO 80302
Ph: 303-413-8500 or 800-794-5355
Fax: 303-449-9640
website: www.hightechhealth.com
e-mail: info@hightechhealth.com

Healing Arts
Spa and Wellness Products and
    Services
Healing Arts Stores, LLC
Cedar Lane
Weston, CT 06883
Ph: 203-226-0248
Fax: 775-655-1936
website: www.healingartsguide.com
e-mail: jed@healingartsguide.com

Inflammation Research Foundation
42 Stanwood Road
Swampscott, MA 01907
Ph: 978-539-0100
Fax: 978-539-0139
website: www.inflammationresearch
    foundation.org
e-mail: info@inflammationresearch
    foundation.org

**The Institute for Functional
    Medicine (IFM)**
4411 Point Fosdick Drive NW, Suite 305
P.O. Box 1697
Gig Harbor, WA 98335
Ph: 800-228-0622
Fax: 253-853-6766
website: www.functionalmedicine.org
e-mail: client_services@fxmed.com

Institute of Heart Math
14700 West Park Ave.
Boulder Creek, CA 95006
Ph: 800-450-9111 or 831-338-8500
Fax: 831-338-8504
website: www.heartmath.org
e-mail: info@heartmath.org

**International Academy of Oral
    Medicine and Toxicology
    (IAOMT)**
8297 Champion's Gate Blvd #193
Champions Gate, FL 33896
Ph: 863-420-6373
Fax: 863-420-6394
website: www.iaomt.org
e-mail: info@iaomt.org

**International Anti-Aging Systems
    (IAS)**
Suite 1
Sark, Gy9 0SF
Channel Islands, Great Britain
Ph: +44 870 151 4144
Fax: +44 709 211-5519 or
        +44 870 151 4145
website: www.antiaging-systems.com
e-mail: ias@antiaging-systems.com

**The International Association for
    Cytobiological Therapies**
Robert-Bosch Strasse 56a
D-69190
Walldorf, Germany
Ph: +49-622763268
Fax: +49-622763301

**International Health, Racquet,
    and Sportsclub Association
    (IHRSA)**
263 Summer Street
Boston, MA 02210
Ph: 800-228-4772 or 617-951-0055
Fax: 617-951-0056
website: www.ihrsa.org
e-mail: info@ihrsa.org

International Spa Association
2365 Harrodsburg Road, Suite A325
Lexington, KY 40504-4326
Ph: 888-651-ISPA (4772) or
    859-226-4326
Fax: 859-226-4445
website: www.experienceispa.com
e-mail: ispa@ispastaff.com

**Medaus Pharmacy and
Compounding Center**
2637 Valleydale Rd. #200
Birmingham, Alabama 35244
Ph: 800-526-9183 or 205-981-2352
Fax: 800-526-9184 or 205-981-2767
website: www.medaus.com
e-mail: info@medaus.com

Nutramedix
900 East Indiantown Road, Suite 301
Jupiter, FL 33477
Ph: 800-730-3130 or 561-745-2917
Fax: 561-745-3017
websites: www.nutramedix.com or
        www.samento.com.ec
e-mail: info@nutramedix.com

Optimum Health International, LLC
257 East Center Street
Manchester, CT 06040
Ph: 800-228-1507
Fax: 860-643-2531
website: www.opthealth.com
e-mail: info@opthealth.com

Purify FIRST
1919 Seventh Street, Suite 100
Boulder, CO 80302
Ph: 303-938-8600
website: www.purifyfirst.com

Superslow Zone
285 West Central Parkway,
    Suite 1726
Altamonte Springs, FL 32714
Ph: 407-937-0050
e-mail: mross@superslowzone.com

The Spa Association
P.O. Box 273283
Fort Collins, CO 80527
Ph: 970-207-4293
Fax: 815-550-2862
website: www.thespaassociation.com
e-mail: info@thespaassociation.com

SpaFinder Magazine
Ph: 212-924-6800 x221
website: www.spafinder.com
e-mail:
    customerservice@spafinder.com

Spa Index
1511 M. Sycamore #104
Hercules, CA 94547
Ph: 877-832-6169
website: www.spaindex.com
e-mail: info@spaindex.com

Zone Café, LLC
1495 Ridgeview Drive, Suite 230
Reno, NV 89509
Ph: 775-673-9663
Fax: 775-825-6447
website: www.zonecafe.com
e-mail: info@zonecafe.com

MEDI-SPAS

Canyon Ranch
8600 E. Rockcliff Road
Tuscon, AZ 85750
Ph: 800-742-9000
website: www.canyonranch.com

Chico Water Cure Spa
6670 Chico Way NW
Bremerton, WA 98312
Ph: 360-692-5554
Fax: 360-698-760
website: www.chicospa.com
e-mail: watercure@chicospa.com

CuisinArt Resort and Spa
P.O. Box 2000
Rendezvous Bay
Anguilla, B.W.I.
Ph: 264-498-2000
Fax: 264-498-2010
website: www.cuisinartresort.com
e-mail: info@cuisinartresort.com

Gurney's Inn Resort, Spa & Conference Center
200 Old Montauk Highway
Montauk, NY 11954
Ph: 631-668-2345
website: www.gurneys-inn.com
e-mail: info@gurneys-inn.com

MeSuá Dermocosmetic Spa
1900 Brickell Avenue
Miami, FL 33129
Ph: 305-854-3666 or 877-77-MESUA
Fax: 305-854-7944
website: www.mesua.com
e-mail: drmesua@mesua.com

Blue Skies Dermatology and Trinity Medi-Spa
23003 Mack Ave, Suite A
Saint Clair Shores, MI 48080
Ph: 586- 778-2410
Fax: 586-778-6221
e-mail: drcalo@blueskies dermatology.com

Tortuga del Sol
Baja-Mexico
(An eco-resort and Zone medi-spa currently under construction)
Ph: 775-771-5443
website: www.tortugadelsol.net
e-mail: info@tortugadelsol.net

Zone Medi-Spa (ACT III)
5050B Meadowood Mall Circle
Reno, NV 89502
Ph: 775-219-6740
Fax: 775-825-6447
website: www.zonemedispa.com

RECOMMENDED PHYSICIANS

David A. Amato, D.O. (Dermatology)
All About Faces @ Community Dermatology
845 Sir Thomas Court, Suite 1
Harrisburg, PA 17109
Ph: 717-652-5800

Mark Baily, M.D./Sharon McQuillan, M.D. (AMA Accredited botox training)
291 Barberry Road
Highland Park, IL 60035
Ph: 800-863-5085
website: www.totalbotox.com

Dr. Mark Breiner, D.D.S.
   (Holistic Dentistry)
5520 Park Avenue, Suite 301
Trumbull, Connecticut 06611
Ph: 203-371-0300
Fax: 203-365-8479
website: www.wholebodydentistry.com
e-mail: info@wholebodydentistry.com

Dr. Stephen Brown (Plastic Surgery)
100 Asylum Avenue
Hartford, CT 06105
Ph: 860-249-0083
website: www.drstevebrown.com
e-mail: info@drstevebrown.com

David Pearlmutter, M.D. (Neurology)
800 Goodlette Road North #270
Naples, FL 34102
Ph: 239-649-7400
website: www.Brainrecovery.com

Nicholas Perricone, M.D.
   (Cosmetic Dermatology)
Clinical Creations Skin
377 Research Parkway
Meriden, CT 06450
Ph: 888-823-7837
Fax: 203-379-0817
website: www.clinicalcreations.com
e-mail: customersupport@clinical
   creations.com

Dr. Mark G. Rubin
   (Cosmetic Dermatology)
153 S. Lasky Drive, Suite 1
Beverly Hills, CA 90212
Ph: 310-556-0119
website: www.markrubin.dermdex.net/

Gary E. Russolillo, M.D.
   (Cosmetic Plastic Surgeon)
970 Farmington Avenue
West Hartford, CT 06107
Ph: 860-521-2200
Fax: 860-521-2605
website: www.germd.com

Smith Dermatology Clinic
   (Dermatology)
5801 E. 4th Street
Tulsa, OK 74135
Ph: 918-664-9881
website: www.smithderm.com
e-mail: Info@SmithDerm.com

Dr. Blake Tearnan, Ph.D.
   (Psychology)
Healthnet Solutions, Inc.
4790 Caughlin Parkway, Suite 160
Reno, NV 89509
Ph: 888-286-9302
website: www.healthnetsolutions.com
e-mail: hns@charter.net

Carl R. Thornfeldt, M.D.
   (Dermatology)
811 NW 12th Street
Fruitland, ID 83619
Ph: 208-452-7450
Fax: 208-452-7550

George Weiss, M.D. (Medical
   Director, Wellness and Longevity
   Medical Group of La Jolla)
7360 Say Avenue
La Jolla, CA 92037
Ph: 858-450-1700
Fax: 858-459-6990
website: www.georgeweissmd.com
e-mail: wellnessdoc@aol.com

References and Related Reading

CHAPTER 1

Cohen, Jay. *Overdose: The Case against the Drug Companies*. New York, NY: Putnam Publishing Group, 2001.

Cousins, Norman. *Anatomy of an Illness*. New York, NY: W.W. Norton, 1979.

Dubos, Rene Jules. *Mirage of Health*. New York, NY: Harper and Row, 1971.

Dunn, Halbert. *High Level Wellness*. Arlington, VA: R.W. Beaty, 1967.

Northrup, Christine. *Women's Bodies, Women's Wisdom*. New York, NY: Bantam Books, 2001.

Sedlar, Jeri and Miners, Rick. *Don't Retire, REWIRE!* New York, NY: Alpha Books, 2002.

Smuts, Jan. *Holism and Evolution*. New York, NY: Viking Press, 1961.

Travis, John. *Wellness Workbook*, 3rd Edition. Berkeley, CA: Celestial Arts, 1981, 1988, 2004.

Healthy People 2,000. U.S. Surgeon General and the Public Health Service. Department of Health and Human Services, Centers for Disease Control and Prevention, Epidemiology Program Office, Division of Public Health Surveillance and Informatics. 1991.

CHAPTER 2
Books

Baker, Sidney. *Detoxification and Healing*. New Canaan, CT: Keats Publishing, 1997.

Bland, Jeffrey. *The 20-Day Rejuvenation Diet Program*. New Canaan, CT: Keats Publishing, 1999.

Breiner, Mark. *Whole Body Dentistry*. Fairfield, CT: Quantum Health Press, 1999.

Fries, James, and Crapo, Lawrence. *Vitality and Aging*. New York, NY: Freeman and Sons, 1981.

Kellas, William. *Surviving the Toxic Crisis: Today's Ultimate Solutions to Chronic Illness*. Encinitas, CA: Comprehensive Health, 1996.

Lemole, Gerald M. *The Healing Diet*. New York, NY: William Morrow, 2000.

Mandell, Marshall, and Scanlon, Lynne Waller. *Doctor Mandell's Five-Day Allergy Relief System*. New York, NY: Pocket Books, 1983.

Ott, John. *Light, Radiation and You: How to Stay Healthy*. Old Greenwich, CT: Devin-Adair, 1982.

Quicksilver Associates, Bronte, Lidia. *The Mercury in Your Mouth*. New York, NY: Quicksilver Press, 1994.

Roberts, Arthur, et al. *Nutraceuticals*. New York, NY: The Berkeley Publishing Group, 2001.

Ziff, Sam. *The Toxic Time Bomb*. Santa Fe, NM: Aurora Press, 1986.

Periodicals

Damstra, T, Page, SW, Herrman, JL, et al. "Persistent organic pollutants: potential health effects?" *Journal of Epidemiology and Community Health* 56(11) (2002):824–825.

Ernst, D, Pecho, E, Wirz, P, et al. "Regular sauna bathing and the incidence of common colds." *Annals of Medicine* 22(4) (1990):225–227.

Goldberg, Burton. "Longevity." *AlternativeMedicine.com* 2001.

Hansen LG. "Persistent organic pollutants in food supplies." *Journal of Epidemiology and Community Health* 56(11) (2002):820–821.

Khara, T, Biro, S, Imamura, M, et al. "Repeated sauna treatment improves vascular endothelial and cardiac function in patients with chronic heart failure." *Journal of the American College of Cardiology* 39(5) (2002):754–759.

Kilburn, KH, Warsaw, RH, Shields, MG. "Neurobehavioral dysfunction in firemen exposed to polychlorinated biphenyls (PCBs): possible improvement after detoxification." *Archives of Environmental Health* 44(6) (1989):345–350.

Kirchheimer, S. "Toxins in 20% of U.S. food supply." *WebMD*. (16 October 2002):1–2.

Krop, J. "Chemical sensitivity after intoxication at work with solvents: response to sauna therapy." *Journal of Alternative and Complementary Medicine* 4(1) (1998):77–86.

Lovejoy, HB, Bell, ZG, Vizena, TR. "Mercury exposure evaluations and their correlation with urine mercury excretion: 4. Elimination of mercury by sweating." *Journal of Occupational Medicine* 15 (1973):590–591.

Schafer, KS, Kegley, SE. "Persistent toxic chemicals in the US food supply." *Journal of Epidemiology and Community Health* 56(11) (2002):813–817.

Schnare, DW, Denk, G, Shields, M, et al. "Evaluation of a detoxification regimen for fat stored xenobiotics." *Medical Hypothesis* 9 (1982):265–282.

Tei, C, Horikiri, Y, Park, JC, et al. "Acute hemodynamic improvement by thermal vasodilation in congestive heart failure." *Circulation* 91(10) (1995):2582–2590.

CHAPTER 3
Books

Agatston, Arthur. *The South Beach Diet*. New York, NY: Random House, 2003.

Cordain, Loren. *The Paleo Diet*. New York, NY: Wiley & Sons, 2002.

Eaton, Boyd. *The Paleolithic Prescription*. New York, NY: HarperCollins, 1988.

Heller, Richard and Rachael. *The Carbohydrate Addict's Diet*. New York, NY: Dutton/Plume, 1991.

Roizen, Michael. *The Real Age Diet*. New York, NY: HarperCollins, 2001.

Sears, Barry. *Enter the Zone*. New York, NY: HarperCollins, 1995.

Sears, Barry. *The Age-Free Zone*. New York, NY: HarperCollins, 1999.

Sears, Barry. *The OmegaRx Zone*. New York, NY: HarperCollins, 2002.

Sinatra, Stephen, and Sinatra, Jan. *Lower Your Blood Pressure in Eight Weeks*. New York, NY: Ballantine, 2003.

Smith, Melissa Diane. *Going Against the Grain*. New York, NY: Contemporary Books, 2002.

Willett, Walter C. *Eat, Drink and Be Healthy*. New York, NY: Simon and Schuster, 2001.

Periodicals

Alarcon de la Lastra, C, Barranco, MD, Motilva, V, Herrerias, JM. "Mediterranean diet and health: biological importance of olive oil." *Current Pharmaceutical Design* 7(10) (2001): 933–950.

Burkitt, DP, Walker, A, Painter, N. "Dietary fiber and disease." *Journal of the American Medical Association (JAMA)* 229 (1974):1068.

de Lorgeril, M, Salen, P, Martin, JL, et al. "Effects of Mediterranean type of diet on the rate of cardiovascular complications in patients with coronary artery disease." *Journal of the American College of Cardiology* 28(5) (1996):1103–1108.

Dumesnil, JG, Turgeon, J, Tremblay, A, et al. "Effect of a low-glycemic index low-fat high-protein diet on the atherogenic metabolic risk profile of abdominally obese men." *British Journal of Nutrition* 86(5) (2001):557–568.

Eaton, Boyd, Konner, Melvin. "Paleolithic nutrition." *New England Journal of Medicine* 312(5) (31 January 1985):283–289.

Kalus, U, Pindur, G, Jung, F, et al. "Influence of the onion as an essential ingredient of the Mediterranean diet on arterial blood pressure and blood fluidity." *Arzneimittelforschung* 50(9) (2000):795–801.

Kouris-Blazos, A, Wahlqvist, ML. "The traditional Greek food pattern and overall survival in elderly people." *Australian Journal of Nutrition and Dietetics* 55(4) (1998):520–523.

Kushi, LH, Lenart, EB, Willett, WC. "Health implications of Mediterranean diets in light of contemporary knowledge. Meat, wine, fats, and oils." *American Journal of Clinical Nutrition* 61suppl (1995):1416S–1427S.

Maxwell, S, Cruickshank, A, Thorpe, D. "Red wine and antioxidants activity in serum." *The Lancet* 344 (1994):193–194.

Renaud, S, de Lorgeril, M. "Wine, alcohol, platelets and the French paradox for coronary heart disease." *The Lancet* 339 (1992):1523–1526.

Weisburger, JH. "Evaluation of the evidence on the role of tomato products in disease prevention." *Proceedings of the Society of Experimental Biological Medicine* 218(2) (1998): 140–143.

Willett, WC, Sacks, F, Trichopoulo, A, et al. "Mediterranean diet pyramid: a cultural model for health eating." *American Journal of Clinical Nutrition* 61suppl (1995):1402S–1406S.

CHAPTER 4
Books

Bates, W. *Better Eyesight Without Glasses*. New York, NY: Pyramid Books, 1975.

Brownell, Kelly D. *LEARN Program for Weight Control*. Dallas, TX: American Health Publishing Co., 1999.

Fries, James. *Aging Well*. New York, NY: Addison Wesley, 1989.

Phillips, Bill. *Body for Life*. New York, NY: HarperCollins, 1999.

Roizen, Michael. *Real Age: Are You as Young as You Can Be?* New York, NY: HarperCollins, 1999.

Rose, Marc, and Rose, Michael. *Save Your Sight.* New York, NY: Warner Books, Inc. 1998.

Sinatra, Stephen, and Sinatra, Jan. *Lower Your Blood Pressure in Eight Weeks.* New York, NY: Ballantine Books, 2003.

Periodical

Sinatra, Stephen, et al. "Effect of continuous passive motion, walking and a placebo intervention on physical and psychological well-being." *Journal of Cardiopulmonary Rehabilitation* 10 (1990): 279–286.

CHAPTER 5
Books

Anderson, Norman. *Emotional Longevity: What Really Determines How Long You Live?* New York, NY: Viking Books, 2003.

Antonovsky, Aaron. *Health, Stress and Coping.* San Francisco, CA: Jossey-Bass, 1979.

Benson, Herbert. *The Relaxation Response.* New York, NY: Hearst Books, 1976.

Borysenko, Joan. *Minding the Body—Mending the Mind.* New York, NY: Bantam Books, 1988.

Brown, Barbara. *Stress and the Art of Biofeedback.* New York, NY: Harper and Row, 1977.

Childre, Doc Lew. *Freeze Frame.* Boulder Creek, CA: California Planetary Publications, 1994.

Cousins, Norman. *Head First.* New York, NY: E.P. Dutton, 1989.

Dossey, Larry. *Healing Words.* San Francisco, CA: HarperCollins, 1993.

Dossey, Larry. *Meaning and Medicine.* New York, NY: Bantam Books, 1991.

Dossey, Larry. *Space, Time, and Medicine.* Boston, MA: Shambhala, 1982.

Eliot, Robert. *Is It Worth Dying For?* New York, NY: Bantam Books, 1984.

Evans, W, and Rosenberg, I. *Biomarkers.* New York, NY: Simon and Schuster, 1991.

Friedman, Meyer. *Type A Behavior and Your Heart.* Greenwich, CT: Fawcett Crest Paperbacks, 1974.

Goleman, Daniel. *Mind-Body Medicine.* New York, NY: Consumer Reports Books, 1993.

Green, Elmer and Green, Alyce. *Beyond Biofeedback.* New York, NY: Delacorte Press, 1977.

Kabat-Zinn, Jon. *Full Catastrophe Living.* New York, NY: Dell Publishing, 1990.

Klatz, R, Goldman, B. Chapter 26: Simpson, Graham. "Worldview and Well-Being." *Anti-Aging Medicine Therapeutics,* Vol II. Chicago, IL: Health Quest Publishers, 1998.

Ornstein, Robert, and Sobel, David. *The Healing Brain.* New York, NY: Simon and Schuster, 1987.

Pelletier, Kenneth. *Holistic Medicine: From Stress to Optimum Health.* New York, NY: Dell Publishing, 1980.

Pelletier, Kenneth. *Mind as Healer, Mind as Slayer.* New York, NY: Delta Books, 1977.

Pert, Candace. *Molecules of Emotion: Why You Feel the Way You Feel.* New York, NY: Scribner, 1997.

Rinpoche, Sogyal. *The Tibetan Book of Living and Dying.* New York, NY: HarperCollins, 1992.

Sapolsky, Robert. *Why Zebras Don't Get Ulcers.* New York, NY: W.H. Freeman and Co., 1994.

Selye, Hans. *Stress of Life.* New York, NY: McGraw Hill, 1956.

Selye, Hans. *Stress Without Distress.* New York, NY: Signet, 1974.

Sinatra, Stephen. *Heartbreak and Heart Disease.* New York, NY: McGraw-Hill, 1996.

Singh Khalsa, Dharma. *Brain Longevity.* New York, NY: Warner Books, 1997.

Spiegel, David. *Living Beyond Limits.* New York, NY: Times Books, 1993.

Temoshok, Lydia. *The Type C Connection.* New York, NY: Random House, 1992.

Watkins, Alan. *Mind-Body Medicine.* London, England: Churchill-Livingstone, 1997.

Periodicals

Curtis, BM, O'Keefe, JH. "Autonomic tone as a cardiovascular risk factor: the dangers of chronic fight or flight." *Mayo Clinic Proceedings* 77 (2002):45–54.

Sinatra, ST, Lowen, A. "Heartbreak and heart disease. The origin and cause of coronary prone behavior." *British Holistic Medicine* 2 (1987):169–171.

Sinatra, ST. "Stress and the heart: behavior interaction and plan for surgery." *Connecticut Medicine* 48 (1984):81–86.

CHAPTER 6
Books

Finch, C. *Longevity, Senescence, and the Genome.* Chicago, IL: University of Chicago Press, 1990.

Gorner, P, Kotulak, R. *Aging on Hold.* Orlando, FL: Tribune Publishing, 1992.

Hayflick, L. *How and Why We Age.* New York, NY: Ballantine Books, 1994.

Klatz, R, and Goldman, R. *The Anti-Aging Revolution.* North Bergen, NJ: Basic Health Publications, 2002.

Periodicals

Bjorksten, J. "The crosslinkage theory of aging." *Comprehensive Therapy* II (1976):65.

Dilman, V, Dean, W. "The neuroendocrine theory of aging." *Florida: Center for Biogerentology* (1992):3–92.

CHAPTER 7
Books

Breiner, M. *Whole Body Dentistry.* Fairfield, CT: Quantum Health Press, 1999.

Lopez, D., Williams, R., Miehlke, K., *Enzymes: The Fountain of Life.* Munich Germany: The Neville Press, 1994.

Sears B. *OmegaRx Zone.* New York, NY: HarperCollins, 2002.

Sinatra, ST, and Peterson, SJ. "Use of Alternative Medicines in Treatment of Cardiovascular

Disease." Frishman, WH, Sonnenblick, EH, Sica, DA (eds). *Cardiovascular Pharmacotherapeutics Manual* 2nd ed. New York, NY: McGraw-Hill, 2004:485–512.

Sinatra Stephen T. *The Coenzyme* Q_{10} *Phenomenon*. New Canaan, CT: Keats Publishing, 1998.

Periodicals

Abou-Raya, S, Naeem, A, Abou-EI, KH, et al. "Coronary artery disease and periodontal disease: is there a link?" *Angiology* 53(2) (2002):141–148.

Actis-Goretta, L, Ottaviani, JI, Keen, CL, et al. "Inhibition of angiotensin converting enzyme (ACE) activity by flavan-3-ols and procyanidins." *Federation of European Biochemical Societies Letters* 555(3) (2003):597–600.

Bertelli, A, Bertelli, AA, Giovanni, L, et al. "Protective synergic effect of coenzyme Q_{10} and carnitine of hyperbaric oxygen toxicity." *International Journal of Tissue Reactions* 12 (1990): 193–96.

Bertelli, A, Ronca, G. "Carnitine and coenzyme Q_{10}: biochemical properties and functions synergism and complementary action." *International Journal of Tissue Reactions* 12 (1990): 183–86.

Bertelli, A, Ronca, R, Ronca, G, et al. "L-Carnitine and Coenzyme Q_{10} protective action against ischemia and reperfusion of working rat heart." *Drugs under Experimental Clinical Research* 18 (1992):43–46.

Burke, BE, Neuenschwander, R, Olson, RD. "Randomized, double-blind, placebo-controlled trial of Coenzyme Q_{10} in isolated systolic hypertension." *The Southern Medical Journal* 94(11) (2001):1112–1117.

Cacciatore, L, Cerio, R, Ciarimboli, M, et al. "The therapeutic effect of L-Carnitine in patients with exercise-induced stable angina: a controlled study." *Drugs under Experimental Clinical Research* 17(4) (1991):225–235.

Chang,WC, Hsu, FL. "Inhibition of platelet aggregation and arachidonate metabolism platelets of procyanidins." *Prostaglandins Leukotrienes Essential Fatty Acids* 38(3) (1989): 181–188.

Danesh, J, Collins, R, Peto, R. "Lipoprotein(a) and coronary artery disease. Meta-analysis of prospective studies." *Circulation* 102(10) (2000):1082–1085.

Duan, W, Landenheim, B, Cutler, RG, et al. "Dietary folate deficiency and elevated homocysteine levels endanger dopaminergic neurons in models of Parkinson's disease." *Journal of Neurochemistry* 80(1) (2002):101–110.

Dumesnil, JG, Turgeon, J, Tremblay, A, et al. "Effect of low glycaemic index-low-fat-high protein diet on the atherogenic metabolic risk profile of abdominally obese men." *British Journal of Nutrition* 86 (2001):557–568.

El Boustani, S, Causse, JE, Descomps, B, et al. "Direct in vivo characterization of delta 5 desaturase activity in humans by deuterium labeling: effects of insulin." *Metabolism* 38 (1989):315–321.

Ernest, E. "Chelation therapy for coronary heart disease: an overview of all clinical investigations." *American Heart Journal* 140 (2002):139–141.

Freeman, DJ, Norrie, J, Caslake, MJ, et al. "C-reactive protein is an independent predictor of risk for the development of diabetes in the West of Scotland Coronary Prevention Study." *Diabetes* 51 (2002):1596–1600.

Ghirlanda, G, Oradei, A, Manto, A, et al. "Evidence of plasma CoQ$_{10}$-lowering effect by HMG-CoA reductase inhibitors: a double-blind, placebo-controlled study." *Journal of Clinical Pharmacology* 33(3) (1993):226–229

GISSI Preventzione Investigators. "Dietary supplementation with n-3 polyunsaturated fatty acids and vitamin E after myocardial infarction: results in the GISSI Preventzione trial." *The Lancet* 354 (1999):447–455.

Gorman, C, Park, A. "The Fires Within." *Time Magazine,* February 23, 2004, 38–46.

Goyette P, Christensen B, Rosenblatt DS, et al. "Severe and mild mutations in cis for the methylenetetrahydrofolate reductase (MTHFRO gene), and description of 5 novel mutations in MTHFR." *American Journal of Human Genetics* 59 (1996):1268–1275.

Hankey, GJ, Eikeboom, JW. "Homocysteine and vascular disease." *The Lancet* 354 (1999):407–413.

Hertog, MG, Feskens, EJ, Hollman, PC, et al. "Dietary antioxidant flavonoids and risk of coronary heart disease: The Zutphen Elderly Study." *The Lancet* 342 (1993):1007–1011.

Kajander, EO, et al. "Nanobacteria: an alternative mechanism for pathogenic intra-and extracellular calcification and stone formation." *Proceedings of the National Academy of Science* 95 (1998):8274–8279.

Kajander, EO, et al. "Nanobacteria from blood, the smallest culturable autonomously replicating agent on Earth." *Proceedings of Society of Photo-Optical Instrumentation Engineers* 3111 (1997):420–428.

Kajander, EO, Ciftcioglu, N, Aho, K, et al. "Characteristics of nanobacteria and their possible role in stone formation." *Urological Research* 31(2) (2003):47–54.

Kajander, EO, Ciftcioglu, N, Miller-Hjelle, MA, et al. "Nanobacteria: controversial pathogens in nephrolithiasis and polycystic kidney disease." *Current Opinions of Nephrological Hypertension* 10(3) (2001):445–452.

Kamikawa, T, Kobayashi, A, Yamashita, T, et al. "Effects of Coenzyme Q$_{10}$ on exercise tolerance in chronic stable angina pectoris." *American Journal of Cardiology* 56 (1985):247–251.

Langsjoen, PH, Langsjoen, AM. "Overview of the use of CoQ$_{10}$ in cardiovascular disease." *Biofactors* 9 (1999):273–284.

Layman, DK, Shiue, H, Cather, C, et al. "Increased dietary protein modifies glucose and insulin homeostasis in adult women during weight loss." *Journal of Nutrition* 133 (2003): 405–410.

Lemaitre, RN, King, IB, Mozaffarian, D, et al. "n-3 polyunsaturated fatty acids, fatal ischemic heart disease, and nonfatal myocardial infarction in older adults: the cardiovascular health study." *American Journal of Clinical Nutrition* 77(2) (2003):279–280.

Libby, P. "Atherosclerosis: the new view." *Scientific American* (May 2002):24–55.

Lichodziejewsta, B, Klos, J, Rezler, J, et al. "Clinical symptoms of mitral valve prolapse are related to hypomagnesemia and attenuated by magnesium supplementation." *American Journal of Cardiology* 79(6) (1997):768–772.

Loesche, WJ. "Periodontal disease: link to cardiovascular disease." *Compendium of Continuing Education of Dentistry* 21(6) (2000):463–466,468,470.

Ludwig, DS. "The glycemic index: physiological mechanism relating to obesity, diabetes, and cardiovascular disease." *Journal of the American Medical Association (JAMA)* 287 (2002): 2414–2423.

Meuier, MT, Ville, F, Jonadet, M, et al. "Inhibition of angiotensin I converting enzyme by flavanolic compounds: in vitro and in vivo studies." *Planta Medica* 53(1) (1987):12–15.

Miller, AL. "The methionine-homocysteine cycle and its effects on cognitive diseases." *Alternative Medicine Review* 8(1) (2003):7–19.

Mokdad, AH, Marks, JS, Stroup, DF, et al. "Actual causes of death in the United States." *Journal of the American Medical Association (JAMA)* 291 (2004):1238–1245.

Morita, H, Taguchi, J, Kuihara, H, et al. "Genetic polymorphism of 5, 10-methylenetetrahydrofolate reductase (MTHFR) as a risk factor of coronary artery disease." *Circulation* 95 (1997):2032–2036.

Morisco, C, Trimarco, B, Condorelli, M. "Effective Coenzyme Q_{10} therapy in patients with congestive heart failure: a long-term multicenter randomized study." *Clinical Investigations* 71(8 Suppl) (1993):S134–136.

Nygard, O, Nordrehaug, JE, Refsum, H, et al. "Plasma homocysteine levels and mortality in patients with coronary artery disease." *New England Journal of Medicine* 337 (1997):230–236.

Pauly, D, Johnson, C, St. Cyr, JA. "The benefits of ribose in cardiovascular disease." *Medical Hypotheses* 60(2) (2003):149–151.

Pauly, D, Pepine, C. "D-Ribose as a supplement for cardiac energy metabolism." *Journal of Cardiovascular Pharmacology* 5(4) (2000):249–258.

Pelikonova, T, Kohout, J, Base, J, et al. "Effect of acute hyperinsulinemia on fatty acid composition of serum lipids in non-insulin dependent diabetics and healthy men." *Clinica Chimica Acta* 203 (1991):329–337.

Pliml, W, von Arnim, T, Stablein, A, et al. "Effects of ribose on exercise-induced ischemia in stable coronary artery disease." *The Lancet* 340 (1992):507–510.

Pradhan, AD, Manson, JE, Rifai, N, et al. "C-Reative protein, interleukin 6, and risk of developing type-2 diabetes mellitus." *Journal of the American Medical Association (JAMA)* 286 (2001):327–334.

Retter, AS. "Carnitine and its role in cardiovascular disease." *Heart Disease* 1 (1999): 108–113.

Ridker, PM, Hennekens, CH, Buring, JE, et al. "C-reactive protein and other markers of inflammation in the prediction of cardiovascular disease in women." *New England Journal of Medicine* 342 (2000):836–843.

Ridker, PM, Rifai, N, Pfeffer, MA, et al. "Inflammation, pravastatin, and the risk of coronary events after myocardial infarction in patients with average cholesterol levels." *Circulation* 98 (1998):839–844.

Salonen, JT, Nyyssonen, K, Korpela, H, et al. "High stored iron levels are associated with excess risk of myocardial infarction in eastern Finnish men." *Circulation* 86(3) (1992): 803–811.

Salonen, JT, Seppanen, K, Nyyssonen, K, et al. "Intake of mercury from fish, lipid peroxidation, and the risk of myocardial infarction in coronary, cardiovascular, and any death in eastern Finnish men." *Circulation* 91(3) (1995):645–655.

Seddon, JM, Gensler, G, Milton, RC, et al. "Association between C-reactive protein and age-related macular degeneration." *Journal of the American Medical Association (JAMA)* 291(6) (2004):704–710.

Seshadri, S, Beiser A, Selhub J, et al. "Plasma homocysteine as a risk factor for dementia and Alzheimer's disease." *New England Journal of Medicine* 346(7) (2002):476–483.

Seymour, RA, Preshaw, PM, Steele, JG. "Oral health and heart disease." *Primary Dental Care* 9(4) (2002):125–131.

Shechter, M, Merz, CN, Paul-Labrador, M, et al. "Oral magnesium supplementation inhibits platelet-dependent thrombosis in patients with coronary artery disease." *American Journal of Cardiology* 84(2) (1999):152–156.

Sinatra, ST. "Alternative medicine for the conventional cardiologist." *Heart Disease* 2 (2000):16–30.

Sinatra, ST. "Care, cancer, and coenzyme Q_{10}." *Journal of the American College of Cardiology* 33(3) (March 1999):897–899.

Sinatra, ST. "Coenzyme Q_{10}, L-Carnitine, apoptosis and the heart." *International Journal of Anti-Aging Medicine* (Winter 2000):15–24.

Sinatra, ST. "Is cholesterol lowering with statins the gold standard for treating patients with cardiovascular risk and disease?" *The Southern Medical Journal* 96(3) (March 2003):220–222.

Sinatra, ST. "Stay in the Sinatra-Smart Zone for Optimum Health." *The Sinatra Health Report.* Potomac, MD: Phillips Health, LLC, May 2003.

Singh, RB, Niaz, MA, Agarwal, P, et al. A randomized, double-blind, placebo-controlled trial of L-Carnitine in suspected acute myocardial infarction. *Postgraduate Medical Journal* 72 (1996):45–50.

Singh, RB, Wander, GS, Rastogi, A, et al. "Randomized, double-blind placebo-controlled trial of Coenzyme Q_{10} in patients with acute myocardial infarction." *Cardiovascular Drugs Therapy* 12 (1998):347–353.

Sullivan, JL. "The iron paradigm of ischemic heart disease." *American Heart Journal* 117(5) (1989):1177–1188.

Tanka, J, Tominaga, R, Yoshitoshi, M, et al. "Coenzyme Q_{10}: The prophylactic effect on low cardiac output following cardiac valve replacement." *Annals of Thoracic Surgery* 33 (1982): 145–151.

Turunen, M, Olsson, J, Dallner, G. "Metabolism and function of Coenzyme Q_{10}." *Biochima et Biophysica Acta-Biomembranes* 1660(1–2) (2004):171–199.

Visser, M, Bouter, LM, McQuillan, GM, et al. "Elevated C-reactive protein levels in overweight and obese adults." *Journal of the American Medical Association (JAMA)* 282 (1999): 2131–2135.

Walter, DH, Fichtlscherer, S, Sellwig, M, et al. "Preprocedural C-reactive protein levels and cardiovascular events after coronary stent implantation." *American Journal of Cardiology* 37 (2001):839–846.

Wegrowski, J, Robert, AM, Moczar, M. "The effect of procyanidolic oligomers on the composition of normal and hypercholesterolemic rabbit aortas." *Biochemical Pharmacology* 33 (21) (1984):3491–3497.

Wolfe, BM, Piche, LA. "Replacement of carbohydrate by protein in a conventional-fat diet reduces cholesterol and triglyceride concentrations in healthy normolipidemic subjects." *Clinical Investigations in Medicine* 22 (1999):140–148.

CHAPTER 8

Books

Crook, Thomas. *The Memory Cure.* New York, NY: Pocket Books, 1999.

Khalsa, Dharma Singh. *Brain Longevity.* New York, NY: Warner Books, 1997.

Kyriazis, Marios. *The Anti-Aging Plan.* London: UK: Element, 2000.

Packer, Lester. *The Antioxidant Miracle.* Hoboken, NJ: John Wiley and Sons, 1999.

Perlmutter, David, *Brain Recovery.Com: Powerful Therapy for Challenging Brain Disorders.* Naples, FL: Perlmutter Inc., 2000.

Perlmutter, David, and Colman, Carol. *The Better Brain Book.* New York, NY: Riverhead Books, August, 2004.

Rath, Matthias. *The Heart.* Santa Clara, CA: MR Publishing, 2001.

Roberts, Arthur. *Nutraceuticals.* New York, NY: The Berkeley Publishing Group, 2001.

Sinatra, Stephen T. *Optimum Health: A Natural Lifesaving Prescription for Your Body and Mind.* New York, NY: Bantam Books, 1997.

Sinatra, Stephen T. *The CoQ$_{10}$ Phenomenon.* Chicago, IL: Keats Publishing, 1998.

Werbach, Melvyn. *Botanical Influences on Illness.* Tarzana, CA: Third Line Press, 1994.

Periodicals

Babizhayev, M, Yermakova, VN, Deyev, AI, et al. "Imidazole containing peptidomimetic NACA as a potent drug for the medicinal treatment of age-related cataract in humans." *Journal of Anti-Aging Medicine.* 3 NI (2000) Mary Ann Liebert Inc., publisher.

Birchall, JD, Chappel, JS, "Aluminum, chemical physiology and Alzheimer's disease." *The Lancet* 2(8618) (1998):1008–1010.

Clarke, R, Smith, AD, Jobst, KA, et al. "Folate, vitamin B$_{12}$ and serum total homocysteine levels in confirmed Alzheimer's disease." *Archives of Neurology* 55 (1998):1449–1455.

Crook, TH, Tinklenberg, J, Yesavage, J. "Effects of phosphatidylserine in age-associated memory impairment." *Neurology* 41 (1991):644–649.

Le Bars, PL, Katz, MM, Berman, N, et al. "A placebo-controlled, double-blind, randomized trial of an extract of Ginkgo biloba for dementia." *Journal of the American Medical Association (JAMA)* 278 (1997):1237–1332.

Maichuk, IuF, Formaziuk, VE, Sergienko, VI. "Development of carnosine eye drops and assessing their efficiency in corneal diseases." *Vestnik Oftalmol* 113(6) (1997):27–31.

Preston, J, et al. "Toxic effects of B-amyloid on immortalized rat brain endothelial cell: protection by carnosine, homocarnosine and B-alanine." *Neuroscience Letters* 242 (1998): 105–108.

Sano, M, et al. "A controlled trial of selegiline, alpha-tocopherol, or both as treatment for Alzheimer's disease." *New England Journal of Medicine* 336(17) (1997):1216–1222.

Shults, CW, Beal, MF, Fontaine, K, et al. "Absorption, tolerability and effects on mitochondrial activity of oral Coenzyme Q_{10} in Parkinsonian patients." *Neurology* 50 (1998): 793–795.

Sinatra, Stephen T. *The Sinatra Health Report.* Potomac, MD: Phillips Health, LLC, 2000–2001.

Sobel, E, Dunn, M, Davanipour, Z, et al. "Elevated risk of Alzheimer's disease among workers with likely electromagnetic field exposure." *Neurology* 47 (1996):1477–1481.

Stao, Y, Asoh, T, Oizumi, K. "High prevalence of vitamin D deficiency and reduced bone mass in elderly women with Alzheimer's disease." *Bone* 23(6) (1998):555–557.

Stewart, WF, Kawas, C, Corrada, M, "Risk of Alzheimer's disease and duration of NSAID use." *Neurology* 48 (1997):626–632.

CHAPTER 9

DHEA

Bologa, L. "DHEA and its sulphated derivative reduce neuronal death and enhance astrocytic differentiation in brain cell cultures." *Journal of Neuroscience Research* 17(3) (1987): 225–234.

Flood J: "DHEA and its sulfate enhance memory retention in mice." *Brain Research* 447(2) (1988):269–278.

Flood, J, Roberts, E. "DHEA sulfate improves memory in aging mice." *Brain Research* 448(1) (1988):178–181.

Leary, M, Zisk, J. "Anti-obesity effect of two different levels of DHEA in lean and obese middle-aged Zucker rats." *International Journal of Obesity* 10(3) (1986):193–204.

Morales, AJ. "Effects of replacement dose of DHEA in men and women." *Journal of Clinical Endocrinology and Metabolism* 78 (1994):1360–1366.

Pearson, D, and Shaw, S. *Life Extension: A Practical Scientific Approach.* New York, NY: Warner Books, 1982.

Regelson, W. "Hormonal intervention." *Annals of New York Academy of Science* 521 (1988): 260–273.

Roberts, E. "Effects of DHEA and its sulphate on brain tissue in culture and on memory in mice." *Brain Research* 406(1-2) (1987):357–362.

Suderland, T. "Reduced plasma DHEA concentrations in Alzheimer's disease." *The Lancet* 2(8662) (1989):570.

Westler, JE, Barlascini, CO, Clore, JN, et al. "DHEA reduces body fat but does not alter insulin sensivity in normal men." *Journal of Clinical Endocrinology and Metabolism* 66(1) (January 1988):57–61.

Yang, Jyh-Yuan, Schwartz, A, Henderson, E. "Inhibition of HIV-1 Latency Reactivation by DHEA and an analog of DHEA." *AIDS Research and Human Retroviruses* 9(8) (1993) Mary Ann Liebart Inc., publisher.

Melatonin

Pierpaoli, Walter. *The Melatonin Miracle.* New York, NY: Simon and Schuster, 1995.

Regelson, William. *The Super Hormone Promise.* New York, NY: Simon and Schuster, 1996.

Rozencwaig, Roman. *The Melatonin and Aging Source Book.* Prescott, AZ: Hohm Press, 1997.

Pregnenolone

Akwa, Y, Young, J, Kabbadj, K, et al. "Neurosteroids; biosynthesis, metabolism and function of pregnenolone and DHEA in the brain." *Journal of Steroidal, Biochemical, and Molecular Biology* 40 (1991):71–81.

Flood, J, Morley, J, Roberts, E. "Memory-enhancing effects in male mice of pregnenolone and steroids metabolically derived from it." *Proceedings of the National Academy of Science USA* 89 (1992):1567–1571.

McGavack, T, Chevally, J, Weissberg, J. "The use of pregnenolone in various clinical disorders." *Journal of Clinical Endocrinology and Metabolism* 11 (1951):559–577.

Maione, S, Berrino, L, Viagliano, S, Leyva, J, et al. "Pregnenolone sulfate increases the convulsants potency of NMDA in mice." *European Journal of Pharmacology* 219(3) (1992): 477–479.

Roberts, E. "Pregnenolone from Selye to Alzheimer and a model of the pregnenolone sulfate binding site on the GABA receptor." *Biochemical Pharmacology* 49 (1995):1–16.

South, J. "Reducing stress and increasing productivity with pregnenolone." *Anti-Aging Bulletin* Volume 3, International Anti-Aging Systems (1996).

Thyroid

Barnes, B, Galtor, L. *Hypothyroidism: The Unsuspected Illness.* New York, NY: Harper Trade, 1976.

Langer, S, Scheer, J. *Solved: The Riddle of Illness.* New Canaan, CT: Keats Publishing, 1984.

Thymus

Fahmy, Z. "Immuno-stimulation therapy with thymus extract in rheumatoid arthritis." *Erfahrungsheilkunde* 31(5) (May 1982):423–427.

Goldstein, A, et al. "Thymosin and the immunopathology of aging." *Federation Proceedings* 33 (1974):2053–2056.

Goss, John, A. *The Thymus Regulator of Cellular Immunity.* Austin, TX: R.G. Landes Co., 1993.

Kelly, K, et al. "A pituitary-thymus connection during aging." *Annals of the New York Academy of Science* 521 (1998):88–98.

Thym-Uvocal, Immunotherapeutic Agent; A 32-page booklet with many references and case histories published by Medalfa AG, Pratteln, Switzerland.

Zatz, M, Goldstein, A. "Mechanism of action of thymosin." *Journal of Immunology* (134) (1985):1032–1038.

Estrogen and Progesterone

Barnes, R, Lobo, R. "Pharmacology of Estrogens." In: Mishell, D, Jr, ed. *Menopause: Physiology and Pharmacology.* Chicago, IL: Year Book Medical Publishers, Inc., 1987.

Follingstad, A. "Estriol the forgotten hormone?" *Journal of the American Medical Association (JAMA)* 239 (1978):29–30.

Heimer, G. "Estriol in the postmenopausal." *Acta Obstetricia et Gynecologica Scandinavica* 139 (1987):1–23.

Isoif, C. "Effects of protracted administration of Estriol on the lower genitourinary tract in postmenopausal women." *Archives of Gynecology and Obstetrics* 251 (1992):115–120.

Lauritzen, C. "Results of a 5-year prospective study of Estriol succinate treatment in patients with climacteric complaints." *Hormone and Metabolic Research* 19 (1987):579–584.

Lee, J. "Is natural progesterone the missing link in osteoporosis prevention and treatment?" *Medical Hypotheses* 35 (1991):316–318.

Lemon, H. "Estriol and prevention of breast cancer." *The Lancet* (1973):546–547.

Lemon, H, Kumar, P, Peterson, C, et al. "Inhibition of radiogenic mammary carcinoma in rats by estriol or tamoxifen." *Cancer* 63 (1989):1685–1692.

Lemon, H, Wotiz, H, Parsons, L, et al. "Reduced Estriol secretion in patients with breast cancer prior to endocrine therapy." *Journal of the American Medical Association (JAMA)* 196 (1966):112–120.

Northrup, Christiane. *The Wisdom of Menopause.* New York, NY: Bantam Books, 2001.

PEPI Trial Writing Group. "Effects of estrogen or estrogen/progestin regimens on heart disease risk factors in postmenopausal women. The premenopausal estrogen/progestin interventions (PEPI) trial." *Journal of the American Medical Association (JAMA)* 273 (1995): 199–208.

Premarin (conjugated estrogen tablets). Wyeth-Ayerst Company. *Physicians' Desk Reference,* 52nd edition. 1998. Montvale, NJ; Medical Economics Company, 3111–3113.

Schliesman, B, Robinson, L. "Serum estrogens: quantitative analysis of the concentration of Estriol compared to Estradiol and Estrone." Meridian Valley Laboratories. 1997; Kent, WA. Data on file.

Sinatra, Stephen. *Heart Sense for Women.* Washington, DC: Regnery Publishing, 2000.

Somers, Suzanne. *The Sexy Years.* New York, NY: Crown Publishing Group, 2004.

Utian, W. "The place of estriol therapy after menopause." *Acta Endocrinologica* 223(suppl) (1980):51–56.

Testosterone

Anderson, RA, Bancroft, J, Wu, FC. "The effects of exogenous testosterone on sexuality and mood of normal men." *Journal of Clinical Endocrinology and Metabolism* 75(6) (December 1992):1503–1507.

AndroGel prescribing information: 2/28/00. Unimed Pharmaceuticals, Inc. Buffalo Grove, IL 60089-1864. In: *Physicians' Desk Reference (PDR),* 2004.

Barrett-Connor, E, Von Muhlen, DG, Kritz-Silverstein, D. "Bioavailable testosterone and depressed mood in older men: the Rancho Bernardo Study." *Journal of Clinical Endocrinology and Metabolism* 84(2) (February 1999):573–577.

Dabbs, JM, Jr. "Salivary testosterone measurements: reliability across hours, days and weeks." *Physiology and Behaviour* 48 (1990):83–86.

Gooren, LJ. "Endocrine aspects of aging in the male." *Molecular and Cellular Endocrinology* 145(1–2) (25 October 1998):153–159.

Nankin, HR, Calkins, J. "Decreased bio-available testosterone in aging and normal men." *Journal of Clinical Endocrinology and Metabolism* 63 (1986):1418.

Rosano, GM, Leonardo, F, et al. "Acute anti-ischemic effect of testosterone in men with coronary artery disease." *Circulation* 99(13) (6 April 1999):1666–1670.

Rudman, D, Drinka, PJ, Wilson, CR, et al. "Relations of endogenous anabolic hormones and physical activity to bone mineral density and lean body mass in elderly men." *Journal of Clinical Endocrinology and Metabolism* 40(5) (May 1994):653–661.

Swerdloff, RS, Wang, C. "Androgen deficiency and aging in men." *Western Journal of Medicine* 159(5) (November 1993):579–585.

Tenover, JL. "Male hormone replacement therapy including andropause." *Endocrinology and Metabolism Clinics of North America (United States)* 27(4) (1998):969–987.

Growth Hormone

"Drug of the decade: human growth hormone." *Ladies Home Journal* 317 (October 1990):91–92.

Hertoghe, Thierry. *The Hormone Solution.* New York, NY: Harmony Books, 2002.

"Human growth hormone could be a blockbuster." *Scientific American* 263 (September 1990):164–166.

"Human growth hormone: the fountain of youth?" *Harvard Medical Report* 17 (1992):1–2.

Klatz, Ronald. *Grow Young with HGH.* New York, NY: HarperCollins Publishers, 1998.

Klatz, Ronald, Goldman, Robert. *The Anti-Aging Revolution.* North Bergen, NJ: Basic Health Publications, 2002.

"Little big drug: human growth hormone." *Economist* 317 (6 October 1990):102.

Rudman, D, Feller, AG, Nagral, HS, et al. "Effects of human growth hormone in men over 60." *New England Journal of Medicine* 323(1) (5 July 1990):1–6.

Rudman, D, Kutmer, MH, Blackston, RD. "Children with normal-vibrant short stature: treatment with HGH for 6 months." *New England Journal of Medicine* 305(3) (16 July 1981):123–131.

CHAPTER 10

Hertzog, MG, et al. "Dietary antioxidants, flavonoids, and the risk of coronary artery heart disease: the Zutphen Elderly Study." *The Lancet* 342 (1993):1000–1011.

Perricone, Nicholas. *The Perricone Prescription.* New York, NY: HarperCollins, 2002.

Purba, M, Blazos, A, et al. "Skin wrinkling: can food make a difference?" *Journal of the American College of Clinical Nutrition* 20 (2001):71–80.

AFTERWORD

Dossey, Larry. *Recovering the Soul*. New York, NY: Bantam Books New Age, 1989.

Dossey, Larry. *Reinventing Medicine*. San Francisco, CA: Harper San Francisco, 1999.

Gebser, Jean. *The Ever Present Origin: The Foundations and Manifestations of the Aperspectival World*. Athens, OH: Ohio University Press, 1985.

APPENDIX A

Antonovsky, Aaron. *Health, Stress and Coping*. San Francisco, CA: Jossey-Bass, 1979.

Bertalanffy, L. Von. *General System Theory Foundations Development Applications*. New York, NY: George Braziller, Inc., 1968.

Dossey, Larry. *Recovering the Soul*. New York, NY: Bantam Books New Age, 1989.

Engel, George L. "The need for a new medical model." *Science* 196 (1977):129–136.

Gebser, Jean. *The Ever Present Origin: The Foundations and Manifestations of the Aperspectival World*. Athens, OH: Ohio University Press, 1985.

Healthy People 2000. U.S. Surgeon General and the Public Health Service. Department of Health and Human Services, Centers for Disease Control and Prevention, Epidemiology Program Office, Division of Public Health Surveillance and Informatics. 1991.

Idler, Ellen, Kasl, Stanislav. "Yale health aging report." *Journal of Gerontology* (15 November 1997).

Jung, Carl, *The Portable Jung*. Joseph Campbell, ed. "Eastern And Western Thinking." New York, NY: Viking Press, 1971:480–502.

Ranjan, "Magic or logic: can 'alternative' medicine be scientifically integrated into modern medical practice?" *Advances in Mind-Body Medicine* 14 (1998):51–61.

Simpson, Graham. *Monograph: Remembering the Future*. http://eternitymedicine.com/english/03_eternity_medicine/mongraph_remembering%20the%20future.htm

Voeglin, Eric. *Collected Works*. Columbia, MO: University of Missouri Press, 2001.

Wilber, K. *Up from Eden: A Transpersonal View of Human Evolution*. Wheaton, IL: Quest Books, 1981.

APPENDIX B

Dispenza, Joseph. *Live Better Longer: The Parcells Center 7-Step Plan For Health and Longevity*. San Francisco, CA: HarperSanFrancisco, 1997.

APPENDIX G

Books

Schmid, Franz. *Cell Therapy: A New Dimension of Medicine*. Thoune, Switzerland: Ott Publishers, 1983.

Schmid, Franz. *Das Down Syndrome*. Musterdorf, Germany: Verlag Hansen and Hansen, 1987.

Periodicals

Kment, A. Obective Demonstration of the Revitalization Effect After Cell Injections. *Cell Research and Cellular Therapy.* Thorne Switzerland: Ott Publishers, 1967.

German Federal Health Gazette 533 (16 May 1961).

Medawar, PB. Immunological tolerance Nobel lecture. *Nature* 189(14) (1961).

Index

About the Authors

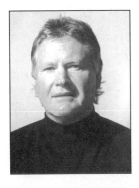

Graham Simpson, M.D., graduated from the University of Witwatersrand Medical School, Johannesburg, S.A. After practicing in South Africa and England, he moved to the United States where he is board certified in internal medicine and emergency medicine. Dr. Simpson, a founding member of the American Holistic Medical Association (AHMA), and a member of the Institute for Functional Medicine, is also a licensed homeopath who has practiced integrative medicine for more than twenty-five years. A published author, he has taught at the University of Nevada, Reno, and is the medical director of the Zone Medi-Spa in Nevada. Dr. Simpson can be contacted at the Zone Café, 1495 Ridgeview Drive, Suite 230, Reno, NV 89509. Ph: 775-673-9663; Fax: 775-825-6447; e-mail: graham@zonecafe.com.

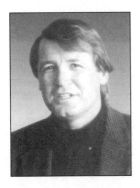

Stephen T. Sinatra, M.D., is a board-certified cardiologist, a certified bioenergetic psychotherapist, and a certified nutrition and antiaging specialist. At his practice in Manchester, CT, Dr. Sinatra integrates conventional medicine with complementary nutritional and psychological therapies to help heal the heart. He is an assistant clinical professor at the University of Connecticut School of Medicine, and is the author of several books, including *Optimum Health, Hearbreak and Heart Disease, Heart Sense For Women*, and *Eight Weeks to Lowering Blood Pressure*. Dr. Sinatra can be contacted at The New England Heart Center, 257 East Center Street, Manchester, CT 06040. Ph: 860-647-9729; Fax: 860-643-2531; e-mail: nehcpiazza@aol.com.

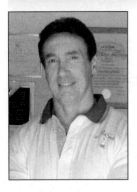

Jorge Suárez-Menéndez, M.D., graduated from the Medical College of Georgia in Augusta—a top medical school in the United States. He continued with his training in general surgery at Mount Sinai Hospital in Miami Beach, Florida; Orlando Medical Center in Orlando, Florida; Shans Hospital at the University of Florida in Gainsville; and Sloan-Kettering Memorial Hospital in New York City. Then, he trained in plastic surgery in Cincinnati, Ohio. Since going into private practice, he has performed more than 20,000 surgeries and has been the chief of plastic surgery at four major hospitals in Miami, Florida. A leading innovator in the cosmeceutical industry, he owns the holistic MeSuá Dermocosmetic Spa in Miami where his therapies include his unique antiaging skin-care product line that combines the best features of modern cosmetic chemistry and ancient beauty traditions. Dr. Suárez-Menéndez has lectured and appeared on TV and radio shows worldwide, and has been written about and quoted in numerous magazines and newspapers. He has also received many international honors and awards of recognition for his continued service in the field of plastic surgery. Dr. Suárez-Menéndez can be contacted at the MeSuá Dermocosmetic Spa, 1900 Brickell Avenue, Miami, FL 33129. Ph: 305-854-3838; email: drmesua@mesua.com.